Lecture Notes in Computer Science　　10541

Commenced Publication in 1973
Founding and Former Series Editors:
Gerhard Goos, Juris Hartmanis, and Jan van Leeuwen

More information about this series at http://www.springer.com/series/7412

Qian Wang · Yinghuan Shi
Heung-Il Suk · Kenji Suzuki (Eds.)

Machine Learning in Medical Imaging

8th International Workshop, MLMI 2017
Held in Conjunction with MICCAI 2017
Quebec City, QC, Canada, September 10, 2017
Proceedings

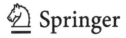 Springer

Editors
Qian Wang
Shanghai Jiao Tong University
Shanghai
China

Yinghuan Shi
Nanjing University
Nanjing
China

Heung-Il Suk
Korea University
Seoul
Korea (Republic of)

Kenji Suzuki
Illinois Institute of Technology
Chicago, IL
USA

ISSN 0302-9743   ISSN 1611-3349   (electronic)
Lecture Notes in Computer Science
ISBN 978-3-319-67388-2   ISBN 978-3-319-67389-9   (eBook)
DOI 10.1007/978-3-319-67389-9

Library of Congress Control Number: 2017952855

LNCS Sublibrary: SL6 – Image Processing, Computer Vision, Pattern Recognition, and Graphics

Printed on acid-free paper

This Springer imprint is published by Springer Nature
The registered company is Springer International Publishing AG
The registered company address is: Gewerbestrasse 11, 6330 Cham, Switzerland

Preface

The 8th International Workshop on Machine Learning in Medical Imaging (MLMI 2017) was held in the Quebec City Convention Centre, Quebec, Canada on September 10, 2017, in conjunction with the 20th International Conference on Medical Image Computing and Computer Assisted Intervention (MICCAI).

Machine learning plays an essential role in the medical imaging field, including computer-assisted diagnosis, image segmentation, image registration, image fusion, image-guided therapy, image annotation, and image database retrieval. Advances in medical imaging bring about new imaging modalities and methodologies, and new machine learning algorithms/applications. Due to large inter-subject variations and complexities, it is generally difficult to derive analytic formulations or simple equations to represent objects such as lesions and anatomy in medical images. Therefore, tasks in medical imaging require learning from patient data for heuristics and prior knowledge, in order to facilitate the detection/diagnosis of abnormalities in medical images.

The main aim of this MLMI 2017 workshop is to help advance scientific research within the broad field of machine learning in medical imaging. This workshop focuses on major trends and challenges in this area, and presents works aimed to identify new cutting-edge techniques and their use in medical imaging. We hope that the MLMI workshop becomes an important platform for translating research from the bench to the bedside.

The range and level of submissions for this year's meeting were of very high quality. Authors were asked to submit full-length papers for review. A total of 63 papers were submitted to the workshop in response to the call for papers. Each of the 63 papers underwent a rigorous double-blind peer review process, with each paper being reviewed by at least two (typically three) reviewers from the Program Committee, composed of 68 well-known experts in the field. Based on the reviewing scores and critiques, the 44 best papers (69%) were accepted for presentation at the workshop and chosen to be included in this Springer LNCS volume. The large variety of machine-learning techniques applied to medical imaging were well represented at the workshop.

We are grateful to the Program Committee for reviewing the submitted papers and giving constructive comments and critiques, to the authors for submitting high-quality papers, to the presenters for excellent presentations, and to all the MLMI 2017 attendees coming to Quebec City from all around the world.

July 2017

Qian Wang
Yinghuan Shi
Heung-Il Suk
Kenji Suzuki

Organization

Workshop Organizers

Qian Wang	Shanghai Jiao Tong University, China
Yinghuan Shi	Nanjing University, China
Heung-Il Suk	Korea University, South Korea
Kenji Suzuki	Illinois Institute of Technology, USA and World Research Hub Initiative, Tokyo Institute of Technology, Japan

Steering Committee

Dinggang Shen	University of North Carolina at Chapel Hill, USA
Pingkun Yan	Philips Research North America, USA
Kenji Suzuki	Illinois Institute of Technology, USA and World Research Hub Initiative, Tokyo Institute of Technology, Japan
Fei Wang	AliveCor Inc., USA

Program Committee

Amin Zarshenas	Illinois Institute of Technology, USA
Antonios Makropoulos	Imperial College London, UK
Arnav Bhavsar	IIT Mandi, India
Biao Jie	University of North Carolina at Chapel Hill, USA
Chong-Yaw Wee	National University of Singapore, Singapore
Chang Liu	Shanghai Jiao Tong University, China
Daoqiang Zhang	NUAA, China
Daniel Rueckert	Imperial College London, UK
Dong Nie	University of North Carolina at Chapel Hill, USA
Elizabeth Krupinski	University of Arizona, USA
Feng Shi	University of North Carolina at Chapel Hill, USA
Francesco Ciompi	Radboud University Medical Center, Netherlands
Gang Li	University of North Carolina at Chapel Hill, USA
Gerard Sanrom	Pompeu Fabra University, Spain
Ghassan Hamarneh	Simon Fraser University, Canada
Guoyan Zheng	University of Bern, Switzerland
Hamid Soltania-Zadeh	Henry Ford Hospital, USA
Hanbo Chen	University of Georgia, USA
Hayit Greenspan	Tel-Aviv University, Israel

Heang-Ping Chan	University of Michigan Medical Center, USA
Holger Roth	Nagoya University, Japan
Hoo-Chang Shin	National Institutes of Health, USA
Ivana Isgum	University Medical Center Utrecht, Netherlands
Janne Nappi	Massachusetts General Hospital, USA
Jianjia Zhang	CSIRO, Australia
Jing Huo	Nanjing University, China
Jong-Hwan Lee	Korea University, South Korea
Jun Shi	Shanghai University, China
Jun Xu	Nanjing University of Information Science and Technology, China
Jun Zhang	University of North Carolina at Chapel Hill, USA
Junchi Liu	Illinois Institute of Technology, USA
Jurgen Fripp	Australian e-Health Research Centre, Australia
Ken'ichi Morooka	Kyushu University, Japan
Kilian Pohl	SRI International, USA
Le Lu	NIH, USA
Lei Wang	University of Wollongong, Australia
Lei Xiang	Shanghai Jiao Tong University, China
Lei Qi	Nanjing University, China
Li Shen	Indiana University School of Medicine, USA
Li Wang	University of North Carolina at Chapel Hill, USA
Lichi Zhang	Shanghai Jiao Tong University, China
Luping Zhou	University of Wollongong, Australia
Marleen de Bruijne	University of Copenhagen, Denmark
Masahiro Oda	Nagoya University, Japan
Mert Sabuncu	Cornell University, USA
Mingxia Liu	University of North Carolina at Chapel Hill, USA
Pierrick Coupé	Université de Bordeaux, France
Philip Ogunbona	University of Wollongong, Australia
Pim Moeskops	Eindhoven University of Technology, Netherlands
Qian Yu	Nanjing University, China
Sanghyun Park	DGIST, South Korea
Sang-Woong Lee	Gachon University, South Korea
Shaoting Zhang	University of North Carolina at Charlotte, USA
Shu Liao	Siemens, USA
Siamak Ardekani	Johns Hopkins University, USA
Simon Warfield	Harvard University, USA
Tianye Niu	Zhejiang University, China
Wenbin Li	Nanjing University, China
Xi Jiang	University of Georgia, USA
Xiang Li	University of Georgia, USA
Xiaofeng Zhu	University of North Carolina at Chapel Hill, USA
Xuhua Ren	Shanghai Jiao Tong University, China

Contents

From Large to Small Organ Segmentation in CT Using Regional Context

Marie Bieth[1,2]([✉]), Esther Alberts[1], Markus Schwaiger[2], and Bjoern Menze[1]

[1] Department of Computer Science,
The Technical University of Munich, Munich, Germany
marie.bieth@tum.de
[2] Clinic for Nuclear Medicine, Klinikum Rechts der Isar,
The Technical University of Munich, Munich, Germany

Abstract. The segmentation of larger organs in CT is a well studied problem. For lungs and liver, state of the art methods reach Dice Scores above 0.9. However, these methods are not as reliable on smaller organs such as pancreas, thyroid, adrenal glands and gallbladder, even though a good segmentation of these organs is needed for example for radiotherapy planning.

In this work, we present a new method for the segmentation of such small organs that does not require any deformable registration to be performed. We encode regional context in the form of anatomical context and shape features. These are used within an iterative procedure where, after an initial labelling of all organs using local context only, the segmentation of small organs is refined using regional context. Finally, the segmentations are regularised by shape voting. On the Visceral Challenge 2015 dataset, our method yields a substantially higher sensitivity and Dice score than other forest-based methods for all organs. By using only affine registrations, it is also computationally highly efficient.

1 Introduction

Precise organs segmentation is necessary in diverse medical applications, including diagnostics, computer-aided interventions and radiotherapy planning. Therefore, the problem is well-studied and multiple methods exist that produce good segmentations for larger organs such as lungs and liver. For these organs, state of the art methods reach Dice Scores (DS) of over 0.9. However, for smaller organs with a higher variability in location or shape (e.g. pancreas, glands), most existing segmentation methods do not yield good results. Locating these organs is nonetheless crucial for example for radiotherapy planning to avoid irradiation with dramatic consequences. It would also be useful to automatically locate normal glandular uptake when segmenting lesions in PET images. In this work,

Electronic supplementary material The online version of this chapter (doi:10.1007/978-3-319-67389-9_1) contains supplementary material, which is available to authorized users.

Q. Wang et al. (Eds.): MLMI 2017, LNCS 10541, pp. 1–9, 2017.
DOI: 10.1007/978-3-319-67389-9_1

we are therefore interested in fully automatic small organ segmentation. To be usable in clinical practice, the method should have a short computation time and a good sensitivity.

The problem of multi-organs segmentation has been addressed with different approaches. Multi-atlas registration methods followed by label fusion such as [13] generally produce better results than patch or voxelwise labelling methods. However, they usually have a higher computation time because each atlas has to be non-linearly registered to the test image. Deep learning has also been successfully used for segmenting larger organs [7] such as kidneys and liver as well as the pancreas [12], but requires large amounts of training data, which is often difficult to obtain. Lately, more time efficient approaches such as Regression Forests [4] for organ localization, Atlas Forests [17] and Vantage Point Forests [6] for organ segmentation have shown good results. In forest-based methods, prior knowledge can be built in the features and high performance can be achieved with smaller training sets and shorter computation times. Taking into account local as well as long-range context in the features has been shown to improve performance. Haar-like [15] and BRIEF features [3] describe the local context based on intensities. Longer-range context can be provided for example by the output of a previous classifier, in an autocontext fashion [11,14], by the use of distances to landmarks [1] or of shape features [8]. The importance of semantic context has also been explored in [9].

Whilst local context is enough to segment larger organs such as lungs, liver or kidneys, it doesn't allow for segmentation of smaller structures of interest for radiotherapy planning that are sometimes only scarcely visible in CT. In this work, we introduce a novel approach for small organs segmentation that makes use not only of local but also of regional context through features that encode semantic knowledge on nearby anatomy similarly to [1] and organ shapes as in [8] and does not require *any* deformable registration (in contrast to [6,17]). By using fast Vantage Point Forests [6] for inference, it has a computation time that is significantly lower than multi-atlas methods and scales well to large data sets. We implement it in an iterative procedure where small organs labellings are iteratively refined by gradually incorporating better context information in the classification process. A final shape voting step ensures spatial consistency. In the following, we present our approach (Sect. 2), evaluate it on the Visceral Challenge 2015 dataset [5] (Sect. 3) and offer conclusions (Sect. 4).

2   Methods

In this section, we detail the different components of our method for small organs segmentation. In the following, we describe our base classifier, the Vantage Point Forest (VPF), how the initial labelling is performed, and how we further use it to refine labellings by employing context-richer descriptors in subsequent iterations. We then describe how to regularise the labelling using shape voting. In all the following, I is the current image and $v = (x_v, y_v, z_v)$ the current voxel. Note that no pre-alignment of the image is performed, and all the voxels in the image volume enter the first classifier.

2.1 Vantage Point Forest

In our work, we chose a clustering approach that is able to consider all features simultaneously and is less prone to overfitting than classical Random Forests [2] that considers only one feature at each node. As a base-classifier, we use the VPF. It is an algorithm for approximate nearest neighbour search whose atomic element, the Vantage Point Tree, was first described by Yianilos [16]. Each tree of the VPF describes a partition of the data space using hyperspheres centered on training data samples. These center-samples are randomly selected during training, and each tree is grown up to a fixed leaf-size. After training, each internal node contains a center-sample and a radius describing a hypersphere and each leaf contains a set of training samples. At test time, each sample is pushed through the trees by determining at each node whether it is located inside or outside the hypersphere and recursively searching either the left or the right subtree until a leaf node is reached. The training samples contained in that leaf are approximate nearest neighbours of the test sample. Heinrich *et al.* [6] showed that using linear nearest neighbour search over the union of the sets returned by all the trees improves the segmentation results for large organs. The distribution of classes of the nearest neighbours is then used as the output of the classifier.

2.2 Initial Labelling

We define the initial labelling as a multi-class segmentation problem. We use a VPF with BRIEF features as weak descriptors to obtain a tentative labelling of large and small organs. A performance close to the state of the art can be obtained for lungs, liver, spleen and kidneys. For small and more variable structures however, incorrect segmentations are obtained, because BRIEF features are not able to describe small organs precisely enough.

BRIEF Features. BRIEF features [3] encode local intensity differences and are computed on a the smoothed image $\tilde{I}$. For v, the nth BRIEF feature f_n^{BRIEF} is:

$$f_n^{\mathrm{BRIEF}}(v) = \mathrm{sign}(\tilde{I}(v + o_{n,1}) - \tilde{I}(v + o_{n,2})) \tag{1}$$

where $o_{n,1}$ and $o_{n,2}$ are randomly chosen offsets. By imposing, for a fixed proportion of the features, $o_{n,2} = 0$, we ensure that not only the relations between neighbouring structures are described, but also their relation to the current voxel.

2.3 Iterated Forest with Regional Context Descriptors

Even though the initial dense segmentation of small organs using VPF with weak descriptors is sub-optimal, the probability maps obtained contain valuable information. In particular, we propose to compute an approximate location $v_o = (x_o, y_o, z_o)$ of each object o to segment using its probability map $\mathcal{P}_o$ obtained from the initial classifier as an average location weighted by $\mathcal{P}_o$:

$$v_o = (x_o, y_o, z_o) = \sum_{v \in I} (x_v, y_v, z_v) \times \mathcal{P}_o(v) / \sum_{v \in I} \mathcal{P}_o(v) \qquad (2)$$

We then define the small organ segmentation problem as a two class problem and restrict it to a box around v_o. The size of that box is computed as the maximum size of the object to segment in training data plus a security margin.

We introduce anatomical context features and shape features to describe the regional context. These descriptors provide richer information than BRIEF features whilst still benefiting from a low computation time. We iteratively perform new labellings as a two-class problem for each object of interest separately, using BRIEF features, anatomical context features and shape features. The latter are described in the next paragraphs and all features are illustrated in Fig. 1. v_o is recomputed after each iteration.

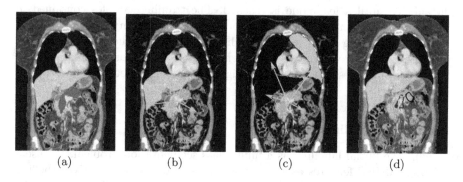

(a)   (b)   (c)   (d)

Fig. 1. Illustration of different types of features: (a) Ground truth for pancreas segmentation (b) BRIEF features: sign of intensity differences between or with nearby voxels are computed (c) Anatomical context features: the initial labelling at nearby voxels is considered (d) Shape features: training shapes at the approximate location of the object of interest are considered. Here, only contours of the shapes are shown.

Anatomical Context Features. We introduce anatomical context features to describe spatial relationships between neighbouring structures. They are related to the *autocontext* method of Tu [14]. Tu uses the probability maps obtained from a classifier as inputs for the next classifier in an iterative process. Here, we consider the labellings of structures segmented in the previous iterations. For v, a labelling L obtained from the previous classifier and a reference label l, the nth anatomical context feature f_n^{anat} is:

$$f_n^{\text{anat}}(v) = (L(v + o_n) == l) \qquad (3)$$

where o_n is a randomly chosen offset.

Shape Features. We introduce shape features as an emulation of regional shape atlases. For each training subject s, a window around the object of interest with label l is selected, yielding a cropped image I_c^s and the corresponding labelling L_c^s. I_c^s is then aligned to I by translation $T_{\to(x_o,y_o,z_o)}$ and affine transformation $Aff_{I_c^s \to I}$. The transformation is then applied to L_c^s to obtain the shape features f_s^{trans} and f_s^{aff}:

$$\begin{cases} f_s^{\text{trans}}(v) = (T_{\to(x_o,y_o,z_o)}(L_c^s)(v) == l) \\ f_s^{\text{aff}}(v) \;\;= (Aff_{I_c^s \to I}(L_c^s)(v) == l) \end{cases} \tag{4}$$

At a local level, affine transformations are complex enough to meaningfully express deformations whilst retaining a lower computational time than deformable registration methods. Because we register a cropped region and not the full image, we chose to restrict the shape features to translations and affine transformations. Our shape features are similar to local multi-atlas features. However, by operating at a local scale and with affine transformations only, they are computationally more efficient.

2.4 Final Shape Voting (SV)

The procedure described above outputs a probability map for each of the organs to segment. It can be discretised by choosing for each voxel the label with the highest probability. However, despite the shape features used in the classification, this approach doesn't ensure an optimal spatial consistency of the resulting segmentation. We propose instead to allow each training structure to vote on the probability map. Each training structure is affinely registered to the corresponding probability map. In each voxel, the number of votes is counted, leading to our final labelling.

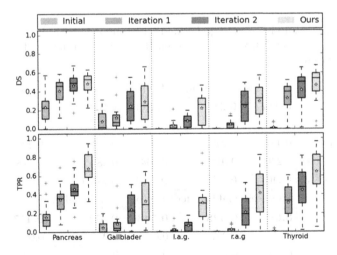

Fig. 2. Evaluation of DS and TPR after the initial labelling, the first iteration, the second iteration and the shape voting.

3   Experiments

We performed segmentation of the pancreas, the gallbladder, the left and right adrenal glands and the thyroid gland in CT images.

Datasets. We evaluated our method on the twenty training images available from the VISCERAL Anatomy 3 dataset [5] for non contrast-enhanced CT. In total, annotations for 20 structures are available, but we chose to concentrate on the small and variable ones, with which other approaches had difficulties. All data was resampled to a 2 mm isotropic resolution. When the ground truth was not available for a particular structure in a subject, the subject was removed of the score calculation for that structure only.

Parameters. Evaluation was performed in a leave-one-out fashion. For each iteration of our method, 15 trees were grown. For the initial labelling, 640 BRIEF features were used. For refining the labelling, we performed two iterations as described in Sect. 2.3. For the first one, 160 BRIEF features were used. For the second one, the liver, lungs, spleen and kidneys were considered as reference organs for the anatomical context features. 128 BRIEF features, 64 anatomical features for each reference organ (384 in total) and 38 shape features (each repeated 3 times, 108 in total) were used. Values for other parameters are provided in the supplementary material.

We compared our method to VPF (15 trees, parameters as in [6]), VPF followed by shape voting (VPF + SV), scale-adaptive Random Forest (saRF) [10] (99 trees) and the best multi-atlas method [13] for small organs of the Visceral Anatomy Challenge at ISBI 2015.

Table 1. Comparison of the average DS and TPR obtained with different methods. Note that the scores for [13] were obtained on the testing and not the training set of the Visceral dataset.

DS	Pancreas	Gallbladder	Thyroid	L. adrenal g.	R. adrenal g.
Ours	**0.481**	**0.288**	**0.463**	**0.220**	**0.294**
VPF	0.234	0.081	0.0	0.0	0.010
VPF + SV	0.447	0.243	0.0	0.0	0.228
saRF	0.246	0.012	0.294	0.08	0.018
Multi-atlas [13]	(0.408)	(0.276)	(0.549)	(0.373)	(0.355)
TPR	Pancreas	Gallbladder	Thyroid	L. adrenal g.	R. adrenal g.
Ours	**0.681**	**0.328**	**0.643**	**0.311**	**0.417**
VPF	0.158	0.047	0.0	0.0	0.005
VPF + SV	0.559	0.233	0.0	0.0	0.238
saRF	0.553	0.010	0.598	0.0	0.013

Results. We evaluated our method using the True Positive Rate (TPR) and the Dice Score (DS). As both for radiotherapy planning and false positive removal in PET, sensitivity is more important than specificity, the TPR is our main guideline. For a segmentation S and a ground truth G, $TPR = |S \cap G|/|G|$ and $DS = 2|S \cap G|/(|G| + |S|)$.

In Fig. 2, we show the influence of each element of our method on its overall performance. It demonstrates that the anatomical context and shape features included in Iteration 2 significantly increased both DS and TPR. In particular, after iteration 1, the adrenal glands were still not found, but the inclusion of anatomical context and shape features allowed to locate them for many subjects. The final shape voting had a limited influence on the DS, but caused a substantial increase in TPR. Examples of segmentations obtained with our method can be seen in Fig. 3.

Table 1 compares the DS and TPR obtained with our method to those obtained by other methods. For the multi-atlas method, the results were obtained on the test dataset whilst for the other methods, they were obtained on the training dataset. Nonetheless, we believe that comparison gives a good orientation so as to their respective performance. For the pancreas and the gallbladder, our method obtained a higher DS than the multi-atlas method (0.073 and 0.012 more respectively). It also obtained a higher DS and TPR than the forest-based methods for all organs, even when using VPF in combination with shape voting.

Note that, in our method, no deformable registrations are performed, which makes it computationally efficient. Typically, feature computation for each iteration for one subject is around one minute (for all organs), and the search of each tree is a matter of seconds.

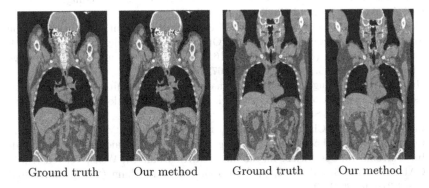

Ground truth   Our method   Ground truth   Our method

Fig. 3. Illustration of the labelling obtained for two subjects. The adrenal glands are shown in green and orange, the pancreas in blue and the thyroid in red. The gallblader is outside of the images. More examples can be found in the supplementary material. (Color figure online)

4 Conclusion

We have presented a novel iterative method for small organ segmentation in CT and introduced the anatomical context and shape features for describing regional context. Through the shape features and the final shape voting, our method has similarities with multi-atlas methods. By using only affine registrations however, it is computationally efficient and still outperforms outperforms other forest-based methods for all small organs.

Acknowledgements. This work was partially funded by the German ministry for education and research (Bundesministerium für Bildung und Forschung) under Grant Agreement No. 01IS12057.

References

1. Bieth, M., Donner, R., Langs, G., et al.: Anatomical triangulation: from sparse landmarks to dense annotation of the skeleton in CT images. In: Proceedings of BMVC, pp. 84.1–84.10 (2015)
2. Breiman, L.: Random forests. Mach. Learn. **45**(1), 5–32 (2001)
3. Calonder, M., Lepetit, V., Ozuysal, M., et al.: BRIEF: computing a local binary descriptor very fast. IEEE Trans. Pattern Anal. Mach. Intell. **34**(7), 1281–1298 (2012)
4. Criminisi, A., Shotton, J., Bucciarelli, S.: Decision forests with long-range spatial context for organ localization in CT volumes. In: MICCAI, pp. 69–80. Citeseer (2009)
5. Göksel, O., Jiménez-del Toro, O.A., Foncubierta-Rodríguez, A., Müller, H.: Overview of the VISCERAL challenge at ISBI 2015. In: Proceedings of the VISCERAL Anatomy Grand Challenge at ISBI (2015)
6. Heinrich, M.P., Blendowski, M.: Multi-organ segmentation using vantage point forests and binary context features. In: Ourselin, S., Joskowicz, L., Sabuncu, M.R., Unal, G., Wells, W. (eds.) MICCAI 2016. LNCS, vol. 9901, pp. 598–606. Springer, Cham (2016). doi:10.1007/978-3-319-46723-8_69
7. Hu, P., Wu, F., Peng, J., et al.: Automatic abdominal multi-organ segmentation using deep convolutional neural network and time-implicit level sets. Int. J. Comput. Assist. Radiol. Surg., 1–13 (2016)
8. Li, Y., Ho, C.P., Chahal, N., Senior, R., Tang, M.-X.: Myocardial segmentation of contrast echocardiograms using random forests guided by shape model. In: Ourselin, S., Joskowicz, L., Sabuncu, M.R., Unal, G., Wells, W. (eds.) MICCAI 2016. LNCS, vol. 9902, pp. 158–165. Springer, Cham (2016). doi:10.1007/978-3-319-46726-9_19
9. Okada, T., Linguraru, M.G., Hori, M., et al.: Abdominal multi-organ segmentation from CT images using conditional shape-location and unsupervised intensity priors. Med. Image Anal. **26**(1), 1–18 (2015)
10. Peter, L., Pauly, O., Chatelain, P., Mateus, D., Navab, N.: Scale-adaptive forest training via an efficient feature sampling scheme. In: Navab, N., Hornegger, J., Wells, W.M., Frangi, A.F. (eds.) MICCAI 2015. LNCS, vol. 9349, pp. 637–644. Springer, Cham (2015). doi:10.1007/978-3-319-24553-9_78

11. Richmond, D., Kainmueller, D., Glocker, B., Rother, C., Myers, G.: Uncertainty-driven forest predictors for vertebra localization and segmentation. In: Navab, N., Hornegger, J., Wells, W.M., Frangi, A.F. (eds.) MICCAI 2015. LNCS, vol. 9349, pp. 653–660. Springer, Cham (2015). doi:10.1007/978-3-319-24553-9_80

12. Roth, H.R., Lu, L., Farag, A., Shin, H.-C., Liu, J., Turkbey, E.B., Summers, R.M.: DeepOrgan: multi-level deep convolutional networks for automated pancreas segmentation. In: Navab, N., Hornegger, J., Wells, W.M., Frangi, A.F. (eds.) MICCAI 2015. LNCS, vol. 9349, pp. 556–564. Springer, Cham (2015). doi:10.1007/978-3-319-24553-9_68

13. del Toro, O.A.J., Müller, H.: Hierarchical multi-structure segmentation guided by anatomical correlations. In: Proceedings of the VISCERAL Challenge at ISBI, pp. 32–36. Citeseer (2014)

14. Tu, Z.: Auto-context and its application to high-level vision tasks. In: CVPR, pp. 1–8. IEEE (2008)

15. Viola, P., Jones, M.: Rapid object detection using a boosted cascade of simple features. In: CVPR, vol. 1, p. I-511, IEEE (2001)

16. Yianilos, P.N.: Data structures and algorithms for nearest neighbor search in general metric spaces. In: SODA, vol. 93, pp. 311–321 (1993)

17. Zikic, D., Glocker, B., Criminisi, A.: Atlas encoding by randomized forests for efficient label propagation. In: Mori, K., Sakuma, I., Sato, Y., Barillot, C., Navab, N. (eds.) MICCAI 2013. LNCS, vol. 8151, pp. 66–73. Springer, Heidelberg (2013). doi:10.1007/978-3-642-40760-4_9

Motion Corruption Detection in Breast DCE-MRI

Sylvester Chiang[1]([✉]), Sharmila Balasingham[2], Lara Richmond[2],
Belinda Curpen[2], Mia Skarpathiotakis[2], and Anne Martel[1]

[1] Department of Medical Biophysics,
University of Toronto, Toronto, ON, Canada
sylvester.chiang@mail.utoronto.ca
[2] Sunnybrook Health Sciences Centre, Imaging Research, Toronto, ON, Canada

Abstract. Motion corruption can result in difficulty identifying lesions, and incorrect diagnoses by radiologists in cases of breast cancer screening using DCE-MRI. Although registration techniques can be used to correct for motion artifacts, their use has a computational cost and, in some cases can lead to a reduction in diagnostic quality rather than the desired improvement. In a clinical system it would be beneficial to identify automatically which studies have severe motion corruption and poor diagnostic quality and which studies have acceptable diagnostic quality. This information could then be used to restrict registration to only those cases where motion correction is needed, or it could be used to identify cases where motion correction fails. We have developed an automated method of estimating the degree of mis-registration present in a DCE-MRI study. We experiment using two predictive models; one based on a feature extraction method and a second one using a deep learning approach. These models are trained using estimates of deformation generated from unlabeled clinical data. We validate the predictions on a labeled dataset from radiologists denoting cases suffering from motion artifacts that affected their ability to interpret the image. By calculating a binary threshold on our predictions, we have managed to identify motion corrupted cases on our clinical dataset with an accuracy of 86% based on the area under the ROC curve. This approach is a novel attempt at defining a clinically relevant level of motion corruption.

Keywords: DCE-MRI · Motion artifacts · Registration · Feature extraction · Convolutional neural networks

1 Introduction

Dynamic contrast-enhanced MRI (DCE-MRI) has been shown to increase the sensitivity of cancer detection in breast screening programs for women at higher risk of breast cancer [3]. In these exams, a single pre-contrast image and a series of post-contrast images are acquired and the degree and rate of contrast-enhancement is used to identify cancer. Motion corruption can create artifacts in subtraction images which may obscure lesions and decrease the diagnostic utility of the images. Automated non-rigid registration [6] can be used to align temporally sequential sequences of DCE-MRI and are commonly used as a pre-processing step in computer aided

© Springer International Publishing AG 2017
Q. Wang et al. (Eds.): MLMI 2017, LNCS 10541, pp. 10–18, 2017.
DOI: 10.1007/978-3-319-67389-9_2

detection algorithms [9]. However there are unique difficulties in registering DCE-MRI images, including the non-rigid deformability of breast tissue, lack of clear landmarks, and the presence of contrast-enhancement. These characteristics can result in the failure of registration resulting in a reduction in image quality [2]. Furthermore, the use of image registration inevitably results in some blurring due to interpolation [2] and this is particularly a problem in clinical breast imaging where the pixels are very anisotropic. Registration also has an associated time penalty with non-rigid registration algorithms running on the order of a single minute to upwards of 15 min [2].

This paper proposes an automated method for motion-corruption detection in DCE-MRI scans. This would allow for an independent assessment of registration quality that is completely separate from any optimization metric in the registration process. This predictive model could also serve in a CAD pipeline to determine the necessity of registration, thereby reducing the associated time penalty and removing the possibility of mis-registration. A unique challenge associated with this task is to identify motion artifacts that are clinically relevant and need to be corrected to allow for proper interpretation. To build this binary model, we first attempted to use a feature extraction approach that has been used for registration quality assessment in other imaging modalities and biological models [1, 5]. We also utilized a deep learning approach to generate binary labels using convolutional neural networks to draw a comparison between the different learning paradigms.

2   Methodology

We propose a two-stage process to detect motion corruption. First, we estimated the average deformation using a regression model trained on unlabeled data. Then we used the output from the regression models to predict a binary categorical label that corresponded to the motion-corruption labels provided by radiologists. We explored supervised learning methods using a traditional feature extraction approach and drew comparisons with a neural network model. Receiver operating characteristic (ROC) curves allowed us to analyze the trade-off between the true positive rate (TPR) and false positive rate (FPR) at different binary thresholds making it more clinically adaptable (see Fig. 1).

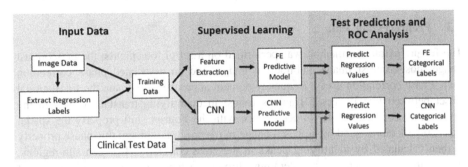

Fig. 1. This is the learning model for our proposed experiment. Regression labels were extracted from the DCE-MRI data and used to train two separate supervised learning models. The test set was then fed to both models to predict regression values which were used to infer a binary label.

2.1 Data Acquisition

In our experiments we work with DCE-MRI data which is acquired at our institution as a set of volumes consisting of a pre-contrast volume and four post-contrast volumes. The post-contrast volumes are acquired approximately 90 s apart to allow for circulation of the contrast agent. The dimension of each volume was $512 \times 512 \times 80$ with an in-plane resolution of approximately 0.35 mm and a slice thickness of 3 mm. Subtraction images were generated by subtracting the pre-contrast image from each of the post-contrast images with each subtraction treated as a separate instance.

To obtain a training dataset we pulled unlabeled volumes from our database of breast MR images and associated radiology reports. Reports with motion-identifying phrases such as "motion corrupted" and "motion artifacts" were queried to collect a sample of motion-corrupted volumes. We then conducted another search filtering out these phrases and selected an equivalent number of volumes to acquire a set of data free of severe motion-corruption. In total we obtained a balanced dataset of 88 DCE-MRI volumes. To validate our results, we acquired a completely separate set of 40 patient MRIs to use as our final test set. These volumes were provided by radiologists asked to submit motion-corrupted cases they recognized in their daily work. To keep a balanced dataset they were requested to submit a case free of motion-related artifacts in conjunction with the motion-corrupted images. There was a high degree of variation within each class, as individual radiologists tolerated different amounts of motion.

2.2 Generating Deformation Estimates for Unlabeled Images

We could not assume that the absence of a comment about motion corruption in the radiology report was sufficient to label an image as being free of motion-corruption. This meant that it was necessary to generate surrogate labels to quantify the deformation present in these images for the purpose of supervised learning. We used the Elastix library to perform 3D b-spline registration on these images and then used Transformix to output the resulting deformation fields. The field contained vectors dictating the pixel shift for the registration, and the Euclidean distance for each vector was calculated and averaged over the entire volume to calculate a single metric. This process allowed us to capture the quantity of deformation in a volume as a continuous variable which we could then use to train a regression model via supervised learning.

2.3 Preprocessing Data

The feature extraction method was performed on a set of four inputs; the pre-contrast image, post-contrast image, subtraction image, and an associated phase correlation map. Phase correlation uses a frequency domain approach to estimate the translational offset between two images [7] and is robust in quantifying translation even in the presence of contrast agents. In accordance with the Fourier shift property the spatial translation is represented by a phase change in the spectral domain; this phase property is then calculated by identifying peaks in the cross-correlation between sub-regions. The map was generated by iterating through patches of the pre-contrast and post-contrast image to calculate a dense phase correlation map.

In our experiments, only one set of pre-contrast and post-contrast images were considered at a time. Different institutions utilize different imaging protocols and may produce a different number of post-contrast images. Creating a model to only use one pre-contrast and one post-contrast image would be more generalizable across institutions and could be more easily adopted. Segmentations were applied to the breast volumes to remove the surrounding air and chest wall which were not significant in the analysis of breast deformation and could have in fact added more irrelevant noise. The DCE-MRI images were acquired as 3D volumes but slices were extracted along the center of each breast to augment the number of instances in our training model.

2.4 Training a Supervised Learning Model

The regression models discussed were trained on the dataset of 88 patients. We augmented our dataset by taking slices from each 3-dimensional volume, in total producing 3180 training instances. This image set was split into an 80% training set and 20% tuning set, with data stratification on a volume level. We compared two different feature extraction approaches in our experiments. The first was based on hand-crafted features that were then used as an input vector for a variety of classical machine learning algorithms. A second approach consisted of utilizing a Convolutional Neural Network (CNN) based on deep learning theory. This type of network contains convolutional layers which act as high-level feature extractors that operate on raw images as input. These extracted features are then fed into a series of dense layers for classification.

Feature Extraction. Features were calculated globally, within the inner volume of the breast, and the edges of the breast near the skin because motion artifacts that occur in particular regions may be more significant. These region masks were generated by eroding segmentations. 15 intensity-based features were calculated for each region, including mean, mode, skew, and negative sum of squares (NSSQ) which was the sum of squares exclusively calculated over negative regions. These features were computed over the subtraction images while mutual information features were calculated using the pre-contrast and post-contrast images.

Texture analysis using gray-level co-occurrence matrices provided a second source of features. Texture measures are highly utilized in computer vision problems within the medical field. This extraction method examined the contrast, correlation and homogeneity of images. These texture features were also applied to the phase correlation maps. In total we generated a set of 52 features from each 2D sample. These features were used as input to machine learning algorithms available through sklearn, specifically Support Vector Machines (SVMs) and tree-based ensemble learning methods.

Convolutional Neural Networks. Deep learning networks are computational models built to learn hierarchal representations of data at different levels of abstraction CNNs have been applied to image classification tasks with a high amount of success, achieving record accuracies [4]. As opposed to dense mappings between individual perceptrons within the hidden layers, CNNs learn a large number of filters that are convolved with a 2D input data. These networks perform well on computer vision problems due to a reduced parameter space and their usage of translationally invariant filters. Another advantage of utilizing CNNs is that image data can generally be directly fed into the network with minimal pre-processing steps, unlike feature extraction which requires a manual exploration of discriminative metrics.

Our architecture was inspired by a simple CNN, AlexNet [4] with two reduced layers to make the network easier to train due to fewer parameters. It consisted of four convolutional layers followed by a dense mapping to two fully-connected layers (Fig. 2). We chose rectified linear units (ReLU) as our activation function, which are lightweight and helped to address the vanishing gradient problem [4]. Dropout was also added as a regularization tool and operates by masking random activations therefore preventing neighboring nodes from clustering together to learn specific representations of image features [8]. The input of the CNN was comprised of 3 channels; the pre-contrast, post-contrast, and phase correlation map which were all downsampled to 256×256 pixels. The neural networks were built using the Theano and Lasagne libraries in Python which allowed for optimized calculations to power the learning process (see Fig. 3).

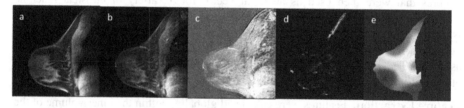

Fig. 2. Visualized input data, pre-contrast image (a), post-contrast image (b), subtraction image with a noticeable motion artifact along the top edge of the breast (c), segmented phase correlation map (d), segmented deformation field (e)

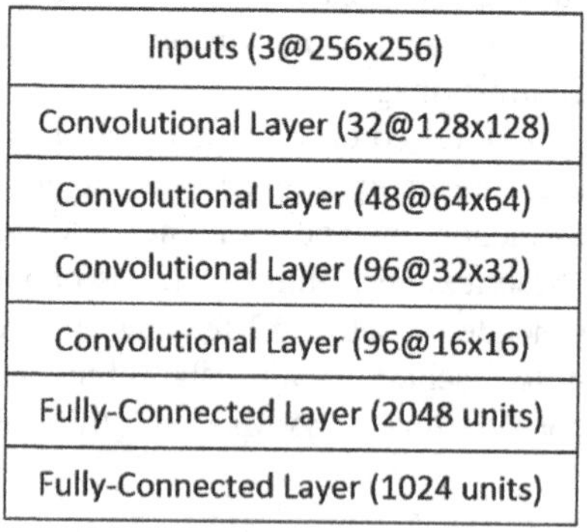

Inputs (3@256x256)
Convolutional Layer (32@128x128)
Convolutional Layer (48@64x64)
Convolutional Layer (96@32x32)
Convolutional Layer (96@16x16)
Fully-Connected Layer (2048 units)
Fully-Connected Layer (1024 units)

Fig. 3. The architecture of the CNN. The first convolutional layer is the product of a (5×5) kernel followed a (2×2) max-pool. The following three layers were convolved by a (3×3) filter again followed a (2×2) max-pool. The activations after the fourth convolutional layer were flattened and mapped to a dense fully-connected layer.

3 Results

3.1 Comparing Learning Models

Both supervised learning methods were trained on the set of 88 patients and then tested on the radiologist-labelled set of 40 DCE-MRI images. The regression values were used to generate thresholds and subsequently infer categorical labels. The sensitivity (TPR) and specificity (1-FPR) at each threshold value were plotted to form an ROC curve representing the accuracy of the predictions compared to our ground truth labels. Averaging the deformation predictions of individual slices to generate a volume-level prediction before constructing the ROC increased the AUC value. The increase in aggregate mean accuracy was likely due to the labelling being performed on a volume basis. Taking the mean value offered a better representation of the 3D volume and as a result predicted the ground truth more accurately. However the results from the hand-crafted features still underperformed compared to the CNN (see Fig. 4).

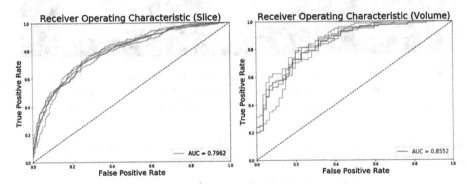

Fig. 4. The ROC curve calculated from the regression values predicted by the CNN. Blue lines represent different randomly initialized neural networks and the red represents the average ROC. The left image shows the curve constructed for every slice and the right curve plots the deformation metric aggregated over volumes (6 slices). (Color figure online)

The same training and testing paradigm was used on the CNN model. The AUC of ROC value was 0.80 ± 0.01 and when averaged over volumes demonstrated an AUC value of 0.86 ± 0.01 (Fig. 5). CNNs achieved a predictive power higher than previous supervised learning methods based on hand-crafted feature extraction. On a 3.6 GHz CPU, phase map preprocessing required on average 5.4 s followed by a forward pass of this CNN which took approximately 0.5 s. These values compared favorably to the Elastix registration time which ran for 140 s per volume on average. The advantage of running this classification model could yield a large potential temporal benefit as this time penalty is incurred for every post-contrast image leading to large processing times (see Table. 1).

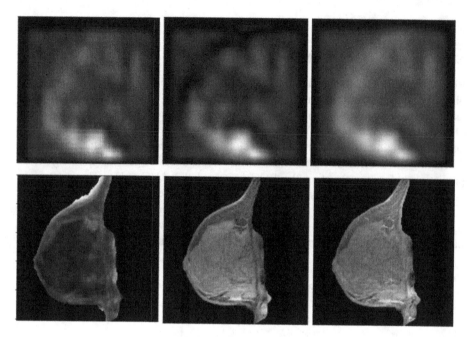

Fig. 5. The top row shows the maximum activations in the first dense layer of the network deconvolved, and the corresponding input images shown on the bottom row. From left to right columns, the images show the phase map, the pre-contrast image, and the post-contrast image.

Table 1. A table of the AUC metric calculated on ROC curves. The left column is calculated for each individual slice and the right column shows the metric per volume.

AUROC (area under the receiver operator characteristic curve)		
Learning method	Per slice	Aggregate mean
Random forest (n = 100)	0.65 ± 0.02	**0.71 ± 0.02**
Random forest (n = 500)	0.65 ± 0.02	**0.71 ± 0.02**
AdaBoost (n = 100)	0.69 ± 0.03	**0.72 ± 0.03**
AdaBoost (n = 500)	0.65 ± 0.03	**0.70 ± 0.05**
SVM	0.72 ± 0.01	**0.77 ± 0.01**
CNN	0.80 ± 0.01	**0.86 ± 0.01**

3.2 Visualizing Neural Networks

While neural network features can be difficult to understand, new visualization methods can help provide visual cues of what the learned features represent. Deconvolution nets project large activations back to the input space to better understand visual features that strongly impact the final classification score. We extracted the maximum activations in various layers and applied a deconvolution using the set of transposed weights learned from the forward pass. This was followed by an unpooling operation [10] to regain an output of the same dimension as the input. The deconvolved images showed that large activations have correspondence with features at the edge of the breast. This provided evidence that even though features internal to the breast had a role in determining the amount of motion, the significant motion artifacts that are noted by clinicians tended to occur at the surface of the breast.

4 Conclusion

In this paper we compared the classical method of utilizing feature extraction to solve classification problems, to more recent deep learning approaches in the domain of registration accuracy. We achieved an accuracy of 0.86 based on the AUC of the ROC curve. We theorize that hand-crafted features rely on intuition and are often influenced by features common throughout the field of medical imaging. CNNs differ by extracting extremely domain-specific features at deeper convolution levels that are represented as a pattern of weights resulting in higher classification performance.

Motion corruption detection in DCE-MRI volumes remains a challenging task but automated assessment of these cases will become more impactful as larger amounts of medical information are processed. In this experiment we explored a preliminary method to predict motion corruption as it pertains to clinical interpretation. The model that we proposed is robust to contrast-enhancement due to the inclusion of phase correlation maps which register translation on sub-regions. We also introduced a method of estimating deformation in an image that is independent of physician subjectivity, and did not require any manual creation of landmarks. Finally we have developed a model to define a level of motion corruption that is relevant to a clinician's ability to diagnose an image, allowing for a more intelligent approach to applying registrations.

References

1. Armato, S.G., et al.: Temporal subtraction in chest radiography: automated assessment of registration accuracy. Med. Phys. **33**(5), 1239 (2006)
2. Klein, A., et al.: Evaluation of 14 nonlinear deformation algorithms applied to human brain MRI registration. Neuroimage **46**(3), 786–802 (2009)
3. Kok, T., et al.: Efficacy of MRI and Mammography for breast-cancer screening in women with a familial or genetic predisposition. Engl. J. Med. **351**(5), 427–437 (2004)
4. Krizhevsky, A., et al.: ImageNet classification with deep convolutional neural networks. Adv. Neural Inf. Process. Syst. 1–9 (2012)
5. Muenzing, S.E.A., et al.: Supervised quality assessment of medical image registration: application to CT lung registration. Med. Image Anal. **16**(8), 1521–1531 (2012)
6. Rueckert, D., et al.: Nonrigid registration using free-form deformations: application to breast MR images. IEEE Trans. Med. Imaging **18**(8), 712–721 (1999)
7. Srinivasa Reddy, B., Chatterji, B.N.: An FFT-based technique for translation, rotation, and scale-invariant registration. IEEE Trans. Image Process. **5**(8), 1266–1271 (1996)

8. Srivastava, N., et al.: Dropout: a simple way to prevent neural networks from overfitting. J. Mach. Learn. Res. **15**, 1929–1958 (2014)
9. Vignati, A., et al.: A fully automatic lesion detection method for DCE-MRI fat-suppressed breast images. SPIE Med. Imaging **7260**, 726026 (2009)
10. Zeiler, M.D., Fergus, R.: Visualizing and understanding convolutional networks. In: Fleet, D., Pajdla, T., Schiele, B., Tuytelaars, T. (eds.) ECCV 2014. LNCS, vol. 8689, pp. 818–833. Springer, Cham (2014). doi:10.1007/978-3-319-10590-1_53

Detection and Localization of Drosophila Egg Chambers in Microscopy Images

Jiří Borovec[(⊠)], Jan Kybic, and Rodrigo Nava

Department of Cybernetics, Faculty of Electrical Engineering,
Czech Technical University in Prague, Prague, Czech Republic
jiri.borovec@fel.cvut.cz

Abstract. *Drosophila melanogaster* is a well-known model organism that can be used for studying oogenesis (egg chamber development) including gene expression patterns. Standard analysis methods require manual segmentation of individual egg chambers, which is a difficult and time-consuming task. We present an image processing pipeline to detect and localize Drosophila egg chambers that consists of the following steps: (i) superpixel-based image segmentation into relevant tissue classes; (ii) detection of egg center candidates using label histograms and ray features; (iii) clustering of center candidates and; (iv) area-based maximum likelihood ellipse model fitting. Our proposal is able to detect 96% of human-expert annotated egg chambers at relevant developmental stages with less than 1% false-positive rate, which is adequate for the further analysis.

Keywords: Drosophila oogenesis · Clustering · Egg segmentation · Ellipse model fitting · Label histograms · Ray features

1 Introduction

The motivation of this work is to provide a tool for automatic analysis of spatial and temporal patterns of gene expression during the egg-chamber development (oogenesis) of the common fruit fly, *Drosophila melanogaster* [1]. Such studies aim to discover the functionality of specific genes, which is of paramount importance in basic biological research with possible therapeutic applications in medicine. The task solved here is a segmentation of individual egg chambers.

Figure 1(a) shows an example of an input fluorescence microscopy image consisting of a chain of egg chambers in different developmental stages. It is a common practice to collect thousands of such images to analyze different genes of interest [2]. Once the individual egg chambers are localized (see Fig. 1(c)), they will be grouped by developmental stage [3], segmented, aligned, and their gene expression detected and analyzed [4]. Previously, most of the analysis was done manually [5,6], which is very time consuming.

Unlike for *Drosophila embryogenesis* [7], to the best of our knowledge, there are no previous works about Drosophila egg chamber detection and localization [6]. A texture-based classification method for egg chamber images was

© Springer International Publishing AG 2017
Q. Wang et al. (Eds.): MLMI 2017, LNCS 10541, pp. 19–26, 2017.
DOI: 10.1007/978-3-319-67389-9_3

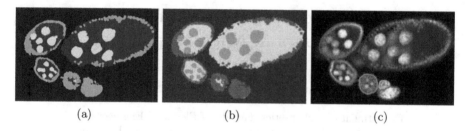

Fig. 1. Illustrative example of a fluorescence microscopy image containing several egg chambers in different processing phases. *(a)* Cell nuclei are shown in magenta and RNA gene expression in green. *(b)* Automatic initial segmentation into four classes: Background (blue), cytoplasm (red), nurse cells (yellow), and follicle cells (cyan). *(c)* Manually delineated egg chambers used for validation. (Color figure online)

described in [8]. The segmentation is not robust enough (Fig. 5) but can be used as the first step of our approach (Fig. 1(b)).

The key contributions of this work are the novel shape and appearance features, label histograms, and orientation invariant ray distances, as well as the area-based maximum likelihood ellipse fitting. For simplicity, we represent the detected egg chambers with ellipses.

2   Methodology

Our proposal uses the cellular structure channel (magenta in Fig. 1(a)). It consists of superpixel-based segmentation (Sect. 2.1), center candidate detection (Sect. 2.2), center candidate clustering (Sect. 2.2), and ellipse model fitting (Sect. 2.3).

2.1   Superpixel Segmentation

We use superpixel segmentation proposed in [8]: First, SLIC superpixels are calculated [9] with an initial size of 15 pixels. For each superpixel, color and texture features are computed. Then, the superpixels are assigned to one of the following four classes (background, follicle cells, cytoplasm, or nurse cells) using a random forest classifier with Graphcut [10] regularization (see Fig. 1(b)).

2.2   Center Detection

In order to detect points within the central part of the egg chambers, we use two sets of features based on label histograms and modified ray features [11]. The center candidates are chosen from superpixel centroids using a random forest classifier. The features are normalized to zero mean and unit variance. For training, superpixels close to a center are considered positive (as measured by the relative distance to the background), superpixels far away as negative, ignoring those in-between (see Fig. 2(a)).

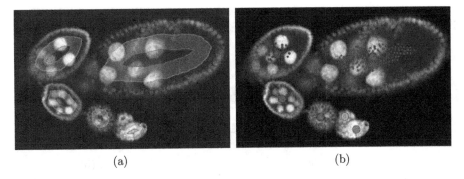

(a)   (b)

Fig. 2. *(a)* A center detector is trained using positive central examples in green and negative far away examples in red, ignoring the intermediate zone in yellow. *(b)* Automatically detected central points clustered using DBSCAN. Each cluster is shown in a different color. The centroids of the clusters are drawn as large dots. (Color figure online)

Label Histograms. Around a given point, a set of N annular regions D_i is defined (see Fig. 3(a)). For each region, a normalized label (class) histogram is computed, counting the number of pixels of each class within each region is counted. The histograms are concatenated.

Ray Features. To describe a shape, we use a simplified version of the ray features [11]. Rays are oriented straight lines cast from the point of interest with a predetermined angular step ω. For each ray i, we measure the distance r_i to the first background-class point in the given direction. To obtain rotational invariance, the vector $R = (r_1, \ldots, r_n)$ is circularly shifted to start with the largest element.

Center Clustering. Detections corresponding to individual eggs are grouped together using density-based spatial clustering (DBSCAN) [12] that handles arbitrarily shaped clusters and naturally detects outliers. The distance threshold parameter of DBSCAN is set to 3× the superpixel size. Each cluster is represented by its mean position c_k (see Fig. 2(b)).

2.3   Ellipse Fitting and Segmentation

We represent each egg by an ellipse (see Fig. 5). The advantages are: a small number of parameters, convexity, and compactness. Given a cluster mean c_k (egg center) and the four-class pixel-level segmentation Y (Sect. 2.1), the ellipse should maximize the likelihood

$$\prod_{i \in \Omega_F} P_F(Y_i) \cdot \prod_{i \in \Omega \setminus \Omega_F} P_B(Y_i) \qquad (1)$$

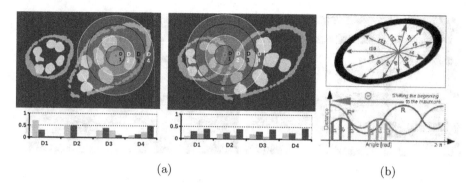

(a)   (b)

Fig. 3. (a) Label histogram descriptor for two different points. A set of annular regions D_i is defined around a reference point, then normalized histograms of label frequencies are computed. (b) Ray descriptor illustration. A set of rays is cast from a reference point to the closest background pixel and the distances r_i are measured. To achieve rotation invariance, we find the maximal element in R (blue curve) and shift it to the beginning to obtain R^* (green curve). (Color figure online)

where Ω_F is the ellipse interior and Ω is the entire image. $P_F(Y_i)$ and $P_B(Y_i)$ are the probabilities that a pixel i inside and outside the egg chamber is classified to a class Y_i, respectively. For the four classes of Y (0-background, 1-follicle cells, 2-cytoplasm, and 3-nurse cells) we have set $P_B(Y_i = 0) = P_F(Y_i \in \{1,2,3\}) = 0.9$ and $P_F(Y_i = 0) = P_B(Y_i \in \{1,2,3\}) = 0.1$. If accurate pixel-level reference segmentation is available, the probabilities P_F and P_B can be obtained from the training data instead.

Using negative log likelihood $g_\bullet = -\log P_\bullet$ and substituting $\sum_{i \in \Omega} g_B(Y_i) = \sum_{i \in \Omega_F} g_B(Y_i) + \sum_{i \in \Omega \setminus \Omega_F} g_B(Y_i)$ we obtain an equivalent problem:

$$\min \sum_{i \in \Omega_F} g_F(Y_i) - g_B(Y_i) \qquad (2)$$

Possible ellipse boundary points are determined by casting rays from the center c_k as described in (Sect. 2.2) and taking the first background point along the ray or the first non-follicle class point after a follicle class point (see Fig. 4(a)). Points on the boundary closer than 5 pixels each other are eliminated to reduce clutter. To obtain a robust fit, we use a random sampling (RANSAC-like) strategy. Ellipses are fitted [13] to randomly selected subsets of 40% of detected boundary points for each center. The best ellipse with respect to Eq. (2) is chosen.

3   Materials and Experiments

Our dataset consists of 4338 2D microscopy slices extracted from 2467 volumes. Experts identified the developmental stage and approximate location for 4853 egg chambers by marking three points on their boundaries. (see red rectangles in Fig. 5). The automatic detection is considered as correct if the detected center is

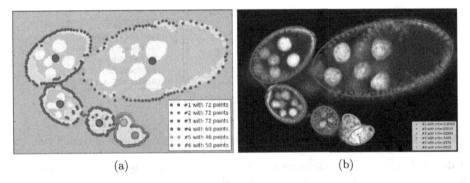

(a)   (b)

Fig. 4. *(a)* Ellipse fitting takes as input the four-class segmentation and cluster centers c_k (shown as large dots). Possible ellipse boundary points are found as end-points of rays cast from each cluster center. *(b)* Fitted ellipses are shown overlaid over the segmentation and original image.

Input image   Initial segmentation   Detected individual eggs

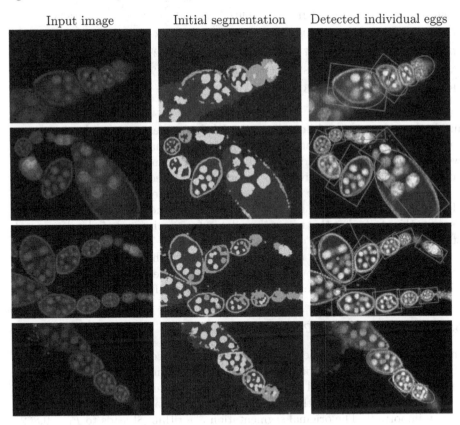

Fig. 5. Input images (left), initial segmentation (middle) followed by the detected centers (cluster means) as dots and the fitted ellipses in green (right). Expert drawn bounding boxes are shown as red rectangles (not all eggs are annotated). (Color figure online)

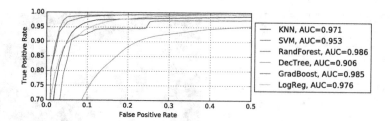

Fig. 6. ROC curves for different classifiers for the center candidate detection task.

Table 1. Egg detection performance of the egg detection task by development stages, in terms of false positives, false negatives, and the number of multiply detected eggs before and after post-processing with ellipse fitting.

Egg chambers	Stage				
	1	2	3	4	5
Number	921	1403	865	834	836
False negatives	306 (33%)	158 (11%)	6 (0.7%)	1 (0.1%)	0 (0.0%)
Multiple detections (MD)	37 (4.0%)	31 (2.2%)	109 (12%)	80 (9.6%)	90 (11%)
MD after ellipse fitting	18 (2.0%)	13 (0.9%)	27 (3.1%)	20 (2.4%)	30 (3.6%)
False positives	43 (0.9%)				

inside the user annotated bounding box. We have reference pixel-level segmentation on a subset of 72 images comprising 196 eggs chambers. The experiments were conducted using 10-fold cross-validation. For quantitative evaluation of the correct identification of individual eggs we use adjusted Rand Score (ARS).

Drosophila egg chamber development can be divided up to 14–15 stages [3]. However, some of them are hard to distinguish and the differences are not relevant for this study. For this reason, our dataset recognizes only 5 developmental stages, numbered 1–5 that correspond to stages 1, 2–7, 8, 9, and 10–12 of [3], respectively. Stage 1 in our notation corresponds to the smallest egg chambers without any distinguishable internal structure (e.g. the smallest egg chamber in Fig. 1(c)) and is of no interest for gene expression analysis.

3.1   Center Detection Performance

In the first group of experiments, we have studied the accuracy of center detection (Sect. 2.2), formulated as a binary classification problem on superpixels. The area under the curve (AUC) and the F_1 measure were evaluated.

The first observation is that the quality of the initial four-class segmentation is very important. The original segmentation algorithm [8] leads to $F_1 = 0.862$. Using a random forest classifier and GraphCut regularization, the performance was improved to $F_1 = 0.916$.

When evaluating the influence of the diameters of the annular regions for the label histogram descriptors (Sect. 2.2), we have discovered that it is important to include both small and large regions. With five regions spanning diameters in range from 10 to 300 pixels, we get $F_1 = 0.916$ and AUC $= 0.988$. Including more regions does not significantly improve the results – with 9 regions, we get $F_1 = 0.923$ and AUC $= 0.989$.

Using a four-class initial segmentation is helpful, with a binary segmentation the performance drops to $F_1 = 0.868$ and AUC $= 0.959$. Concerning ray features (Sect. 2.2), the best performance is obtained for an angular step of $5°\sim15°$. Larger angular steps lead to a loss of details, smaller angular steps increase the descriptor variability.

Using both ray features and label histograms is better, yielding AUC $= 0.987$ and $F_1 = 0.930$, than using them separately, with AUC $= 0.986$ and $F_1 = 0.928$ for the label histogram only and AUC $= 0.972$ and $F_1 = 0.884$ for the ray features only.

Finally, we show the ROC curve for several different classifier algorithms (Fig. 6). We have chosen the random forest classifier which is among the best performing methods and is fast at the same time.

3.2 Egg Chamber Detection

The second part of the experiments evaluates, how many eggs are detected and how many detections are really eggs. The experts marked a subset of 4853 egg chambers with three boundary points (as described above) and a stage label. The results are shown in Table 1. The performance on the smallest stage 1 egg chambers is not important for our purposes. Stage 2 is the most challenging. For the rest, less than 1% of eggs are missed. There is also less then 1% of false positives, which were counted manually for all stages combined, as the stage information is not available for false detections. The most frequent mistake is to detect one egg chamber twice, which can be easily corrected by post-processing— if two ellipses overlap more then 50% of pixels, we keep only the larger one. We show the number of multiple detections both before and after this post-processing.

We also evaluate the performance of ellipse approximation on a pixel-level annotated subset of 72 images containing about 250 egg chambers. With respect to a watershed segmentation [14] using the distance from the background class as a feature, we improved the mean ARS from 0.755 to 0.857 and the mean Jaccard index from 0.571 to 0.674.

Figure 5 shows examples of successful results, including a few corrected multiple detections and a few undetected egg chambers. Note that the user annotation is neither complete nor accurate, which makes the evaluation challenging.

4 Conclusions

We presented a complete pipeline for Drosophila egg chamber detection and localization by ellipse fitting in microscopic images. Our contributions include novel label histogram features, the rotation invariant ray features, and area-based maximum likelihood ellipse fitting. The performance is completely adequate for the desired application—it is important that the number of false positives is small but false negatives are not a problem, as long as a sufficiently high number of egg chambers is detected.

In the future, a specialized model could be created for the earliest developmental stages to reduce the number of misses.

Acknowledgments. This work was supported by Czech Science Foundation projects no. 14-21421S and 17-15361S, and Mexican agency CONACYT with the postdoctoral scholarship no. 266758. The images were provided by Pavel Tomancak's group, MPI-CBG, Germany.

References

1. Bastock, R., St. Johnston, D.: *Drosophila* oogenesis. Curr. Biol. **18**, R1082–R1087 (2008)
2. Parton, R.M., Vallés, A.M., Dobbie, I.M., Davis, I.: Isolation of Drosophila egg chambers for imaging. Cold Spring Harb. Protoc. (2010). doi:10.1101/pdb.prot5402
3. Jia, D., Xu, Q., Xie, Q., Mio, W., Deng, W.M.: Automatic stage identification of Drosophila egg chamber based on DAPI images. Sci. Rep. **6**, 18850 (2016)
4. Borovec, J., Kybic, J.: Binary pattern dictionary learning for gene expression representation in *Drosophila* imaginal discs. In: Chen, C.-S., Lu, J., Ma, K.-K. (eds.) ACCV 2016. LNCS, vol. 10117, pp. 555–569. Springer, Cham (2017). doi:10.1007/978-3-319-54427-4_40
5. Tomancak, P., et al.: Global analysis of patterns of gene expression during Drosophila embryogenesis. Genome Biol. **8**, R145 (2007)
6. Jug, F., Pietzsch, T., Preibisch, S., Tomancak, P.: Bioimage informatics in the context of Drosophila research. Methods **68**, 60–73 (2014)
7. Castro, C., Luengo-Oroz, M., Douloquin, L., et al.: Image processing challenges in the creation of spatiotemporal gene expression atlases of developing embryos. IEEE Eng. Med. Biol. Soc. (EMBC) **2011**, 6841–6844 (2011). https://www.ncbi.nlm.nih.gov/pubmed/22255910
8. Nava, R., Kybic, J.: Supertexton-based segmentation in early Drosophila oogenesis. In: IEEE International Conference on Image Processing (ICIP), pp. 2656–2659 (2015)
9. Achanta, R., et al.: SLIC superpixels compared to state-of-the-art superpixel methods. IEEE PAMI **34**, 2274–2282 (2012)
10. Boykov, Y., Veksler, O.: Fast approximate energy minimization via graph cuts. IEEE Pattern Anal. Mach. Intell. **23**, 1222–1239 (2001)
11. Smith, K., Carleton, A., Lepetit, V.: Fast ray features for learning irregular shapes. In: IEEE 12th International Conference on Computer Vision, pp. 397–404 (2009)
12. Ester, M., Kriegel, H.P., Sander, J., Xu, X.: A density-based algorithm for discovering clusters in large spatial databases with noise. In: International Conference on Knowledge Discovery and Data Mining, pp. 226–231 (1996)
13. Halir, R., Flusser, J.: Numerically stable direct least squares fitting of ellipses. Cent. Eur. Comput. Graph. Visual. **98**, 125–132 (1998)
14. Chen, Q., Yang, X., Petriu, E.: Watershed segmentation for binary images with different distance transforms. IEEE HAVE **2**, 111–116 (2004)

Growing a Random Forest with Fuzzy Spatial Features for Fully Automatic Artery-Specific Coronary Calcium Scoring

Felix Durlak[1]([⊠]), Michael Wels[1], Chris Schwemmer[1], Michael Sühling[1], Stefan Steidl[2], and Andreas Maier[2]

[1] Siemens Healthcare GmbH, Forchheim, Germany
felix.durlak.ext@siemens-healthineers.com
[2] Pattern Recognition Lab, Friedrich-Alexander-Universität, Erlangen-Nürnberg, Germany

Abstract. The amount of coronary artery calcium (CAC) is a strong and independent predictor of coronary heart disease (CHD). The standard routine for CAC quantification is to perform non-contrasted coronary computed-tomography (CCT) on a patient and present the resulting image to an expert, who then uses this to label CAC in a tedious and time-consuming process. To improve this situation, we present an automatic CAC labeling system with high clinical practicability. In contrast to many other automatic calcium scoring systems, it does not require additional cardiac computed tomography angiography (CCTA) data for artery-specific labeling. Instead, an atlas-based feature approach in combination with a random forest (RF) classifier is used to incorporate fuzzy spatial knowledge from offline data. Overall detection of CAC volume on a test set with 40 patients yields an F_1 score of 0.95 and 1.00 accuracy for risk class assignment. The intraclass correlation coefficient is 0.98 for the left anterior descending artery (LAD), 0.88 for the left circumflex artery (LCX), and 0.98 for the right coronary artery (RCA). The implemented system offers state-of-the-art accuracy with a processing time ($< 30\,\mathrm{s}$) by magnitudes lower than comparable systems to be found in the literature.

1 Introduction

Coronary heart disease (CHD) is a major cause of death in the USA [3] and other western countries. Therefore, early detection and risk assessment of CHD is of high interest in order to offer an effective therapy to the patient. A strong and independent predictor of CHD is the amount of coronary artery calcium (CAC) [1]. An artery-specific CAC score is preferred over a total score because it is more informative in predicting CHD that is related to one specific artery and therefore has a higher clinical value [4]. The common clinical standard examination for CAC quantification, also called calcium scoring, is based on ECG-gated non-contrasted cardiac computed tomography (CCT).

On top of CCT, cardiac computed tomography angiography (CCTA) is often performed for detecting non-calcified plaques and severe coronary stenosis, which

© Springer International Publishing AG 2017
Q. Wang et al. (Eds.): MLMI 2017, LNCS 10541, pp. 27–35, 2017.
DOI: 10.1007/978-3-319-67389-9_4

may indicate minimally invasive intervention. However, CCTA requires an additional image acquisition with ionizing radiation and contrast agent injection and thus increases both the overall health risk and expenses. So for the task of overall CAC quantification of asymptomatic patients it is advantageous and sufficient to only use CCT data.

At the moment, many commercially available calcium scoring tools only offer manual or semi-automated CAC labeling and thus require a substantial amount of user interaction for CAC quantification. To manually examine and to label possible CAC candidates in a CCT image, an experienced expert inspecting every slice is required. Hence, the process is time-consuming and the results may be subject to considerable intra- and inter-observer variability which in turn may result in lower accuracy regarding the final risk assessment.

An automatic system can be used to overcome such drawbacks by either assisting or replacing the expert. In that way, it can reduce the clinical staff's workload, accelerate CAC quantification and improve diagnostic accuracy. In this effort, Wolterink et al. [6] created the orCaScore framework for testing and comparing different algorithmic approaches for such systems. While the results of this evaluation seem promising, the presented methods often come with major drawbacks regarding clinical application. Four out of five methods [6] require an additional CCTA image, which is not the regular case in the context of calcium scoring, where – as mentioned above – only a CCT image according to a well-defined protocol is acquired. Two of the systems are semi-automatic [6] and therefore require an operator to be present. The method that does not require CCTA or user interaction has an average runtime of 20 min per examination [6]. All these factors make clinical application of the proposed solutions impractical.

We therefore present a system with a clinically acceptable runtime (< 30 s) for fully automatic CAC scoring, which uses an atlas-based feature approach to build a classifier capable of artery-specific CAC segmentation without the need for CCTA images of the present patient. Separate probabilistic atlases for the aorta and the three main coronary branches encoding rough spatial knowledge are built from CCTA images offline. The pericardium in the CCT image is segmented and utilized as reference structure for atlas registration and to reduce the search space of possible CAC candidates. The remaining CAC candidates are characterized by multiple intrinsic and extrinsic features with the latter focusing on incorporating fuzzy spatial information, for example from the atlases. For final artery-specific CAC detection a random forest (RF) is used, which is particularly known to be able to cope with possibly ambiguous and – considered isolatedly – less discriminative features by combining many weak learners into one strong classifier. Assigning an artery label to present CAC is helpful for deriving an accurate artery-specific CAC score, which – as mentioned in the beginning – increases the diagnostic value over a general CAC score [4].

2   Material and Methods

2.1   Data

The data used for atlas creation, training, and evaluation of the classifier has been provided by the orCaScore framework [6]. It consists both of CCT and CCTA data of patients from four different hospitals and scanners of four different vendors. The training set contains volumetric images of 32 patients and provides one ground truth image per patient in form of segmented and artery-specific labeled CAC in 3D. It was labeled as belonging to either the left anterior descending coronary artery (LAD), left circumflex coronary artery (LCX), or right coronary artery (RCA). If CAC was found in the left main coronary artery, it was also labeled as LAD. The labeling was performed as a consensus reading of two experts. The test set includes images of 40 patients without accompanying ground-truth. The CCTA data of the training set is used offline to extract the coronary arteries and the aorta for the creation of probabilistic atlases. These atlases are the basis for deriving fuzzy spatial features for CAC detection.

2.2   CAC Candidates

After loading a CCT image, the pericardium is segmented by applying a model-based detection framework with data-driven post-refinements through marginal space learning [10]. It is used to reduce our search space for CAC to the volume inside of the resulting mask. In this way, we avoid possible false positives (FP) later on in the classification step. According to the orCaScore challenge's standards, the image is then thresholded to only include voxels with an attenuation value > 130 Hounsfield units (HU). In order to form CAC lesion candidates, region growing with recursive connected component labeling for groups of voxels (3D 6-connectivity) is applied, which merges voxels in the thresholded image into singular lesions. Candidates with a volume $\leq 1.5\,\mathrm{mm}^3$ are not further considered because they are likely caused by image noise [6]. The resulting candidates, which still possibly include noise and non-CAC high-density lesions such as valvular and aortic calcifications, are then subject to feature-based multi-class classification through an RF. A prerequisite for feature computation from these candidates is the availability of roughly aligned probabilistic atlases, which offer fuzzy information about the general positions of aorta, LAD, LCX, and RCA.

2.3   Atlas Creation

For our approach of artery-specific CAC labeling without requiring CCTA data of the examined patient to work, probabilistic atlases which incorporate fuzzy knowledge about the location of the aorta and the coronary arteries relative to the pericardium are built offline. In contrast to the method used by Shahzad et al. [4], our atlas creation procedure is fully automatic so that no manual annotations are required. We use CCTA images to extract the aorta and the

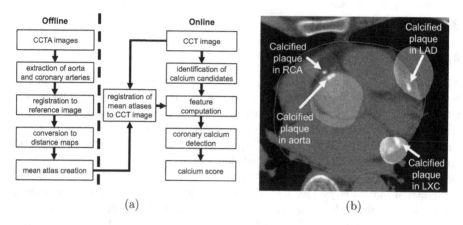

(a)   (b)

Fig. 1. (a) Flowchart visualizing the creation and use of mean atlases for CAC scoring. (b) Slice of a CCT scan showing calcified plaques at four different locations and the overlay of the anatomically corresponding averaged distance maps. The overlays for LAD, LCX, and RCA in this image only show voxels of the mean atlases with Euclidean distance $< 10\,\text{mm}$ (for the aorta: $< 2.5\,\text{mm}$). The thin enclosing line indicates the segmented pericardial boundary. The RCA and aorta calcifications in this image are a good example for CAC candidate locations that are difficult for a classifier to distinguish.

main coronary artery centerlines (LAD, LCX, RCA) into distinct volumes and use them to create mean probabilistic atlases for the aorta, LAD, LCX, and RCA. The role of these atlases in the overall system can be seen in Fig. 1a.

The segmentation of the relevant anatomical structures is based on existing algorithms. The aorta is segmented by marginal space learning [7] using a part-based aorta model [8], which is robust to missing aorta parts in the image occurring due to truncation. The major coronary arteries are extracted by a model-driven algorithm [9], which exploits their spatial relation to the automatically segmented heart chambers in order to use a vessel-specific region-of-interest as constraint for the centerline refinement. We then use the resulting main coronary centerlines to generate individual atlases from them.

The extraction results of all CCTA images are registered to another fixed CCTA image, which was randomly selected beforehand as a reference image in order to transform all segmentation results into one common coordinate system. For this transformation, the pericardium in every image is segmented using the method of Zhong et al. [10]. Principal component analysis (PCA) is then applied to the segmented pericardium of the reference image for finding the center of mass and the eigenvector corresponding to the biggest eigenvalue. Each of the CCTA images for atlas creation is processed in the same manner. Using the results from the PCA, we perform a rigid registration. While the rigid registration in some cases may not yield optimal pericardium shape matching, it is fast and robust enough to map the aorta and coronary arteries to a valid region of interest for atlas creation.

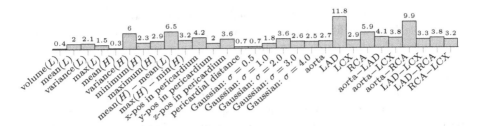

Fig. 2. List of all 29 features and their importance in percent for the RF trained on the training set. The letter L stands for voxels of a lesion itself and H for voxels of its hull. Section 2.4 offers detailed description of all features.

After registration, the transformed aorta region and centerlines of the main coronary artery branches are converted to Euclidean distance maps [2] which encode the spatial distance to the specified object in every voxel of the image. With these individual atlases A_{aorta}^i, A_{LAD}^i, A_{RCA}^i, A_{LCX}^i with $i \in \{1, \ldots, N\}$, the mean atlases A_{aorta}^{mean}, A_{LAD}^{mean}, A_{RCA}^{mean}, A_{LCX}^{mean} are built by averaging over all N images. In Fig. 1b they are visualized in a CCT slice together with CAC at different locations. Later on, these atlases will be used as features quantifying the probability for a voxel of being close to the aorta, LAD, LCX, or RCA. This fuzzy spatial knowledge combined with other features is sufficient for the RF to reliably detect and label CAC according to the corresponding artery branches.

2.4   Feature Generation

For every CAC candidate 29 features are computed, which are listed in Fig. 2. Many of them incorporate spatial information to enable artery-specific CAC classification. Other research also shows the importance of spatial information. For example, location features are used as additional input for a convolutional neural network to identify possible CAC lesion candidates for the final classification step [5]. Without these localization features, the Convolutional Neural Net was not able to differentiate between bony structures and actual CAC. This is consistent with our observations that reliable CAC detection and especially artery-specific labeling is almost impossible without incorporating spatial knowledge into the classification process. Therefore, our approach is to use – amongst others – multiple fuzzy location-based features. We distinguish between appearance-based intrinsic features that are derived from the HU values of the CCT image and location-based extrinsic features which incorporate spatial knowledge that is not available in the CCT image alone.

Appearance Features. In order to better identify noise, which generally has a smaller lesion size than CAC, the volume of the lesion is used as a feature.

Some other features are based on the intensity values of a lesion candidate or its surrounding voxels. Because of the standardized scanning protocol of calcium scoring, absolute HU values are assumed – at least to some extend – to be comparable between different patients. We compute the mean, variance, and maximum of the candidate's voxel intensities. The mean and maximum values for CAC are usually higher than for noise and lower than for bony structures.

Furthermore, we want to capture characteristics of the voxel intensities surrounding a lesion and compare it to some of the lesion's characteristics. This helps in gathering information about the spatial image properties and the tissue in which the lesion is located. For example, a high variance can indicate a noisy area. Therefore, we create a lesion hull represented by the set of voxels $H = \{h^1, \dots, h^M\}$ with M being the number of hull voxels. With respect to the set of lesion voxels $L = \{l^1, \dots, l^N\}$ with N being the number of lesion voxels, every possible combination of a voxel h^i with $i \in [1, M]$ and a lesion voxel l^j with $j \in [1, N]$ has to fulfill the properties $|h_x^i - l_x^j| \leq 1$, $|h_y^i - l_y^j| \leq 1$, and $|h_z^i - l_z^j| \leq 1$. Also, $H \cap L = \emptyset$ must hold. For the voxel intensities of H we compute $\mathrm{mean}(H)$, $\mathrm{variance}(H)$, $\mathrm{minimum}(H)$, $\mathrm{maximum}(H)$ and $\mathrm{maximum}(H) - \mathrm{minimum}(H)$. Additionally, $\mathrm{mean}(H) - \mathrm{mean}(L)$ is computed.

For capturing morphological information of the lesion and its surroundings, we apply convolutions of five differently sized Gaussian kernels with standard deviations 0.5 mm, 1.0 mm, 2.0 mm, 3.0 mm, and 4.0 mm to the image. The resulting intensities at the voxel position of the candidate's maximum intensity prior to filtering is then used as a feature. To improve runtime performance, the Gaussian filter is approximated by a recursive infinite impulse response filter.

Location Features. An axis-aligned bounding box is computed from the pericardium and used for computing the (x, y, z)-position of the candidate's center of gravity relative to the borders of the bounding box. In this way, the relative coordinates of a candidate in the pericardium can be used as spatial features.

Also, an Euclidean distance map is generated from the pericardium to get the distance of the candidate's center of gravity p to the pericardial surface. This distance helps gathering fuzzy spatial knowledge about the lesion and can be helpful in identifying regions with a high probability for CAC occurrence. In the same manner, the values of the mean atlases $A_{\mathrm{aorta}}^{\mathrm{mean}}(p)$, $A_{\mathrm{LAD}}^{\mathrm{mean}}(p)$, $A_{\mathrm{RCA}}^{\mathrm{mean}}(p)$, $A_{\mathrm{LCX}}^{\mathrm{mean}}(p)$ at this position are used as a feature. Furthermore, features are generated from the differences between the atlases: $A_{\mathrm{aorta}}^{\mathrm{mean}}(p) - A_{\mathrm{LAD}}^{\mathrm{mean}}(p)$, $A_{\mathrm{aorta}}^{\mathrm{mean}}(p) - A_{\mathrm{LCX}}^{\mathrm{mean}}(p)$, $A_{\mathrm{aorta}}^{\mathrm{mean}}(p) - A_{\mathrm{RCA}}^{\mathrm{mean}}(p)$, $A_{\mathrm{LAD}}^{\mathrm{mean}}(p) - A_{\mathrm{LCX}}^{\mathrm{mean}}(p)$, $A_{\mathrm{LAD}}^{\mathrm{mean}}(p) - A_{\mathrm{RCA}}^{\mathrm{mean}}(p)$, $A_{\mathrm{RCA}}^{\mathrm{mean}}(p) - A_{\mathrm{LCX}}^{\mathrm{mean}}(p)$. All these spatial features are not only important for detecting CAC, but also and especially for assigning the correct coronary artery label to the lesion.

3   Experiments and Results

We have evaluated our system, which has been implemented in MeVisLab 2.8 (64 Bit), on a regular workstation with Intel Xeon Processor E5-1620V2 (4×3.70 GHz) and 8 GB RAM. For CAC classification we used the RF implementation of OpenCV 2.4.13. The CAC detection for one patient typically took 10 s, no patient took more than 30 s.

Table 1. Volume-based results of different methods evaluated on the test set. Method labels and the corresponding results are taken from Wolterink et al. [6]. The best values in each column are shown in boldface.

Abbreviations: Fully Automatic (AUT), Sensitivity (SENS), Total (TOT), Positive Predictive Value (PPV), F_1 Score (F_1), Two-way Intraclass Correlation Coefficient for Absolute Agreement (ICC), Linearly Weighted Cohen's Kappa for Risk Group Assignment (κ Risk)

Method	CCTA Needed	AUT	Typical runtime	SENS TOT	PPV TOT	F_1 TOT	ICC TOT	ICC LAD	ICC LCX	ICC RCA	κ risk
Ours	No	Yes	10 s	0.93	**0.97**	0.95	**0.99**	0.98	0.88	**0.98**	**1.00**
A	Yes	Yes	80 min	0.85	0.94	0.89	0.97	0.98	0.95	0.90	0.88
B	Yes	No	8 min	**0.99**	0.95	**0.97**	**0.99**	**1.00**	**1.00**	0.96	0.98
C	Yes	Yes	2 min	0.95	0.94	0.94	0.98	0.94	0.87	0.96	0.96
D	Yes	No	3 min	0.57	0.69	0.62	0.60	0.33	0.57	0.51	0.80
E	No	Yes	20 min	0.94	0.96	0.95	**0.99**	0.98	0.98	0.96	**1.00**

For applying our method to the test set, an RF was trained on the complete training set with the following parameters: number of trees $t = 40$, tree depth $d = 20$, samples for split $s = 20$, features for split $f = 5$. They were derived through grid search optimization via cross-validation with the following search space: $t \in \{30, 40, 50, 60, 70, 80\}$, $d \in \{5, 10, 15, 20, 25, 30\}$, $s \in \{15, 20, 25, 30, 35, 40\}$, $f \in \{2, 3, 4, 5, 6, 7, 8, 9\}$. The parameter grid was designed heuristically, based on the OpenCV documentation, our experience, and with overall runtime in mind. For training of the final RF, the relative feature importance is given in Fig. 2. The bar chart shows the high feature importance of the atlas-based features relative to the other ones. The trained RF was then used for the test set. The segmentation results were sent to the organizers of the orCaScore challenge [6] for evaluation. Our results are listed in Table 1 together with results of other researches, who have applied their methods to the same data set. Details to these methods and their evaluation are published by Wolterink et al. [6].

4   Discussion and Conclusions

The feature importance displayed in Fig. 2 clearly shows the significance of the atlas-based fuzzy spatial features. Features derived from the lesion hull also show a great impact for correct classification. Lesion intensity features have the lowest importance for the RF. This indicates that they are not characteristic for CAC of a particular artery branch and also have a low influence on the distinction between CAC and non-CAC lesions.

Looking at our results, we notice that the ICC for CAC volume of the LCX is lower than the ICC for CAC volume of the other arteries. This indicates detection problems of LCX CAC in some rare cases. Since the total volume's ICC is 0.99, we can assume that CAC in these cases was not missed, but labeled as LAD instead of LCX, or vice-versa, because of their close proximity. The influence of this misclassification is higher on the LCX volume's ICC than on the LAD volume's ICC because total LAD CAC volume is higher [6].

The total volume's ICC of 0.99 indicates great accuracy for general CAC scoring and consequently risk class assignment, which was correct for every patient in the test set ($\kappa = 1.00$). This underpins the clinical practicability of our system for CAC scoring.

Over all, our results are on par with the top performing methods tested on the orCaScore framework [6]. However, unlike most other methods, our approach for artery-specific calcium scoring does not require an additional CCTA image acquisition. For this purpose, we trained an RF classifier that mostly relies on multiple fuzzy spatial features. The resulting classification system has shown state-of-the-art accuracy for CAC quantification. On top of that, the system is fully automatic, fast (runtime < 30 s) and therefore conceptually applicable in clinical practice to reduce overall expenses for calcium scoring.

References

1. Becker, A., Leber, A., Becker, C., Knez, A.: Predictive value of coronary calcifications for future cardiac events in asymptomatic individuals. Am. Heart J. **155**(1), 154–160 (2008)
2. Danielsson, P.E.: Euclidean distance mapping. Comput. Graph. Image Process. **14**(3), 227–248 (1980)
3. Go, A.S., et al.: Executive summary: heart disease and stroke statistics-2014 update. Circulation **129**(3), 399–410 (2014)
4. Shahzad, R., van Walsum, T., Schaap, M., Rossi, A., Klein, S., Weustink, A.C., de Feyter, P.J., van Vliet, L.J., Niessen, W.J.: Vessel specific coronary artery calcium scoring: an automatic system. Acad. Radiol. **20**(1), 1–9 (2013)
5. Wolterink, J.M., Leiner, T., Viergever, M.A., Išgum, I.: Automatic coronary calcium scoring in cardiac CT angiography using convolutional neural networks. In: Navab, N., Hornegger, J., Wells, W.M., Frangi, A.F. (eds.) MICCAI 2015. LNCS, vol. 9349, pp. 589–596. Springer, Cham (2015). doi:10.1007/978-3-319-24553-9_72
6. Wolterink, J.M., Leiner, T., de Vos, B.D., Coatrieux, J.L., Kelm, B.M., Kondo, S., Salgado, R.A., Shahzad, R., Shu, H., Snoeren, M., Takx, R.A.P., van Vliet, L.J., van Walsum, T., Willems, T.P., Yang, G., Zheng, Y., Viergever, M.A., Isgum, I.: An evaluation of automatic coronary artery calcium scoring methods with cardiac CT using the OrCaScore framework. Med. Phys. **43**(5), 2361–2373 (2016)
7. Zheng, Y., Barbu, A., Georgescu, B., Scheuering, M., Comaniciu, D.: Four-chamber heart modeling and automatic segmentation for 3-D cardiac CT volumes using marginal space learning and steerable features. IEEE Trans. Med. Imaging **27**(11), 1668–1681 (2008)
8. Zheng, Y., et al.: Automatic aorta segmentation and valve landmark detection in C-arm CT: application to aortic valve implantation. In: Jiang, T., Navab, N., Pluim, J.P.W., Viergever, M.A. (eds.) MICCAI 2010. LNCS, vol. 6361, pp. 476–483. Springer, Heidelberg (2010). doi:10.1007/978-3-642-15705-9_58

9. Zheng, Y., Tek, H., Funka-Lea, G.: Robust and accurate coronary artery center-line extraction in CTA by combining model-driven and data-driven approaches. In: Mori, K., Sakuma, I., Sato, Y., Barillot, C., Navab, N. (eds.) MICCAI 2013. LNCS, vol. 8151, pp. 74–81. Springer, Heidelberg (2013). doi:10.1007/978-3-642-40760-4_10

10. Zhong, H., Zheng, Y., Funka-Lea, G., Vega-Higuera, F.: Automatic heart isolation in 3D CT images. In: Menze, B.H., Langs, G., Lu, L., Montillo, A., Tu, Z., Criminisi, A. (eds.) MCV 2012. LNCS, vol. 7766, pp. 165–180. Springer, Heidelberg (2013). doi:10.1007/978-3-642-36620-8_17

Atlas of Classifiers for Brain MRI Segmentation

Boris Kodner[1,2(✉)], Shiri Gordon[1,2], Jacob Goldberger[3],
and Tammy Riklin Raviv[1,2]

[1] Department of Electrical and Computer Engineering,
Ben-Gurion University of the Negev, Beersheba, Israel
borisv@post.bgu.ac.il
[2] The Zlotowski Center for Neuroscience,
Ben-Gurion University of the Negev, Beersheba, Israel
[3] Faculty of Engineering, Bar-Ilan University, Ramat Gan, Israel

Abstract. We present a conceptually novel framework for brain tissue segmentation based on an *Atlas of Classifiers* (AoC). The AoC allows a statistical summary of the annotated datasets taking into account both the imaging data and the corresponding labels. It is therefore more informative than the classical probabilistic atlas and more economical than the popular multi-atlas approaches, which require large memory consumption and high computational complexity for each segmentation. Specifically, we consider an AoC as a spatial map of voxel-wise multinomial logistic regression (LR) functions learned from the labeled data. Upon convergence, the resulting fixed LR weights (a few for each voxel) represent the training dataset, which might be huge. Segmentation of a new image is therefore immediate and only requires the calculation of the LR outputs based on the respective voxel-wise features. Moreover, the AoC construction is independent of the test images, providing the flexibility to train it on the available labeled data and use it for the segmentation of images from different datasets and modalities.

The proposed method has been applied to publicly available datasets for the segmentation of brain MRI tissues and is shown to outreach commonly used methods. Promising results were obtained also for multimodal, cross-modality MRI segmentation.

1 Introduction

The prevalence of Magnetic Resonance Imaging (MRI) nowadays for clinical purposes and research contributes to an exponential growth in MRI datasets available. This in turn, accelerates the development of automatic and semi-automatic tools for image analysis and brain tissue segmentation in particular. Despite over two decades of efforts, brain parcellation into gray matter (GM), white matter (WM) and cerebrospinal fluid (CSF) remains a difficult problem due to low SNR, partial volume effect, bias field and other imaging artifacts. Additional information, mainly spatial, is therefore required, where image intensities and gradients are not sufficiently discriminative.

Bayesian approaches for brain MRI segmentation [1,3,7,16] are based on the observation that the image intensity distribution can be modeled, with

© Springer International Publishing AG 2017
Q. Wang et al. (Eds.): MLMI 2017, LNCS 10541, pp. 36–44, 2017.
DOI: 10.1007/978-3-319-67389-9_5

good approximation, by a mixture of Gaussians. Prior probabilities are usually obtained by averaging aligned manual annotations. These priors, also called probabilistic atlases, define the spatial probability that a voxel at that particular location belongs to a particular brain tissue.

While the classical atlas-based methods have shown to yield successful segmentation results and are applied in commonly used tools, such as FreeSurfer [3], SPM [1], Fast-FSL [18] and Slicer EM segmenter [10], a main concern is that a single atlas may not capture the large heterogeneity of structural brain images. To address this issue the multi-atlas segmentation (MAS) approach emerged, see [6] and references therein. The fused atlas is specific to a target image as it is based on its similarity to each image (or image patches) in the database. Numerous MAS methods were proposed, based on different global, local and non-local similarity measures and a variety of fusion techniques. The flexibility of adapting the atlas to the test images comes at the price of large memory storage, keeping an entire database along with the associated labels, and high computational complexity as the pairwise similarities between a test image and each of the training instances, or (more economically) clusters in the training set [14], are considered.

Machine learning (ML) approaches for segmentation, e.g. Support Vector Machines (SVM), Random Forests (RF) [15,17] and recently deep neural networks (DNN), e.g. [9,19] use comprehensive set of features to discriminate between the different tissues. These methods provide promising segmentation results, yet at the cost of long and computationally expensive training process, which requires either huge annotated datasets or smart data augmentation.

We hereby propose a conceptually new form of atlas termed an *atlas of classifiers* (AoC), which enables the abstraction of possibly huge datasets with very few parameters for each voxel. Each classifier is a multinomial logistic regression (LR) function. The weights of the LR functions are determined during training (based on the available labeled data) via gradient ascent processes that aim to maximize a regularized objective function. Once the training phase is completed the classifiers' parameters remain fixed. Multi-class soft segmentation of a new image is performed promptly, by simply applying to each of the image voxels the associated multinomial LR function. Note that unlike common ML approaches, the classifiers are voxel-specific and not class-specific. Solving large number of voxel-wise optimization problems with very few parameters (features) each, significantly facilitates and accelerates the entire training process.

In this paper, the partition of brain MRIs into tissues is considered, yet, the proposed paradigm is general and not tailored to a specific application. To allow multi-modal and cross modality segmentation, rather than using the image intensities directly, each voxel is associated with an intensity-based feature vector. These voxel-wise vectors are key components both in the segmentation process, as inputs to the objective function of the LR weights, and for the alignment of the training data into a common-space for the generation of the atlas.

The rest of the paper is organized as follows. In Sect. 2 we present the atlas of classifiers. Promising experimental results for IBSR18 and IBSR20 [11] as well as cross-modality segmentation for MRBrainS13 multi-modal data are presented in Sect. 3. We conclude in Sect. 4.

2   The Atlas of Classifier Approach

Let $\{I_n\}_{n=1}^N$, where $I_n : \Omega \to \mathbb{R}^D$ denote N unimodal ($D = 3$) or multimodal ($D = 4$) training images. Let $\mathcal{I}_n \triangleq \{f^m(I_n)\}_{m=1}^M$, define M features or filters associated with I_n. We denote by $\mathcal{Y}_1, \ldots, \mathcal{Y}_N$ the corresponding labeling functions such that $\mathcal{Y}_n : \Omega \to \{1, \ldots, L\}$ partitions the image domain of I_n into L disjoint regions of interest (ROIs), $\Omega_1, \ldots, \Omega_L$. Our goal can be formulated as follows: given a labeled training set, find the segmentation of a test image I_{TEST} by solving the following maximum a posteriori (MAP) problem:

$$\hat{\mathcal{Y}}_{\text{TEST}} = \arg\max_{\mathcal{Y}_{\text{TEST}}} p(\mathcal{Y}_{\text{TEST}}|\mathcal{I}_{\text{TEST}}, \mathcal{I}_1, \ldots, \mathcal{I}_N, \mathcal{Y}_1, \ldots, \mathcal{Y}_N). \tag{1}$$

Let V represents the 3D image size. The proposed AoC allows a statistical summary of the training sets represented by $V \times M \times L$ parameters, regardless of the number of scanned subjects ($N >> M$) and modalities. For comparison, the multi-atlas approach requires voxel-wise storage of $V \times N \times L$ for unimodal data.

2.1   AoC Model Overview

The AoC concept is illustrated in Fig. 1. The training phase (light blue background) is performed once for a given database of MRI scans and the respective label maps. Each of the raw images is mapped into a feature space which, together with the associated labels, contributes to the generation of the voxel-wise LR functions that represent the atlas, see Fig. 2. The training involves an iterative process in which the LR weights are learned. Segmentation of a test image (light red background) is performed by its mapping to a feature space followed by a straight forward calculation of the MAP segmentation by the atlas's LR functions (Softmax regression).

2.2   Multi-Class Segmentation

Softmax regression (or multinomial LR) is a multi-class (MC) classifier [2]. Consider a set of labeled training data associated with a voxel $\mathbf{x}$, i.e. $\{\{\mathcal{I}_n(\mathbf{x}), \mathcal{Y}_n(\mathbf{x})\}\}_{n=1}^N$ where $\mathcal{I}_n(\mathbf{x}) = \{f^m(I_n(\mathbf{x}))\}_{m=1}^M \triangleq f_{\mathbf{x}n}$. This training data, can be compactly represented by a set of $(M + 1)$-dimensional vectors $\mathbf{w}_{\mathbf{x}}^{\text{MC}} = \{\mathbf{w}_{\mathbf{x}}^l\}_{l=1}^L$, where $\mathbf{w}_{\mathbf{x}}^l = \{w_{\mathbf{x}}^{l,0}, w_{\mathbf{x}}^{l,1}, \ldots, w_{\mathbf{x}}^{l,M}\}$ and $w_{\mathbf{x}}^{l,0}$ is a bias parameter.

Given the scalar product $\mathbf{w}_{\mathbf{x}}^l f_{\mathbf{x}} \triangleq w_{\mathbf{x}}^{l,0} + w_{\mathbf{x}}^{l,1} f_{\mathbf{x}}^1 + \ldots + w_{\mathbf{x}}^{l,M} f_{\mathbf{x}}^M$, the multinomial LR is defined as follows:

$$p(\mathcal{Y}_*(\mathbf{x}) = y_l | I_*) = h_l(\mathbf{w}_{\mathbf{x}}^{\text{MC}}, f_{\mathbf{x}}) = \frac{\exp(\mathbf{w}_{\mathbf{x}}^l f_{\mathbf{x}})}{\sum_{j=1}^L \exp(\mathbf{w}_{\mathbf{x}}^j f_{\mathbf{x}})} \quad \text{for } l \in \{1, \ldots, L\} \tag{2}$$

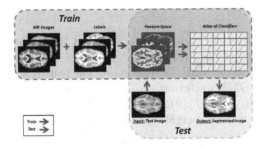

Fig. 1. An overview on the Atlas of Classifier method: In the training phase (light blue background) the MR images are projected into the feature space and are used, along with the associated label maps, to train voxel-wise classifiers. In the test phase (light red background), the test image is projected to a feature space and segmented using the trained classifiers. (Color figure online)

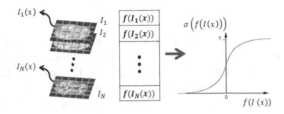

Fig. 2. Training of a classifier. Given a set of labeled images $I_1, \ldots, I_N$, a classifier associated with a voxel $\mathbf{x}$ is trained based on functions of the image intensities at that voxel $\{f(I_n(\mathbf{x}))\}_{n=1}^{N}$ and the respective labels.

where, $\mathcal{Y}_*(\mathbf{x}) \in \{y_1, \ldots, y_L\}$, is a multi-class labeling of a voxel $\mathbf{x}$ in the given input image I_*. Thus, voxel-wise appilcation of the multinomial LRs provides soft segmentations of the examined ROIs. A hard segmentation is obtained by assigning each voxel to the class with maximum probability. The weights $\mathbf{w}_{\mathbf{x}}^{\text{MC}}$ are obtained by maximizing the following objective function:

$$J(\mathbf{w}_{\mathbf{x}}^{\text{MC}}) = \frac{1}{N} \sum_n \log p(\mathcal{Y}_{\mathbf{x}n} | f_{\mathbf{x}n}, \mathbf{w}_{\mathbf{x}}^{\text{MC}}) - \frac{\lambda_R}{2} \| \mathbf{w}_{\mathbf{x}}^{\text{MC}} \|^2, \qquad (3)$$

where λ_R is an hyperparameter that weights the L_2 regularization term. $J(\mathbf{w}_{\mathbf{x}}^{\text{MC}})$ is concave thus using gradient ascent algorithm we are guaranteed to converge to the global optimum. The LR weights update, of each class $l = 1, \ldots L$, for each $\mathbf{x} \in \Omega$, is determined by the following gradient ascent expression:

$$\mathbf{w}_{\mathbf{x}}^{l} \leftarrow \mathbf{w}_{\mathbf{x}}^{l} + \alpha \left(\frac{1}{N} \sum_n \left(1_{\{\mathcal{Y}_{\mathbf{x}n}=l\}} - h_l(\mathbf{w}_{\mathbf{x}}^{\text{MC}}, f_{\mathbf{x}n}) \right) f_{\mathbf{x}n} - \lambda_R \mathbf{w}_{\mathbf{x}}^{l} \right), \qquad (4)$$

where α defines the learning rate and $1_{\{\mathcal{Y}_{\mathbf{x}n}=l\}} = 1$ when $\mathcal{Y}_{\mathbf{x}n} = l$ and 0 otherwise.

2.3   Features

Intensity distribution of each image I_n is modeled by a mixture of Gaussians (GMM) with parameters $\theta_n = \{\kappa_{i,n}, \mu_{i,n}, \sigma_{i,n}\}_{i=1}^M, M = 3$, where each Gaussian represents a different tissue: CSF, WM and GM. The feature space of an image I_n is determined by its GMM such that each of its voxels $\mathbf{x}$ is represented by a feature vector $\{\mathcal{L}(\kappa_{i,n}, \mu_{i,n}, \sigma_{i,n} | I_n(\mathbf{x}))\}_{i=1}^M$. The GMM is learned using a maximum a-posteriori version of the expectation maximization algorithm (MAP-EM) [4] that incorporates prior knowledge (obtained by utilizing the training label maps) about the intensity distribution of each tissue (across the images), to guide the EM algorithm. This representation significantly improves the performance of our classifiers and the accuracy of the preceding registration process (to be detailed next) as compared to using the original intensities as features. It also allows multi-modal, cross-modality segmentation, see Table 2.

2.4   Registration

To form the AoC all training images and the associated annotations should be aligned to a common space. This common space is chosen to be the domain of an image $I_{\hat{n}}$, that its label map $\mathcal{Y}_{\hat{n}}$ is the one with the highest sum of pairwise Dice Similarity Coefficients (DSC) with respect to all other training labels. Let $\mathcal{I}_{\hat{n}} = \{f^m(I_{\hat{n}})\}_{m=1}^M$ denote the vectorized representation in the feature space of $I_{\hat{n}}$. The transformation $R_{k \to \hat{n}}$ of the source image coordinates I_k to the target image domain can be calculated by solving the following minimization problem:

$$\hat{R}_{k \to \hat{n}} = \underset{R_{k \to \hat{n}}}{\arg \min} D_{\mathrm{SIM}}(\mathcal{I}_{\hat{n}}, R_{k \to \hat{n}} \circ \mathcal{I}_k), \qquad (5)$$

where D_{SIM} is the sum of squared differences between the target and the source image features. In practice, for the AoC construction, rather than calculating a multi-channel similarity measure, we perform $M = 3$ registration processes for each annotated image by a pair-wise comparison of each feature separately: $D_{\mathrm{SIM}}(f^m(I_{\hat{n}}), R_{k \to \hat{n}} \circ f^m(I_k))$. This allows to augment the data since three pairs of feature and label maps are obtained for every training image. In addition, the aligned label maps are no longer discrete, therefore $1_{\{\mathcal{Y}_{\mathbf{x}n}=l\}}$ in Eq. (4) is replaced by a 'soft label' $\tilde{\mathcal{Y}}_{\mathbf{x},n}^l \in [0,1]$. In the test phase, the voxel-wise multinomial LR weights $\mathbf{w}_{\mathbf{x}}^{\mathrm{MC}}$ are registered, by a non-parametric transformation $R_{\hat{n} \to \mathrm{TEST}}$, to the image domain of the test image [13]. This ensures that the test image features are not distorted throughout the registration process. Moreover, registration of the atlas weights $\mathbf{w}_{\mathbf{x}}^{\mathrm{MC}}$ serves as an additional regularization, as the weights are spatially smoothed due to interpolation.

3   Experimental Results

We evaluated the AoC on the IBSR18 and IBSR20 data sets from the Internet Brain Segmentation Repository (see http://www.nitrc.org and [11]). To demonstrate multi-modal and cross-modality segmentation, we used the MRBrainS13 challenge dataset [8]. In all cases, the AoC was generated in a leave-one-out (LOO) manner excluding the test image from the atlas construction.

Unimodal experiments: Both IBSR18 (18 scans, $256 \times 256 \times 128$) and IBSR20 (20 scans, $256 \times 256 \times 60$) datasets consist of MRI T1-weighted volumetric images of normal subjects and manual labels for three tissue types (CSF, GM, WM). IBSR18 dataset is provided following skull stripping and bias correction via CMA routines. We used the SPM8 package (http://www.fil.ion.ucl.ac.uk/spm) for bias correction of the IBSR20. Image intensities were normalized to improve contrast between tissues. Figure 3 visually demonstrates the process of training the multinomial LR weights, for the bias and the GM, WM intensity features. Note that as the training proceeds, the spatial contrast between the weights representing different tissues is enhanced. Also note that voxels at different anatomical locations that belong to the same tissues, may have different weight combinations. This motivates the construction of a spatial map of classifiers rather than using a single classifier for each tissue. We compared our AoC method to four other segmentation methods: GMM-EM [5], MAP-EM [4], the GMM-based unified registration-segmentation algorithm from the SPM8 package [1] and the FAST algorithm from the FSL package [18]. The intensity distribution parameters of the training images were obtained using the ground-truth labels. The calculated parameters were used to initialize the GMM-EM and as priors for the MAP-EM of the test images. SPM8 toolbox was used with probabilistic atlases calculated from the IBSR datasets, for fair comparison. Segmentation accuracy was calculated per tissue using the DSC. Training run-time for IBSR datasets (after registration) is approximately 10 min (50–70 iterations), using unoptimized Matlab code. Segmentation of a new image takes 4 s on average, excluding the registration of the atlas to the feature domain. Table 1 summarizes the performance of the different methods. The proposed AoC method outperforms the other examined algorithms for both data sets, presenting the highest mean DSC measures and the lowest standard deviations, Refer also to [12] for the DSC measures obtained by other methods applied to these IBSR datasets, *without* annotation correction.

Table 1. DSC results for IBSR18 and IBSR20 data sets (mean ± standard deviation).

Data set	Type	GMM	MAP-EM	SPM8	FSL	AoC
IBSR18	WM	77.61±6.73	85.89 ± 2.90	89.03 ± 1.12	87.12 ± 3.04	**90.87 ± 2.02**
	GM	86.27 ± 2.98	88.46 ± 3.01	85.19 ± 3.01	78.59 ± 2.50	**92.37 ± 2.09**
	CSF	69.06 ± 8.50	72.34 ± 5.04	59.28 ± 6.60	53.31 ± 5.53	**75.62 ± 4.19**
IBSR20	WM	68.04 ± 14.68	76.83 ± 11.86	81.11 ± 6.29	80.10 ± 7.54	**84.35 ± 4.72**
	GM	77.30 ± 18.64	84.79 ± 5.13	88.92 ± 3.69	69.64 ± 6.38	**90.94 ± 2.67**
	CSF	28.47 ± 11.05	36.52 ± 14.67	55.99 ± 17.92	14.07 ± 4.88	**79.48 ± 4.23**

We also tested the AoC for the segmentation of the IBSR20 images while performing the training with the IBSR18 dataset and obtained the following

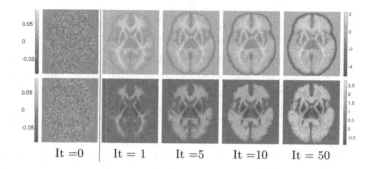

| It =0 | It = 1 | It =5 | It =10 | It = 50 |

Fig. 3. Spatial maps of three Softmax weights $\mathbf{w}_{\mathbf{x}}^{l}$ of the WM class: the bias (first row) and WM (second row) intensity features, as captured during the training process based on IBSR18 dataset after 0, 1, 5,10 and 50 iterations. Left colorbars refer to the left-most images, right colorbars to the other images in the row.

Table 2. DSC results (mean ± standard deviation) for MRBrainS13 challenge training data. The columns represent the two modalities used for training. Rows represent modalities used for the test.

	Type	T1 and T1 IR	T1 and T2 FLAIR	T1 IR and T2 FLAIR
T1	WM	83.65 ± 3.80	83.83 ± 3.75	80.93 ± 3.78
	GM	78.56 ± 2.85	80.66 ± 3.28	72.54 ± 2.68
	CSF	83.91 ± 1.60	85.59 ± 1.69	79.28 ± 2.26
T1 IR	WM	79.68 ± 4.28	79.96 ± 4.28	77.96 ± 4.14
	GM	71.35 ± 2.08	74.69 ± 2.93	69.11 ± 2.26
	CSF	79.48 ± 2.37	81.57 ± 1.78	78.15 ± 2.64
T2 FLAIR	WM	62.85 ± 1.86	63.55 ± 1.60	65.00 ± 0.96
	GM	67.93 ± 2.29	66.73 ± 1.92	68.38 ± 2.27
	CSF	81.94 ± 2.12	81.71 ± 2.09	80.83 ± 2.13

DSC measures: 82.90 ± 5.50 for WM; 88.23 ± 4.08 for GM and 55.62 ± 14.79 for CSF. Although the results are not optimal for this dataset, the method still performs better than some of the other tested methods, demonstrating one of its main benefit – the usability of a single-shot training of one dataset for the segmentation of different datasets.

Multi-modal, cross-modality experiments: We tested the proposed AoC on the training MRBrainS13 challenge data set [8], which contains five sets of multi-modal MRI scans: T1, T1-IR and T2-FLAIR. The AoC was trained (LOO) on bi-modal scans and was tested on unimodal, including cross-modality scans, see Table 2. We find the results very promising given the extremely small training and the fact that both T1-IR and T2-FLAIR imaging (unlike T2) drastically changes the intensity distribution of the tissues, affecting the compatibility between the train and the test feature space.

4   Discussion

A novel approach for brain MRI segmentation, which replaces the "traditional" probabilistic atlas with an *atlas of classifiers* is presented. The atlas of classifiers, is a spatial map, defined on the image domain, in which each voxel is represented by a small set of weights, learned from a much larger set of annotated scans, that defines a multinomial LR function. Each of these voxel-wise Softmax functions is more informative than the spatial probability of that voxel, obtained by averaging the training label maps, regardless of the intensity images. On the other hand, unlike existing voxel-wise classification approaches, the spatial location of each voxel does matter. Consider for example the LR weight maps, displayed in Fig. 3. Voxels of the same tissues may have different weight combinations depending on the anatomy. In contrast to the atlas fusion framework, the AoC construction is completely independent of the test images. In fact, we demonstrate comparable segmentation results for test images acquired at significantly different settings with respect to the training.

Mapping the image intensities into a feature space based on their probability distributions allows to combine the benefits of machine learning with the prior knowledge on the underlying anatomy and imaging. The *atlas of classifiers* can be viewed as a *light weight* neural network or a grid of artificial neurons. Its structure allows inputs as big as whole images, gaining the full contextual spatial information, which cannot be preserved using image patches. Moreover, the excellent performances obtained with a very modest training procedure- a single batch with less than twenty annotated images, a relatively small set of parameters and no back-propagation, manifest its great advantage.

Acknowledgments. This study was partially supported by the Israel Science Foundation (1638/16 T.R.R) and IDF Medical Corps (T.R.R.).

References

1. Ashburner, J., Friston, K.J.: Unified segmentation. Neuroimage **26**(3), 839–851 (2005)
2. Bishop, C.M.: Pattern recognition. Mach. Learn. **128**, 1–58 (2006)
3. Fischl, et al.: Whole brain segmentation: automated labeling of neuroanatomical structures in the human brain. Neuron **33**(3), 341–355 (2002)
4. Goldberger, J., Greenspan, H.: Context-based segmentation of image sequences. TPAMI **28**(3), 463–468 (2006)
5. Gupta, L., Sortrakul, T.: A gaussian-mixture-based image segmentation algorithm. Pattern Recogn. **31**(3), 315–325 (1998)
6. Iglesias, J.E., Sabuncu, M.R.: Multi-atlas segmentation of biomedical images: a survey. MEDIA **24**(1), 205–219 (2015)
7. Leemput, V., et al.: Automated model-based tissue classification of MR images of the brain. TMI **18**(10), 897–908 (1999)
8. Mendrik, et al.: MRBrainS challenge: Online evaluation framework for brain image segmentation in 3T MRI scans. Comput. Intelll. Neurosci. **2015**, 16 (2015)

9. Moeskops, P., et al.: Automatic segmentation of MR brain images with a convolutional neural network. TMI **35**(5), 1252–1261 (2016)

10. Pohl, K.M., et al.: A hierarchical algorithm for MR brain image parcellation. TMI **26**(9), 1201–1212 (2007)

11. Rohlfing, T.: Image similarity and tissue overlaps as surrogates for image registration accuracy: widely used but unreliable. TMI **31**(2), 153–163 (2012)

12. Valverde, S., et al.: Comparison of 10 brain tissue segmentation methods using revisited IBSR annotations. J. Magn. Res. Imaging **41**(1), 93–101 (2015)

13. Vercauteren, T., et al.: Diffeomorphic demons: efficient non-parametric image registration. NeuroImage **45**, S61–S72 (2009)

14. Wachinger, C., Golland, P.: Spectral label fusion. In: Ayache, N., Delingette, H., Golland, P., Mori, K. (eds.) MICCAI 2012. LNCS, vol. 7512, pp. 410–417. Springer, Heidelberg (2012). doi:10.1007/978-3-642-33454-2_51

15. Wang, L., et al.: LINKS: learning-based multi-source integration framework for segmentation of infant brain images. NeuroImage **108**, 160–172 (2015)

16. Wells, W.M., et al.: Adaptive segmentation of MRI data. TMI **15**(4), 429–442 (1996)

17. Yaqub, M., et al.: Investigation of the role of feature selection and weighted voting in random forests for 3-d volumetric segmentation. IEEE Trans. Med. Imaging **33**(2), 258–271 (2014)

18. Zhang, Y., et al.: Segmentation of brain MR images through a hidden markov random field model and the expectation-maximization algorithm. TMI **20**(1), 45–57 (2001)

19. Zhang, W., et al.: Deep convolutional neural networks for multi-modality isointense infant brain image segmentation. NeuroImage **108**, 214–224 (2015)

Dictionary Learning and Sparse Coding-Based Denoising for High-Resolution Task Functional Connectivity MRI Analysis

Seongah Jeong[1]([envelope]), Xiang Li[2], Jiarui Yang[2], Quanzheng Li[2], and Vahid Tarokh[1]

[1] School of Engineering and Applied Sciences (SEAS),
Harvard University, 29 Oxford Street, Cambridge, MA 02138, USA
sej293@g.harvard.edu
[2] Department of Radiology, Massachusetts General Hospital
and Harvard Medical School, Boston, MA 02114, USA

Abstract. We propose a novel denoising framework for task functional Magnetic Resonance Imaging (tfMRI) data to delineate the high-resolution spatial pattern of the brain functional connectivity via dictionary learning and sparse coding (DLSC). In order to address the limitations of the unsupervised DLSC-based fMRI studies, we utilize the prior knowledge of task paradigm in the learning step to train a data-driven dictionary and to model the sparse representation. We apply the proposed DLSC-based method to Human Connectome Project (HCP) motor tfMRI dataset. Studies on the functional connectivity of cerebro-cerebellar circuits in somatomotor networks show that the DLSC-based denoising framework can significantly improve the prominent connectivity patterns, in comparison to the temporal non-local means (tNLM)-based denoising method as well as the case without denoising, which is consistent and neuroscientifically meaningful within motor area. The promising results show that the proposed method can provide an important foundation for the high-resolution functional connectivity analysis, and provide a better approach for fMRI preprocessing.

Keywords: Functional magnetic resonance imaging (fMRI) · Denoising · Dictionary learning · Sparse coding · Connectivity

1 Introduction

Functional magnetic resonance imaging (fMRI) enables the inference of functional connectivity among different brain regions [1–5] and the early diagnosis of various brain disorders [6,7]. However, the functional connectivity analysis based on the fMRI data is limited in accuracy and reliability due to the inherently low signal-to-noise ratio (SNR) of fMRI signals which results from the high intrinsic noise and small magnitude of Blood Oxygen Level Dependent (BOLD) signals. To address this issue, the preprocessing to reduce the noise and improve the

© Springer International Publishing AG 2017
Q. Wang et al. (Eds.): MLMI 2017, LNCS 10541, pp. 45–52, 2017.
DOI: 10.1007/978-3-319-67389-9_6

SNR is typically carried out either by improving the sample size (i.e. group-wise study with multiple subjects), or via filtering [1–4,8,9], e.g., Gaussian low pass (GLP)-based filter [8] and non-local means (NLM)-based filter [9].

In this work, we develop a novel denoising framework for task fMRI (tfMRI) data to enable the high-resolution functional connectivity analysis via dictionary learning and sparse coding (DLSC)-based method. The proposed method exploits the sparsity of the underlying fMRI signals, by which the temporal dynamics at each voxel can be represented as a sparse combination of basis functions to characterize global brain dynamics [10,11]. In order to overcome the limitations of the current unsupervised DLSC-based fMRI studies such as absence of the interpretation of the output and loss of statistical power, we utilize the prior knowledge of task paradigm in the learning step to train a data-driven dictionary and to model the sparse representation [12]. We apply the proposed DLSC-based denoising method to the tfMRI data acquired during motor task from Human Connectome Project (HCP) [13]. It is observed that the proposed denoising method can exert more pronounced effects on the connectivities with high correlation, but less pronounced effects on the connectivities with low correlation which are estimated from the raw signals, in comparison to the baseline method. This allows us to obtain a more distinct spatial connectivity pattern and to achieve the high-resolution functional connectivity analysis.

2   Methods

In this section, we first briefly describe the HCP motor tfMRI dataset [13], and then provide the detailed description of the proposed denoising framework.

2.1   Dataset

In this work, we use the minimally preprocessed fMRI data (TR = 720 ms, TE = 33.1 ms, 2 × 2 × 2 mm voxel) from 50 subjects provided in HCP Q1 release [13]. The details for data acquisition and experiment design can be found in [13]. The tfMRI data are obtained during motor task, where the participants are informed with visual cues to tap their left or right fingers, squeeze their left or right toes, and move their tongue. This task is verified to be able to identify the effector corresponding to the specific activation individually in [3,4]. Each run consists of 13 blocks with 2 tongue movements, 2 right and 2 left hand movements, 2 right and 2 left foot movements and three 15 s fixation blocks, where each block lasts 12 s and is preceded by a 3 s visual cue. The number of frames or time samples for each subject is 284 and the total run duration is 214 s.

2.2   Dictionary Learning and Sparse Coding (DLSC)-Based Denoising

The proposed DLSC-based denoising method aims at representing the fMRI signal at each voxel as a sparse linear combination of dictionary basis functions

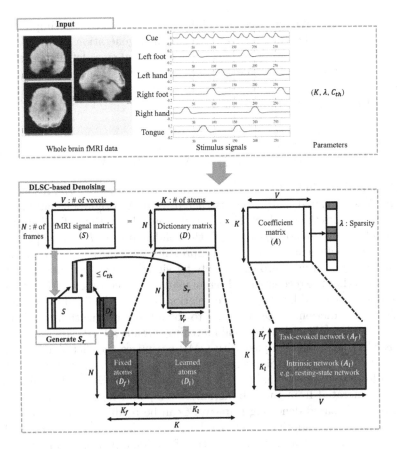

Fig. 1. The framework of the DLSC-based denoising method.

or atoms characterizing global brain dynamics. Unlike the existing unsupervised DLSC-based fMRI studies, we utilize the prior knowledge of task paradigm in the learning step to train the data-driven dictionary and to develop the sparse coding as illustrated in Fig. 1.

Specifically, for each subject, we factorize the $N \times V$ fMRI signal matrix S, with N being the number of frames and V being the number of voxels, into $S = DA$, where D is the $N \times K$ dictionary matrix with K being the number of atoms and A is the corresponding $K \times V$ coefficient matrix. In the proposed DLSC-based scheme, we consider two different sets of dictionary atoms such as fixed atoms and learned atoms. Accordingly, the dictionary matrix D is composed as $D = [D_f \ D_l]$, where the sub-dictionary matrices D_f and D_l consist of the K_f fixed atoms and the K_l learned atoms, respectively, which correspond to the sub-coefficient matrices A_f and A_l constructing the coefficient matrix $A = [A_f; A_l]$. The fixed atoms are predefined as the task stimulus curves which are generated by the convolution of a Statistical Parametric Mapping (SPM)

[14] canonical hemodynamic response function (HRF) and the simple boxcar stimulus function indicating each occurrence of a generation event. Here, we consider the six different stimulus curves for the visual cues, left hand, left foot, right hand, right foot and tongue movements in Fig. 1. The learned atoms are trained in unsupervised way with the reconstructed signal matrix S_r by solving the following minimization problem:

$$\underset{D_l, A^*}{\text{minimize}} \quad \|S_r - D_l A^*\|_F^2 \tag{1a}$$

$$\text{s.t.} \quad \|a_v^*\|_0 \leq \lambda, \quad v = 1, \ldots, V_r, \tag{1b}$$

where $\|\cdot\|_F$ and $\|\cdot\|_0$ indicate the Frobenius norm and the zero norm, respectively; S_r is the $N \times V_r$ signal matrix reconstructed from the original signal matrix S which only includes the voxels with the correlation value with the fixed atoms less than predefined threshold C_{th} to satisfy the condition $V_r \geq K_l$; $A^* = [a_1^* \cdots a_{V_r}^*]$ is the $K_l \times V_r$ coefficient matrix; and λ represents the sparsity constraint on the maximum number of non-zero coefficients for signal at each voxel of the matrix S_r. It is noted that the reconstructed signal matrix S_r is considered for mitigating the malfunction caused by the intra-correlation between the fixed dictionary D_f and the learned dictionary D_l. In order to solve the minimization problem (1), K-SVD algorithm [15] and orthogonal matching pursuit (OMP) [16] are adopted, where K-SVD algorithm coupled with OMP optimizes the dictionary D_l in an iterative and alternative fashion with the sparse coding A^*. Then, the coefficient matrix A for the original signal matrix S is determined with the final dictionary matrix D generated from the sub-dictionaries D_f and D_l by using OMP. The proposed DLSC-based denoising framework can be readily applied to the other tfMRI datasets, e.g., emotion, gambling, language, relational, social and working memory tasks [13], but also used with other functional neuroimaging methods.

For the DLSC-based denoising method, the parameter tuning for the dictionary size K, the sparsity λ and the threshold C_{th} is required which affects the denoising performance. However, since there is no gold criterion for the choice of these parameters, we perform a grid-search for finding the best parameter combinations with $K = 300$ to 500, with step of 100, $\lambda = 5$ to 50, with step of 5, and $C_{th} = 0.1$ to 0.4, with step of 0.1, and finally choose $(K, \lambda, C_{th}) = (400, 40, 0.1)$ based on visual inspection of resulting connectivity performance.

3   Results

In this work, we focus on the cerebrocerebellar circuits involved in somatomotor networks to analyze the validity of proposed method. To this end, the ground truth functional connectivity as reported in [3,4] between three cerebellar seed regions for the foot (F), hand (H) and tongue (T) tasks and six cerebral regions ($M1_F$, $S1_F$, $M1_H$, $S1_H$, $M1_T$ and $S1_T$) related to the corresponding seed regions in the left and right hemisphere are considered (see, Fig. 2). Each region consists of a single surface vertex (4×4 mm) centering at the MNI coordinate tabulated in [3,4], and the visualization is performed via BrainNet [17]. For comparison,

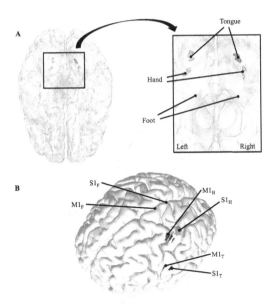

Fig. 2. Cerebrocerebellar circuits involved in somatomotor networks. A: Cerebellar seed regions corresponding to foot, hand and tongue tasks. B: $M1_F$, $S1_F$, $M1_H$, $S1_H$, $M1_T$ and $S1_T$ in the left cerebral cortex.

the temporal non-local mean (tNLM)-based denoising method [9] is adopted which can achieve significant performance improvement in comparison to the linear filter-based denoising. The tNLM-based method effectively substitutes the spatial similarity weighting in standard NLM with a weighting that is based on the correlation between time series. For the tNLM-based denoising method, we set the distance parameter = 11 and the smoothing level = 0.72 following [9] to empirically provide good results with reasonable computational cost.

The group-averaged functional connectivity maps for the raw data (black solid line) and the denoised data by using tNLM-based method (black dashed line) and our proposed DLSC-based method (red solid line) are visualized for the foot, hand and tongue tasks in Fig. 3. The functional connectivity is evaluated by computing the Pearson's correlation coefficient between contralateral cerebral and cerebellar regions and averaged across the hemispheres. Fisher's r-to-z transformation and its inverse transformation are further applied to promote the normality of the distribution of correlations.

In Fig. 3, it is observed that our novel denoising framework can strengthen the connectivity between the seed regions associated with each particular movement and the corresponding M1 and S1 regions, that is, the connectivities at $M1_F$ and $S1_F$ for foot task, $M1_H$ and $S1_H$ for hand task, and $M1_T$ and $S1_T$ for tongue task can be strikingly pronounced by the proposed DLSC-based denoising method. Furthermore, the emphasis effect of the DLSC-based method is more significant on the connectivities with high correlation, but less on the connectivities with low

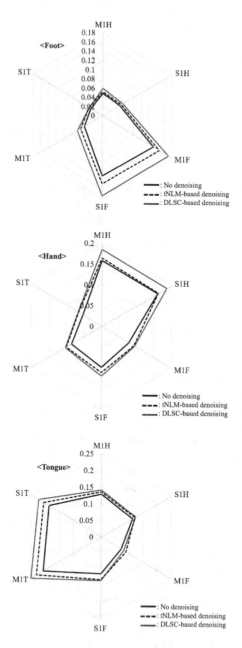

Fig. 3. Quantitative measures of functional connectivity strength of unprocessed data (black solid line), tNLM-based denoised data (black dashed line) and DLSC-based denoised data (red solid line) for cerebellar anterior lobe seed regions linked to the foot, hand and tongue representations (Color figure online)

correlation estimated from the raw signals, which is consistent across the tasks and subjects. This can provide the neuroscientifically meaningful within motor area to enable the high-resolution functional connectivity analysis, which cannot be attained by the tNLM-based denoising method nor with no denoising method applied. For example, the highest connectivity emphasis effect of the tNLM-based method is on M1$_T$ and M1$_F$ in the hand movement of Fig. 3. In addition, the DLSC-based method shows the strongest connectivity patterns for all motor tasks than the tNLM-based method. We believe that, from these important observations, the proposed DLSC-based denoising method can effectively recover the disrupted functional connectivity by artifacts and noise, and therefore have the potential to discover the previously hidden spatial connectivity pattern.

4 Discussion

In this work, we have studied a DLSC-based denoising framework for the high-resolution tfMRI functional connectivity analysis by using the sparseness of the underlying hemodynamic signals in brain. Unlike the traditional unsupervised DLSC-based fMRI studies, we utilize the prior knowledge of task paradigm in the learning step to train the dictionary and to develop the sparse coding. The denoising effect of the proposed framework is evaluated by applying it to the publicly available HCP motor tfMRI dataset. Studies on the functional connectivity between cerebellar seed regions and cerebral regions in somatomotor networks show the significant denoising performance of the proposed scheme, in comparison to tNLM-based denoising method as baseline scheme as well as no denoising case. It is observed that the DLSC-based denoising method can exert more pronounced effects on the connectivities with high correlation, but less pronounced effects on the connectivities with low correlation estimated from the raw signals, which is consistent and neuroscientifically meaningful within motor area. This shows the capability of the proposed DLSC-based denoising framework to provide a more distinct spatial pattern and accordingly to enable the high-resolution functional connectivity analysis.

References

1. Biswal, B., Yetkin, F.Z., Haughton, V.M., Hyde, J.S.: Functional connectivity in the motor cortex of resting human brain using echoplanar MRI. Magn. Reson. Med. **34**(4), 537–541 (1995). doi:10.1002/mrm.1910340409
2. Fox, M.D., Raichle, M.E.: Spontaneous fluctuations in brain activity observed with functional magnetic resonance imaging. Nat. Rev. Neurosci. **8**(9), 700–711 (2007). doi:10.1038/nrn2201
3. Yeo, B.T., Krienen, F.M., Sepulcre, J., Sabuncu, M.R., Lashkari, D., Hollinshead, M., Roffman, J.L., Smoller, J.W., Zöllei, L., Polimeni, J.R., Fischl, B.: The organization of the human cerebral cortex estimated by intrinsic functional connectivity. J. Neurophysiol. **106**(3), 1125–1165 (2011). doi:10.1152/jn.00338.2011

4. Buckner, R.L., Krienen, F.M., Castellanos, A., Diaz, J.C., Yeo, B.T.: The organization of the human cerebellum estimated by intrinsic functional connectivity. J. Neurophysiol. **106**(5), 2322–2345 (2011). doi:10.1152/jn.00339.2011

5. Jeong, S., Li, X., Farhadi, H., Li, Q., Tarokh, V.: fMRI signal denoising by dictionary learning for high-resolution functional connectivity inference. In: 23rd Annual Meeting of the Organization for Human Brain Mapping (OHBM), Vancouver, Canada (2017)

6. Wee, C.Y., Yap, P.T., Zhang, D., Denny, K., Browndyke, J.N., Potter, G.G., Welsh-Bohmer, K.A., Wang, L., Shen, D.: Identification of MCI individuals using structural and functional connectivity networks. Neuroimage **59**(3), 2045–2056 (2012). doi:10.1016/j.neuroimage.2011.10.015

7. Jie, B., Zhang, D., Gao, W., Wang, Q., Wee, C.Y., Shen, D.: Integration of network topological and connectivity properties for neuroimaging classification. IEEE Trans. Biomed. Eng. **61**(2), 576–589 (2014). doi:10.1109/TBME.2013.2284195

8. Wink, A.M., Roerdink, J.B.: Denoising functional MR images: a comparison of wavelet denoising and Gaussian smoothing. IEEE Trans. Med. Imaging **23**(3), 374–387 (2004). doi:10.1109/TMI.2004.824234

9. Bhushan, C., Chong, M., Choi, S., Joshi, A.A., Haldar, J.P., Damasio, H., Leahy, R.M.: Temporal non-local means filtering reveals real-time whole-brain cortical interactions in resting fMRI. PLoS ONE **11**(7), e0158504 (2016). doi:10.1371/journal.pone.0158504

10. Lv, J., Jiang, X., Li, X., Zhu, D., Chen, H., Zhang, T., Zhang, S., Hu, X., Han, J., Huang, H., Zhang, J.: Sparse representation of whole-brain fMRI signals for identification of functional networks. Med. Image Anal. **20**(1), 112–134 (2015). doi:10.1016/j.media.2014.10.011

11. Lv, J., Jiang, X., Li, X., Zhu, D., Zhang, S., Zhao, S., Chen, H., Zhang, T., Hu, X., Han, J., Ye, J.: Holistic atlases of functional networks and interactions reveal reciprocal organizational architecture of cortical function. IEEE Trans. Biomed. Eng. **62**(4), 1120–1131 (2015). doi:10.1109/TBME.2014.2369495

12. Zhao, S., Han, J., Lv, J., Jiang, X., Hu, X., Zhao, Y., Ge, B., Guo, L., Liu, T.: Supervised dictionary learning for inferring concurrent brain networks. IEEE Trans. Med. Imaging **34**(10), 2036–2045 (2015). doi:10.1109/TMI.2015.2418734

13. Barch, D.M., Burgess, G.C., Harms, M.P., Petersen, S.E., Schlaggar, B.L., Corbetta, M., Glasser, M.F., Curtiss, S., Dixit, S., Feldt, C., Nolan, D.: Function in the human connectome: task-fMRI and individual differences in behavior. Neuroimage **80**, 169–189 (2013). doi:10.1016/j.neuroimage.2013.05.033

14. Statistical Parametric Mapping: UCL, England. http://www.fil.ion.ucl.ac.uk/spm/software/spm12

15. Aharon, M., Elad, M., Bruckstein, A.: K-SVD: an algorithm for designing overcomplete dictionaries for sparse representation. IEEE Trans. Sig. Process. **54**(11), 4311–4322 (2006). doi:10.1109/TSP.2006.881199

16. Pati, Y.C., Rezaiifar, R., Krishnaprasad, P.: Orthogonal matching pursuit: recursive function approximation with applications to wavelet decomposition. In: 27th Asilomar Conference on Signals, Systems and Computers, pp. 40–44. IEEE Press, Pacific Grove, CA (1993). doi:10.1109/ACSSC.1993.342465

17. Xia, M.L., Wang, J., He, Y.: BrainNet viewer: a network visualization tool for human brain connectomics. PLoS ONE **8**(7), e68910 (2013). doi:10.1371/journal.pone.0068910

Yet Another ADNI Machine Learning Paper? Paving the Way Towards Fully-Reproducible Research on Classification of Alzheimer's Disease

Jorge Samper-González[1,2], Ninon Burgos[1,2], Sabrina Fontanella[1,2],
Hugo Bertin[3], Marie-Odile Habert[3], Stanley Durrleman[1,2],
Theodoros Evgeniou[4], Olivier Colliot[1,2(✉)],
and the Alzheimer's Disease Neuroimaging Initiative

[1] INRIA Paris, ARAMIS Project-team, 75013 Paris, France
[2] Sorbonne Universités, UPMC Univ Paris 06, Inserm, CNRS,
Institut du Cerveau Et la Moelle (ICM), AP-HP - Hôpital Pitié-Salpêtrière,
75013 Paris, France
olivier.colliot@upmc.fr
[3] Sorbonne Universités, UPMC Univ Paris 06, Inserm, CNRS, LIB, AP-HP,
75013 Paris, France
[4] INSEAD, Bd de Constance, 77305 Fontainebleau, France

Abstract. In recent years, the number of papers on Alzheimer's disease classification has increased dramatically, generating interesting methodological ideas on the use machine learning and feature extraction methods. However, practical impact is much more limited and, eventually, one could not tell which of these approaches are the most efficient. While over 90% of these works make use of ADNI an objective comparison between approaches is impossible due to variations in the subjects included, image pre-processing, performance metrics and cross-validation procedures. In this paper, we propose a framework for reproducible classification experiments using multimodal MRI and PET data from ADNI. The core components are: (1) code to automatically convert the full ADNI database into BIDS format; (2) a modular architecture based on Nipype in order to easily plug-in different classification and feature extraction tools; (3) feature extraction pipelines for MRI and PET data; (4) baseline classification approaches for unimodal and multimodal features. This provides a flexible framework for benchmarking different feature extraction and classification tools in a reproducible manner. Data management tools for obtaining the lists of subjects in AD, MCI converter, MCI non-converters, CN classes are also provided. We demonstrate its use on all (1519) baseline T1 MR images and all (1102) baseline FDG PET images from ADNI 1, GO and 2 with SPM-based feature extraction pipelines and three different classification techniques (linear SVM, anatomically regularized SVM and multiple kernel learning SVM). The highest accuracies achieved were: 91% for AD vs CN, 83% for MCIc vs CN, 75% for MCIc vs MCInc, 94% for AD-Aβ+ vs CN-Aβ- and 72% for MCIc-Aβ+ vs MCInc-Aβ+. The code will be made publicly available at the time of the conference (https://gitlab.icm-institute.org/aramislab/AD-ML).

© Springer International Publishing AG 2017
Q. Wang et al. (Eds.): MLMI 2017, LNCS 10541, pp. 53–60, 2017.
DOI: 10.1007/978-3-319-67389-9_7

1 Introduction

Alzheimer's disease (AD) accounts for over 20 million cases worldwide. Biological and brain imaging markers of AD contain information about complementary processes of the disease progression: in anatomical MRI the atrophy due to gray matter loss, hypometabolism in fluorodeoxyglucose (FDG) PET, the accumulation of amyloid-beta protein in the brain tissue in amyloid PET imaging, as well as concentrations of tau and amyloid-beta proteins in cerebrospinal fluid through lumbar puncture. A major interest is then to analyze those markers to identify AD at an early stage.

To this end, a large number of machine learning approaches have been proposed (see [4,14,16] for a review). Such approaches differ by: (1) brain image processing pipelines, (2) feature extraction and selection; (3) machine learning algorithms (classification and/or regression methods). Furthermore, while initial efforts had made use of a single imaging modality (usually anatomical MRI) [10,12,15,18,19], a large number of works have proposed to combine multiple modalities (MRI and PET neuroimaging, fluid biomarkers) [1,2,6,7,9,17]. In particular, the combination of anatomical MRI and FDG PET is the most common.

Validation and comparison of such approaches require a large number of patients with multimodal data and followed over time. The vast majority (over 90%) of published works use the publicly available Alzheimer's Disease Neuroimaging Initiative (ADNI). However, objective comparison between their results is impossible because they use: (i) different subsets of patients (with unclear specification of selection criteria); (ii) different preprocessing pipelines (and thus it is not clear if the superior performance comes for the classification or the preprocessing); (iii) different evaluation metrics; (iv) different cross-validation procedures. At the end, it is very difficult to conclude which methods perform the best and even if a given modality provides useful additional information. As a result, the practical impact of these works has remained very limited.

Comparison papers [11,12] and challenges [3,5] have been an important step towards objective evaluation of machine learning methods, by allowing to benchmark different approaches on the same dataset and with the same preprocessing. Nevertheless, such studies provide a "static" assessment of approaches. Evaluation datasets are used in their current state at the time of the study, whereas new patients are continuously included in studies such as ADNI. Similarly, they are limited to the classification and preprocessing methods that were used at the time of the study. It is thus difficult to complement them with new approaches.

In this paper, we propose a framework for reproducible evaluation of machine learning algorithms in AD and demonstrate its use on multimodal classification of PET and MRI data of the ADNI database. Specifically, our contributions are three-fold: (i) a framework for management of ADNI data and their continuous update with new subjects; (ii) a modular set of preprocessing pipelines, feature extraction and classification methods, that provide a baseline for benchmarking of different components; (iii) a large-scale evaluation of the added value of the combination of anatomical MRI and FDG PET on 967 patients. By providing a fully automatic conversion into BIDS format, we offer a huge saving of time to users, compared to simply making public the list of used subjects. This is particularly true for complex multimodal datasets like ADNI (with plenty of incomplete data, multiple instances of a given modality and complex metadata). Such a standardized data curation also allows future inclusion of other datasets in a transparent way, perfect for external validation (e.g. the Australian Imaging Biomarker and Lifestyle study, AIBL).

Currently, we include relatively standard T1 and (FDG and AV45) PET pipelines and voxel-based SVM classification. The idea is not to impose their use, but to provide a set of baseline tools against which new methods can be easily compared. Researchers working on novel methods can then easily replace a given part of the pipeline (e.g. feature extraction, classification) with their own approach, and evaluate the added value of this specific new component over the baseline approach provided.

2 Material and Methods

In order to serve methodological developments and to provide a common framework for evaluation and comparison of methods, we developed a unified set of tools for data management, image preprocessing, feature extraction and classification. Data management tools allow to easily update the dataset as new subjects become available in ADNI. Processing and classification tools have been designed in a modular way using Nipype library to allow the development and testing of other methods as replacement for a given step. Then, the impact of each method in the results can be objectively measured. A simple command line interface is provided and the code can also be used as a Python library.

2.1 Dataset

ADNI, together with follow ups ADNI GO and ADNI2, is a publicly available database. Overall, it comprises over 300 patients with AD, over 850 patients with mild cognitive impairment (MCI) and over 350 control subjects. An important difficulty with ADNI lies in the organization of the public database. Imaging data, in the state it is downloaded, lacks of a clear structure, and there are multiple image acquisitions for a given visit of a subject. The complementary image information is contained in numerous csv files, making the exploration of the database and subject selection very complicated.

2.2 A Standardized Data Structure

To organize the data, we selected the Brain Imaging Data Structure (BIDS) [8], a community standard to store multiple neuroimaging modalities. Being based on a file hierarchy, rather than a database management system, BIDS can be easily deployed in any environment. For ADNI, among the multiple scans for a visit, we selected a single scan by imaging modality for each subject. In the case of

T1 scans, gradwarp and B1-inhomogeneity corrected images were selected when available, otherwise the original image was selected. When repeated MRI were available for a single session, the higher quality scan (as identified in ADNI csv files) was chosen. 1.5T images were preferred for ADNI-1 since they are available for a larger number of patients. For PET scans, the co-registered averaged across time frames images were selected.

Very importantly, we provide the code that performs these selections in a fully automated way. The code receives as input a folder containing the download of all ADNI data (in their raw format) and creates a BIDS organized version (T1 MRI, FDG and AV-45 PET). This allows direct reproducibility by other groups without having to redistribute ADNI data, which is not allowed. We also provide tools for subject selection according to desired imaging modalities, time of follow up and diagnose, which make possible to use the same groups with the largest possible number of subjects across studies. Finally, we propose a BIDS-inspired standardized structure for all outputs of the experiments.

2.3   Preprocessing and Feature Extraction Pipelines

Two pipelines for processing anatomical T1 MRI and PET images were developed. Pipelines have a modular structure based on Nipype allowing to easily connect and/or replace components. For anatomical T1 MRI, SPM12 was used to perform tissue segmentation (GM, WM, CSF) based on the Unified Segmentation procedure. Next, a DARTEL template is created for all the subjects and a registration to MNI space (DARTEL to MNI) is carried on each of them. The result is that all the images are in a common space, providing a voxel-wise correspondence across subjects. For PET images, we perform a registration of PET data onto the corresponding T1 image in native space. An optional partial volume correction (PVC) step is included using different tissue maps from the T1 in native space. Then the registration into MNI space using the same transformation as for the corresponding T1 and the generation of a parametric image by normalization to a reference region (the reference region is eroded pons for FDG PET, eroded pons and cerebellum combined for amyloid PET) and masking of non-brain regions are performed.

2.4   Classification Methods

The obtained images for all the subjects and for each modality lie in a common space so they can be analyzed voxel-wise. The currently implemented classifiers use voxel-as-features (i.e. GM maps for T1 MRI and parametric FDG PET images). Other types of features such as regional features could be easily implemented in the future. We implemented different classifiers for unimodal (T1 MRI or FDG PET) and multimodal classification.

Unimodal Classification. *Linear SVM.* The first method included to classify single modality images is a linear SVM. For the specified modality, a linear kernel is calculated using the inner product for each pair of images (using all the voxels) for the provided subjects. This kernel is used as input for the generic SVM (makes use of scikit-learn library[1]). Given its simplicity it is useful as a baseline to compare the performance of methods.

Spatially and Anatomically Regularized SVM. The L2 regularization of the standard SVM does not take into account the spatial and anatomical structure of brain images. As a result, the solutions are not easily interpretable (the obtained hyperplanes are highly scattered). To overcome this issue, we implement a classifier that combines a spatial regularization and an atlas based anatomical regularization by using the Fisher metric as proposed by [13]. The spatial proximity takes into account the distance between voxels while anatomical proximity is defined as if two voxels belong to the same atlas defined region or tissue (in our case GM, WM and CSF probability maps). This approach was initially proposed by [13] in the case of T1 MRI. Here, we extend it to FDG PET images. The implementation of this approach provides a baseline classifier with interpretable maps that can be used for comparison of other methods.

Multimodal Classification. For multimodal classification, we included a simple implementation of Multiple Kernel Learning (MKL) for the case of two modalities. A kernel is obtained from the linear combination of two kernels obtained for each imaging modality separately, and then provided as input to the SVM: $K_{\text{T1-FDG}} = \alpha K_{\text{T1}} + (1 - \alpha)K_{\text{FDG}}, \quad 0 \leq \alpha \leq 1$.

Parameter α that maximizes the balanced accuracy is determined by cross validation. This parameter weights the initial kernels into the combined kernel and therefore represents the contribution of each imaging modality into the classification result.

2.5   Validation

Cross-Validation. To assess classification performance without bias, it is important to carefully perform cross-validation (CV). In particular, CV must not only concern the training of the classifier, but also the optimization of hyperparameters. While the former is usually dealt with correctly, the latter has not always been appropriately performed in the literature. Here, we implemented two nested CV procedures for hyperparameter optimization and classifier training. By default, a 10-fold CV is implemented in our framework, and an input parameter lets the user select the number of desired folds.

Metrics. As output of the classification, we report AUC, accuracy, balanced accuracy, sensitivity, specificity and in addition the predicted class for each subject so that the user could calculate any other metric with this information. Also, an image with the SVM weights for each feature is provided. Such weights live in the same space as the MRI and PET images and can thus be used to visualize the brain regions that contributed to the classification.

---

[1] http://scikit-learn.org.

3   Results

We applied the preprocessing pipelines to all (1519) baseline T1 MR images and all (1102) baseline FDG PET images from ADNI 1, GO and 2. Subjects were grouped as AD(239), MCI converter(164), MCI non converter(309) or CN(255), according to diagnosis determined for 36 months of follow up (967 subjects in total). Another grouping was done also taking into account amyloid imaging as AD-Aβ+(125), MCIc-Aβ+(81), MCIc-Aβ-(5), MCInc-Aβ+(105), MCInc-Aβ-(131) and CN-Aβ-(111).

Classification for AD vs CN, MCIc vs CN and MCIc vs MCInc, AD-Aβ+ vs CN-Aβ- and MCIc-Aβ+ vs MCInc-Aβ+ classification tasks was performed using voxel-based linear SVM and spatially and anatomically regularized SVM for each modality separately (T1 and FDG PET). Also the multiple-kernel SVM was used on the combination of linear and regularized kernels for T1 and FDG PET obtained in the previous step. Classification results were averaged over 10 runs. Results can be observed in Table 1.

Table 1. Classification results (mean of 10 runs)

IMAGE TYPE	CLASSIFIER	TASK	AUC	BAL ACC	SENS	SPEC
T1	Linear SVM	AD vs CN	94.2%	88.8%	92.8%	84.8%
		MCIc vs CN	85.5%	80.5%	66.8%	89.3%
		MCIc vs MCInc	73.8%	66.5%	64.9%	69.3%
		AD-Aβ+ vs CN-Aβ−	93.6%	87.9%	90.5%	85.5%
		MCIc-Aβ+ vs MCInc-Aβ+	73.6%	65.8%	69.8%	60.3%
FDG PET	Linear SVM	AD vs CN	96.7%	91.1%	95%	87.2%
		MCIc vs CN	89.1%	83.5%	74.7%	89.2%
		MCIc vs MCInc	80.5%	75.2%	78.5%	69.4%
		AD-Aβ+ vs CN-Aβ−	98.6%	94.4%	95.6%	93.4%
		MCIc-Aβ+ vs MCInc-Aβ+	80.8%	72.8%	77%	67%

Overall, the use of FDG PET provided better results than T1 in general (balanced accuracy of 91% for AD vs CN, 83% for MCIc vs CN, 75% for MCIc vs MCInc, 94% for AD-Aβ+ vs CN-Aβ- and 72% for MCIc-Aβ+ vs MCInc-Aβ+), but it significantly outperforms it in the case of conversion prediction (MCIc vs MCInc and MCIc-Aβ+ vs MCInc-Aβ+ tasks) (Fig. 1).

The combination of different modality kernels confirms this result, providing as best linear combination the case when only FDG PET data was selected, giving no weight to GM kernel.

The use of amyloid imaging to refine groups improved the classification results only for FDG PET in the case of AD-Aβ+ vs CN-Aβ- and not in every task as expected.

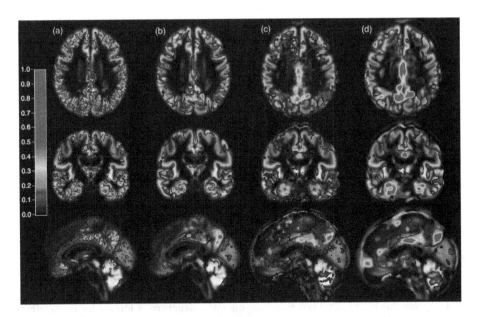

Fig. 1. Normalized w^{opt} coefficients ≥ 0 for AD vs CN: (a) T1 linear SVM, (b) T1 regularized SVM, (c) FDG PET linear SVM, (d) FDG PET regularized SVM

4   Conclusions

We proposed a framework for reproducible machine learning experiments on automatic classification using the ADNI database. It features a standardized data management and a modular architecture for preprocessing, feature extraction and classification. Of note, the dataset can be continuously updated as more data become available. We provide processing pipelines for T1 MRI and PET images as well as classification tools for unimodal and multimodal data.

We applied this framework to classify T1 MRI and FDG PET data. We demonstrate that FDG PET imaging provides superior accuracy over T1 MRI when predicting Alzheimer's disease conversion in MCI patients. Furthermore, combination of both modalities did not result in superior accuracy over FDG PET alone. However, more sophisticated combinations may lead to improvements. The use of amyloid imaging to refine groups of subjects didn't improve results in general, but it might be due to the significantly lower subject counts. The classification accuracy for AD vs CN and MCIc vs CN are in line with the state of the art. Nevertheless, there are some papers that report higher accuracy for prediction of conversion. Our lower accuracy might be due to the fact that we used all available patients, avoiding cherry-picking effects.

The code associated to this work will be made available at the time of the conference. We believe that it will be a useful tool for the community to progress towards more reproducible results in this field.

References

1. Jie, B., et al.: Manifold regularized multitask feature learning for multimodality disease classification. Hum. Brain Mapp. **36**(2), 489–507 (2015)
2. Zhang, D., et al.: Multimodal classification of Alzheimer's disease and mild cognitive impairment. NeuroImage **55**(3), 856–867 (2011)
3. Bron, E., et al.: Standardized evaluation of algorithms for computer-aided diagnosis of dementia based on structural MRI: the CADDementia challenge. NeuroImage **111**, 562–579 (2015)
4. Falahati, F., et al.: Multivariate data analysis and machine learning in Alzheimer's disease with a focus on structural magnetic resonance imaging. J. Alzheimer's Dis. JAD **41**(3), 685–708 (2014)
5. Allen, G., et al.: Crowdsourced estimation of cognitive decline and resilience in Alzheimer's disease. Alzheimer's Demen. **12**(6), 645–653 (2016)
6. Yun, H.J., et al.: Multimodal discrimination of Alzheimer's disease based on regional cortical atrophy and hypometabolism. PLoS ONE **10**(6), e0129250 (2015)
7. Young, J., et al.: Accurate multimodal probabilistic prediction of conversion to Alzheimer's disease in patients with mild cognitive impairment. NeuroImage Clin. **2**, 735–745 (2013)
8. Gorgolewski, K., et al.: The brain imaging data structure, a format for organizing and describing outputs of neuroimaging experiments. Sci. Data **3**, 160044 (2016)
9. Gray, K., et al.: Random forest-based similarity measures for multi-modal classification of Alzheimer's disease. NeuroImage **65**, 167–175 (2013)
10. Liu, M., et al.: Ensemble sparse classification of Alzheimer's disease. NeuroImage **60**(2), 1106–1116 (2012)
11. Sabuncu, M., et al.: Clinical prediction from structural brain MRI scans: a large-scale empirical study. Neuroinformatics **13**(1), 31–46 (2015)
12. Cuingnet, R., et al.: Automatic classification of patients with Alzheimer's disease from structural MRI: a comparison of ten methods using the ADNI database. NeuroImage **56**(2), 766–781 (2011)
13. Cuingnet, R., et al.: Spatial and anatomical regularization of SVM: a general framework for neuroimaging data. IEEE Trans. Pattern Anal. Mach. Intell. **35**(3), 682–696 (2013)
14. Haller, S., et al.: Principles of classification analyses in mild cognitive impairment (MCI) and Alzheimer disease. Journal of Alzheimer's disease: JAD **26**(Suppl. 3), 389–394 (2011)
15. Kloppel, S., et al.: Automatic classification of MR scans in Alzheimer's disease. Brain J. Neurol. **131**(3), 681–689 (2008)
16. Rathore, S., et al.: A review on neuroimaging-based classification studies and associated feature extraction methods for Alzheimer's disease and its prodromal stages. NeuroImage **155**, 530–548 (2017)
17. Teipel, S., et al.: The relative importance of imaging markers for the prediction of Alzheimer's disease dementia in mild cognitive impairment - Beyond classical regression. NeuroImage Clin. **8**, 583–593 (2015)
18. Tong, T., et al.: Multiple instance learning for classification of dementia in brain MRI. Med. Image Anal. **18**(5), 808–818 (2014)
19. Fan, Y., et al.: Spatial patterns of brain atrophy in MCI patients, identified via high-dimensional pattern classification, predict subsequent cognitive decline. NeuroImage **39**(4), 1731–1743 (2008)

Multi-factorial Age Estimation from Skeletal and Dental MRI Volumes

Darko Štern[1,2], Philipp Kainz[1], Christian Payer[2], and Martin Urschler[1,2(✉)]

[1] Ludwig Boltzmann Institute for Clinical Forensic Imaging, Graz, Austria
martin.urschler@cfi.lbg.ac.at
[2] Institute for Computer Graphics and Vision,
Graz University of Technology, Graz, Austria

Abstract. Age estimation from radiologic data is an important topic in forensic medicine to assess chronological age or to discriminate minors from adults, e.g. asylum seekers lacking valid identification documents. In this work we propose automatic multi-factorial age estimation methods based on MRI data to extend the maximal age range from 19 years, as commonly used for age assessment based on hand bones, up to 25 years, when combined with wisdom teeth and clavicles. Mimicking how radiologists perform age estimation, our proposed method based on deep convolutional neural networks achieves a result of 1.14 ± 0.96 years of mean absolute error in predicting chronological age. Further, when fine-tuning the same network for majority age classification, we show an improvement in sensitivity of the multi-factorial system compared to solely relying on the hand.

Keywords: Forensic age estimation · Multi-factorial method · Convolutional neural network · Random forest · Information fusion

1 Introduction

Age estimation of living individuals lacking valid identification documents currently is a highly relevant research field in forensic and legal medicine. Its main application comes from recent migration tendencies, where it is a legally important question to distinguish adult asylum seekers from adolescents who have not yet reached age of majority. Widely used radiological methods for forensic age estimation in children and adolescents take into account complementary biological development of skeletal [3,12] and dental structures [2]. This allows an expert to examine progress in physical maturation related to closing of epiphyseal gaps and mineralization of wisdom teeth. Despite biological variation among subjects of the same chronological age (CA), hand bones are the most suitable anatomical site to follow physical maturation in minors, since epiphyseal gaps start closing at different times, with distal bones finishing earlier and e.g. the radius

D. Štern—This work was supported by the Austrian Science Fund (FWF): P 28078-N33.

© Springer International Publishing AG 2017
Q. Wang et al. (Eds.): MLMI 2017, LNCS 10541, pp. 61–69, 2017.
DOI: 10.1007/978-3-319-67389-9_8

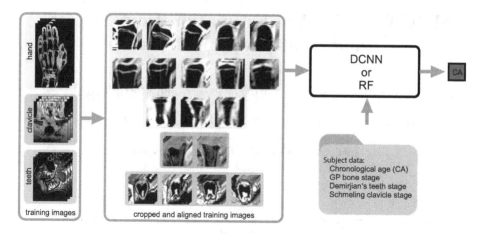

Fig. 1. Overview of our automatic multi-factorial age estimation framework. MRI volumes of hand, clavicle and wisdom teeth are cropped according to locations of age-relevant anatomical landmarks. A random forest (RF) or a deep convolutional neural network (DCNN) performs the nonlinear mapping between appearance information and chronological age.

bone finishing at an age of about 18 years. However, the age range of interest for forensic age estimation is between 13 and 25 years. Therefore, additional anatomical sites are required in a multi-factorial approach to allow an extension of the age estimation range up to 25 years.

The established X-ray imaging based multi-factorial approach [7] for estimation of biological age (BA) uses the Greulich-Pyle (GP) method [3] based on representative hand images of different age groups of a sample population, the Demirjian method [2] involving characteristic stages of wisdom teeth development, and the staging method of Schmeling [8] for assessing clavicle bone maturation. No standardized method exists for the combination of different sites, but, for majority age estimation, guidelines propose to use the minimum age of the most developed anatomical site as seen in a reference population [7].

Besides the lack of a standardized method for combining individual estimates, radiological methods also suffer from intra- and inter-observer variability when determining, from each anatomical site, the stages that define minimum age. While the use of more objective, automated image analysis for age estimation from X-ray data of the hand was already shown in [9,13], no such approaches yet exist for orthopantomograms of the teeth or computed tomography images of the clavicle bones. A novel trend in forensic age estimation research is to replace X-ray based methods with magnetic resonance imaging (MRI), because legal systems in most countries disallow the application of ionizing radiation on healthy subjects. Recently, automatic methods for age estimation based on MRI data were developed [10,11], nevertheless with the hand they also solely investigate a single anatomical site. To the best of our knowledge no automatic image analysis method for multi-factorial age estimation, irrespectively of the imaging modality, has been presented yet.

In this work, we investigate novel methods for multi-factorial age estimation from MRI data of hand bones, clavicles and wisdom teeth (see Fig. 1). Inspired by how radiologists perform staging of different anatomical sites, our methods automatically fuse the age-relevant appearance information from individual anatomical structures into a single chronological age. We compare a random forest (RF) based method [1] with two deep convolutional neural network (DCNN) architectures [4]. The first DCNN is trained on CA and the second one fine-tuned on CA after pre-training it using skeletal and dental age as BA estimates determined by an expert. The proposed methods are evaluated on an MRI database of 103 images by performing experiments assessing CA estimates in terms of regression, as well as distinction of minority/majority age, defined as having passed the 18th birthday, in terms of classification. Our results demonstrate the increase in accuracy and decrease in uncertainty when using the multi-factorial approach as compared to relying on a single anatomical structure.

2   Method

Following the established radiological staging approach involving different anatomical sites in a multi-factorial setup, after cropping of age-relevant structures we perform age estimation from cropped wisdom teeth, hand, and clavicle bones, either by the use of an RF or a DCNN architecture.

Cropping of age-relevant structures: Differently to [9], where a large data set of whole X-ray images is used for age estimation, our motivation for cropping age-relevant structures is to simplify the problem of regressing age from appearance information, such that it is also applicable for smaller data sets. Therefore, automated landmark localization methods as presented in [5] or [6] could be used to localize, align and volumetrically crop age-relevant anatomical structures from skeletal and dental 3D MRI data (see Fig. 1). From hand MRI we crop the same thirteen bones that are also used in the TW2 RUS method [12], similar to [10]. Four wisdom teeth are extracted from the dental MRI data using the locations of the centers of each tooth, and in clavicle MRI data the two clavicle bones are cropped based on four landmarks on the manubrium and two on each clavicle.

RF framework: Starting from the easily extensible framework for hand MRI age estimation proposed in [11], we additionally incorporate the selection of teeth and clavicle bones into each node of an RF. Thus, we allow the RF to select from which anatomical structure it extracts the features that are relevant for modeling the mapping between image appearance information and CA. After training it for regression of CA from all three anatomical sites, we denote this method RF-CA. Additionally, we train the same framework for majority age classification (RF-MAJ), and to compare to previous work [10], we also train an RF using BA as a regression target solely from the hand MRI data (RF-BA-HAND).

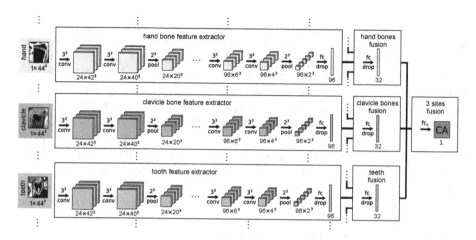

Fig. 2. DCNN architecture for multi-factorial age estimation.

DCNN architecture: Identical feature extraction blocks consisting of convolution (conv) and pooling (pool) stages are used for individual cropped input volumes. Fusion is performed for anatomical sites separately giving a final representation of extracted features. Estimated CA is obtained by combining the extracted features from the three sites with a fully connected (fc) layer.

The details of our individual identical DCNN blocks [4] are shown in Fig. 2, where we connect three stages consisting of two convolution and one max-pooling layer together with Rectified Linear Units (*ReLUs*) as nonlinear activation functions. Each block finishes with a fully connected layer, leading to a dimensionality reduced feature representation consisting of 96 outputs for each cropped input volume. Thus, we require another fully connected layer to fuse feature representations into a single feature vector for the different structures at each anatomical site. Finally, all three sites are fused with a fully connected layer to form a single continuous CA regression target. To reduce overfitting, we include drop-out regularization with a ratio of 0.5 into all fully connected layers except the last layer which solely has a single output. We denote this network DCNN-CA using CA as regression target. Since our network architecture is mimicking how radiologists perform staging of different anatomical sites, it readily supports the use of the assigned stages representing BA to pre-train the network weights of each individual site. This can be achieved by decoupling the last fully connected layer fc_o from the network and adding individual fully connected layers with a single output for each anatomical site. By training these individual networks with their respective radiological stage (e.g. DCNN-BA-HAND), we expect to achieve a better initialization of network weights compared to training DCNN-CA from scratch solely on CA. Fine-tuning of the pre-trained network on CA leads to our network DCNN-CA-RFND. Further, we use the same pre-trained network to directly predict whether a subject is an adult or a minor by fine-tuning network parameters for a classification target instead (DCNN-MAJ).

For training, we associate each training sample $s_n, n \in \{1, .., N\}$, consisting of thirteen cropped hand bone volumes $s_{n,h}^j, j \in \{1, .., 13\}$, 4 wisdom teeth $s_{n,w}^k, k \in \{1, .., 4\}$ and 2 clavicle regions $s_{n,c}^l, l \in \{1, 2\}$, with a regression target y_n^A. Depending on whether it is used for pre-training or for direct training/fine-tuning, here A is either chronological age CA or biological age BA defined as the average assigned radiological stage of the components of each anatomical site. Optimizing a DCNN architecture ϕ with parameters $\mathbf{w}$ is performed by applying stochastic gradient descent to minimize an L_2 loss on the regression target y^A:

$$\hat{\mathbf{w}} = \arg\min_{\mathbf{w}} \frac{1}{2} \sum_{n=1}^{N_s} ||\phi(s_n; \mathbf{w}) - y_n^A||^2. \tag{1}$$

For estimating whether a subject is a minor (m) or an adult (a) with DCNN-MAJ, we use the legally relevant chronological majority age threshold of 18 years to separate our subjects into two groups $\{m, a\}$. As an optimization function for this classification task we apply softmax computed as multinomial logistic loss:

$$\hat{\mathbf{w}} = \arg\min_{\mathbf{w}} \sum_{n=1}^{N_s} \sum_{j \in \{m,a\}} -y_n^j \log \frac{e^{\phi_j(s_n; \mathbf{w})}}{\sum_{k \in \{m,a\}} e^{\phi_k(s_n; \mathbf{w})}}. \tag{2}$$

To distinguish whether introducing multiple sites is beneficial for discriminating minors from adults, we apply the same classification loss for classification based solely on hand bones. Additionally, this network DCNN-MAJ-HAND facilitates a comparison with previous work on hand bone age estimation [10].

3   Experimental Setup and Results

Material: We apply our proposed method on a dataset of $N = 103$ 3D MRIs of the left hand, the upper thorax and the jaw, respectively. The three volumes for each subject were prospectively acquired from male Caucasian volunteers with known CA ranging between 13.01 and 24.89 years (mean $\pm$ std: 19.1 ± 3.5 years, 44 subjects were minors below 18 years) in a single MRI scan session. CA of subjects was calculated as difference between birthday and date of the MRI scan. T1-weighted 3D gradient echo sequences were used for acquiring the hand and clavicle data (resolutions of $0.45 \times 0.45 \times 0.9$ and $0.9 \times 0.9 \times 0.9$ mm^3), while teeth were scanned using a proton density weighted turbo spin echo sequence ($0.59 \times 0.59 \times 1.0$ mm^3).

Regarding biological ages y_n^{BA} as determined by a board-certified radiologist as well as a dentist, for the hand volumes the GP standard [3] y_n^{GP} was used, the wisdom teeth were assessed using the Demirjian system [2] y_n^{DM}, and finally the clavicles were rated with the Schmeling system [8] y_n^{SM}.

Experimental Setup: A cross-validation with four folds was used to compute results for all experiments. In each cross-validation round, one fourth of the available datasets were used for testing, while the remaining subjects were

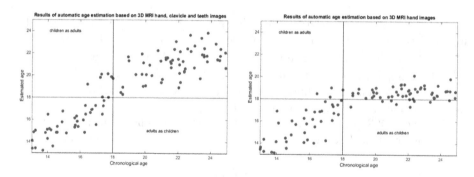

Fig. 3. Regression results for chronological age estimation based on DCNN-CA-RFND (left) and DCNN-CA-HAND restricted to hand MRI data (right).

used to generate training datasets for the RF and DCNN methods. To allow a meaningful evaluation over the given age range, the test sets were chosen by sampling according to the approximately uniform age distribution of our data, where random sampling required that at least two datasets from each bin were chosen for each fold. During training of both RF and DCNN, images were augmented on-the-fly by translating, rotating, scaling and shifting intensities of the cropped volumes. The size of cropped volumes after resampling with trilinear interpolation was $44 \times 44 \times 44$ pixels for all anatomical sites, respectively. We implemented our RF as a regression forest consisting of 100 trees, maximal tree depth of 20, and the number of candidate features/thresholds per node was set to 100/10, respectively. For the DCNN the *Caffe* framework[1] was used. Optimization was done with stochastic gradient descent with a maximum of $2 \cdot 10^4$ iterations, mini-batch size 1, momentum 0.99, and learning rate 10^{-5}. To evaluate our CA regression results, we compute mean and standard deviation of absolute errors between predicted and ground truth age. Classification experiments are evaluated by inspecting confusion matrices (TP, TN, FP, FN) and assessing accuracy (ACC), specificity (SPEC) and sensitivity (SENS), with the latter indicating the percentage of subjects classified as minors who are actually minors.

Results: For estimating biological age from the hand, absolute deviation results are 0.62 ± 0.58 for RF-BA-HAND and 0.33 ± 0.31 years for DCNN-BA-HAND. The mean absolute error of predictions compared to CA are 1.93 ± 1.26 for RF-CA, 1.3 ± 1.13 for DCNN-CA, and 1.14 ± 0.96 years for DCNN-CA-RFND. Regarding majority age classification, Table 1 shows the confusion matrix as well as accuracy, sensitivity and specificity results for the compared methods.

---

[1] Y. Jia, GitHub repository, https://github.com/BVLC/caffe/.

Table 1. Classification results for the majority age experiments (N = 103).

	TP	TN	FP	FN	ACC	SENS	SPEC
DCNN-MAJ	39 (37.9%)	55 (53.4%)	4 (3.9%)	5 (4.8%)	91.3%	88.6%	93.2%
DCNN-MAJ-HAND	36 (35.0%)	57 (55.3%)	2 (1.9%)	8 (7.8%)	90.3%	81.8%	96.6%
RF-MAJ	21 (20.4%)	58 (56.3%)	1 (1.0%)	23 (22.3%)	76.7%	47.7%	98.3%
RF-MAJ-HAND	25 (24.3%)	59 (57.3%)	0 (0.0%)	19 (18.4%)	81.6%	56.8%	100%

4 Discussion and Conclusion

Motivated by the lack of a standardized way of fusing age estimates from multiple complementary anatomical sites, and with the aim to reduce observer variability, we proposed two automated methods for age estimation of the living from MRI data in the age range of 13 to 25 years. It is for the first time that such a large age range was studied by an automatic approach. To verify that our proposed methods achieve state-of-the-art results on a reduced age range between 13 and 19 years, we first compared them with previous work from [10], based solely on hand MRIs for estimation of BA provided as bone age stages by a radiologist. For RF-BA-HAND, we achieved a mean absolute error of 0.62 ± 0.58 years on our data set, while the best RF result in [10] was 0.52 ± 0.60 years, but required a pre-processing step. Without any pre-processing but training directly on image intensity, our result of DCNN-BA-HAND (0.33 ± 0.31 years) was better than the overall best results of 0.36 ± 0.30 years reported in [10]. However, results should be interpreted carefully, since different data sets were used.

Due to biological variation of subjects at the same chronological age, estimation of CA as required in forensic medicine is a much harder task compared to regression of BA. Our main contribution in this work is the extension of the maximal age range for CA regression from 19 years, as possible with solely using hand images, to 25 years, when including data from three anatomical sites. This extension is clearly visible by comparing the scatter plots from DCNN-CA-RFND and DCNN-CA-HAND in Fig. 3. The plot corresponding to the extended age range regression further confirms that after the development of the hand has finished, uncertainty in estimating CA increases since less age relevant features are available. Compared to training DCNN-CA from scratch on chronological age, pre-training of the DCNN-CA-RFND network on the radiological staging results of the individual anatomical sites improved the mean absolute CA regression error from 1.3 ± 1.13 to 1.14 ± 0.96 years. Leading to a much higher error of 1.93 ± 1.26 years, we found that RF-CA was not able to achieve competitive age estimation results for the whole age range by selecting intensity features from all three anatomical sites, while the DCNNs superior feature extraction capabilities proved to be more powerful despite the low amount of training data.

A specific challenge in forensic age estimation is majority age classification of asylum seekers lacking valid identification documents, under the ethical constraint that legal authorities need to avoid misclassifications of minors as adults, i.e. requiring high sensitivity. While the RF based methods do not show competitive classification results, our DCNN-MAJ-HAND network that uses majority age as a binary classification target achieves a classification accuracy of 90.3%, while misclassifying 8 out of 44 minor subjects as adults (see Table 1). Refining the pre-trained multi-factorial network combining all three anatomical sites on majority classification (DCNN-MAJ) improves classification accuracy to 91.3%. More importantly, the number of misclassified minors is reduced to 5 out of 44, an improvement in sensitivity which greatly impacts the involved subjects to their advantage.

A limitation of our results is the low number of 103 studied subjects, so generalization of these results has to be done carefully until a larger set has been evaluated. Additionally, our method was evaluated on volumes cropped using manually annotated landmarks instead of predictions from a landmark localization algorithm. However, since our training stage involved random translational and rotational transformations in the data augmentation step, we expect the same performance using accurate and robust localization algorithms like [5,6].

In conclusion, we have demonstrated with our proposed DCNN method that multi-factorial age estimation based on the three anatomical sites (hand, wisdom teeth, clavicle) can be used to automatically estimate chronological age in the living, extending the age range up to 25 years. However, caution has to be taken when it is used for deciding whether a subject is a minor or an adult.

References

1. Breiman, L.: Random forests. Mach. Learn. **45**, 5–32 (2001)
2. Demirjian, A., Goldstein, H., Tanner, J.M.: A new system of dental age assessment. Hum. Biol. **45**(2), 211–227 (1973)
3. Greulich, W.W., Pyle, S.I.: Radiographic Atlas of Skeletal Development of the Hand and Wrist, 2nd edn. Stanford University Press, Stanford (1959)
4. LeCun, Y., Bottou, L., Bengio, Y., Haffner, P.: Gradient-based learning applied to document recognition. Proc. IEEE **86**(11), 2278–2324 (1998)
5. Lindner, C., Bromiley, P.A., Ionita, M.C., Cootes, T.F.: Robust and accurate shape model matching using random forest regression-voting. IEEE Trans. Pattern Anal. Mach. Intell. **37**(9), 1862–1874 (2015)
6. Payer, C., Štern, D., Bischof, H., Urschler, M.: Regressing heatmaps for multiple landmark localization using CNNs. In: Ourselin, S., Joskowicz, L., Sabuncu, M.R., Unal, G., Wells, W. (eds.) MICCAI 2016. LNCS, vol. 9901, pp. 230–238. Springer, Cham (2016). doi:10.1007/978-3-319-46723-8_27
7. Schmeling, A., Geserick, G., Reisinger, W., Olze, A.: Age estimation. Forensic Sci. Int. **165**(2–3), 178–181 (2007)
8. Schmeling, A., Schulz, R., Reisinger, W., Muehler, M., Wernecke, K.D., Geserick, G.: Studies on the time frame for ossification of the medial clavicular epiphyseal cartilage in conventional radiography. Int. J. Leg. Med. **118**(1), 5–8 (2004)
9. Spampinato, C., Palazzo, S., Giordano, D., Aldinucci, M., Leonardi, R.: Deep learning for automated skeletal bone age assessment in X-ray images. Med. Image Anal. **36**, 41–51 (2017)

10. Štern, D., Payer, C., Lepetit, V., Urschler, M.: Automated age estimation from hand MRI volumes using deep learning. In: Ourselin, S., Joskowicz, L., Sabuncu, M.R., Unal, G., Wells, W. (eds.) MICCAI 2016. LNCS, vol. 9901, pp. 194–202. Springer, Cham (2016). doi:10.1007/978-3-319-46723-8_23
11. Štern, D., Urschler, M.: From individual hand bone age estimation to fully automated age estimation via learning-based information fusion. In: 2016 IEEE 13th International Symposium on Biomedical Imaging, pp. 150–154 (2016). doi:10.1109/ISBI.2016.7493232
12. Tanner, J.M., Whitehouse, R.H., Cameron, N., Marshall, W.A., Healy, M.J.R., Goldstein, H.: Assessment of Skeletal Maturity and Predicion of Adult Height (TW2 Method), 2nd edn. Academic Press, London (1983)
13. Thodberg, H.H., Kreiborg, S., Juul, A., Pedersen, K.D.: The BoneXpert method for automated determination of skeletal maturity. IEEE Trans. Med. Imaging **28**(1), 52–66 (2009)

Automatic Classification of Proximal Femur Fractures Based on Attention Models

Anees Kazi[1](✉), Shadi Albarqouni[1], Amelia Jimenez Sanchez[1],
Sonja Kirchhoff[2], Peter Biberthaler[1,3], Nassir Navab[1,4], and Diana Mateus[1]

[1] Computer Aided Medical Procedures,
Technische Universität München, Munich, Germany
anees.kazi@tum.de
[2] Institute of Clinical Radiology, Ludwig Maximilian University, Munich, Germany
[3] Department of Trauma Surgery, Klinikum Rechts der Isar,
Technische Universität München, Munich, Germany
[4] Whiting School of Engineering, Johns Hopkins University, Baltimore, USA

Abstract. We target the automatic classification of fractures from clinical X-Ray images following the Arbeitsgemeinschaft Osteosynthese (AO) classification standard. We decompose the problem into the localization of the region-of-interest (ROI) and the classification of the localized region. Our solution relies on current advances in multi-task end-to-end deep learning. More specifically, we adapt an attention model known as Spatial Transformer (ST) to learn an image-dependent localization of the ROI trained only from image classification labels. As a case study, we focus here on the classification of proximal femur fractures. We provide a detailed quantitative and qualitative validation on a dataset of 1000 images and report high accuracy with regard to inter-expert correlation values reported in the literature.

1 Introduction

In daily clinical routine fractures of the skeleton are classified based on X-ray imaging. fracture different treatment options follow the classification. For several bones concurrent fracture classification systems exist, e.g. for the proximal femur the Jensen or the system, regrouping fractures specified by characteristics such as general and relative location and number of fracture parts, among others (*cf.* Fig. 1). The AO classification system has been claimed to be more reproducible than other classification systems [8]. However, a recent study [4] revealed that even for this system, inter and intra-expert variability are still high, especially for less experienced physicians or when considering a more fine grained classification.

The problem of automatic fracture classification has gained interest only recently, both for pelvic and spinal Computed Tomography volumes [2,13], as well as for wrist and femur X-rays [1,3]. The focus has been on bottom-up approaches starting from the segmentation of the bone, achieved either with

© Springer International Publishing AG 2017
Q. Wang et al. (Eds.): MLMI 2017, LNCS 10541, pp. 70–78, 2017.
DOI: 10.1007/978-3-319-67389-9_9

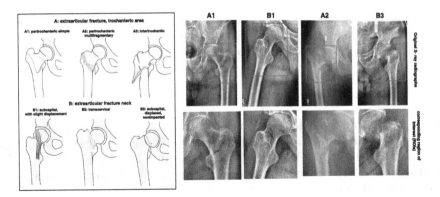

Fig. 1. (**left**) AO classification system for proximal femur fractures. (**right-top**) Example images with classification label. (**right-bottom**) Cropped regions of interest.

simple thresholding and region growing operations [2] or more sophisticated random forests algorithms [9], and sometimes also relying on prior statistical shape models [3,13]. Finally, the goal has been the classification into fracture/normal classes [3] or detection of the fracture lines [2,13].

This work aims at the classification of the X-Ray images of proximal femur according to the AO standard. The problem is very challenging due to the low SNR and great variability of the images. Furthermore, fracture lines have unpredictable shape, poor contrast and may resemble other structures in the image irrespective of the fracture class. To the best of our knowledge, only the work of Bayram *et al.* [1] has targeted the classification of the femur shaft fractures, which is similar but simpler to ours, as no clutter is present. Furthermore, the method relies on a prior segmentation of the bone, and the extraction of high-level features such as the number and area of fragments, prone to errors. Here instead, we model the problem in an end-to-end fashion by means of Convolutional neural networks (CNN), avoiding the need of prior-segmentations, feature design and fine detail annotations.

AO fracture classification depends upon the detailed information of the fracture lines only visible at high resolutions. For this reason, we model the problem in the framework of deep attention models [6,7], capable of finding a Region of Interest (ROI) from the image content. In particular, we rely on the recently introduced Spatial Transformer (ST) [7], which embeds within a classifier the unsupervised learning of a ROI-localization task. STN is a differentiable model to localize and crop a ROI that provides an elegant treatment of the gradient propagation from the classification towards the localization task.

We report results on a clinical dataset of ∼1000 X-ray images of proximal femurs. We discuss and evaluate different architecture configurations including our adaption of the Spatial Transformers, which allows for better convergence of the model. We also study the capability of the method to perform the classification of the images at different levels of the AO hierarchy. From the application perspective, our contribution is a CAD system with high classifications accuracies as compared to inter-expert correlations reported in the literature. From the technical point of view, this is to the best of our knowledge, the first study of deep attention techniques for the classification of medical images.

2   Method

We design a computer-aided tool for automatic classification of fractures from X-ray images. Our objective is to model a classifier that assigns a class label $y \in \{\text{normal}, A1, A2, A3, B1, B2, B3\}$ to an incoming X-ray image $\mathbf{I} \in \mathbb{R}^{H \times W}$. We decompose the problem into the localization of the ROI and the classification of the localized ROI.

The *localization task* $g(\cdot)$ estimates the ROI's spatial parameters $\mathbf{p}$ from the image content $\mathbf{I}$, that is,

$$\hat{\mathbf{p}} = g(\mathbf{I}; \omega_g),$$

where ω_g are the localization model parameters. In practice, $\mathbf{p} = \{t_r, t_c, s\}$ describes a bounding box of scale s centered at (t_r, t_c). Given $\mathbf{p}$, we define a warping function $\mathcal{W}_{\mathbf{p}}(\cdot)$ mapping the image content inside the ROI to a canonical grid $\mathcal{G}$ of size $H' \times W'$. Applying the warp to the input image $\mathbf{I}' = \mathcal{W}_{\mathbf{p}}(\mathbf{I})$ results in an image $\mathbf{I}' \in \mathbb{R}^{H' \times W'}$ of the cropped and resampled ROI.

The *classification* task $f(\cdot)$ takes as input the ROI $\mathbf{I}'$ and predicts a class:

$$\hat{y} = f(\mathbf{I}'; \omega_f),$$

where ω_f are the classification model parameters. Inspired by the recent success of Spatial Transformation Network (STN) [7], we propose a deep attention model that integrates both tasks within a single framework.

2.1   Attention Model

We model the supervised classification task $f(\mathbf{I}'; \omega_f)$ with a CNN to minimize the primary classification objective function, *i.e.* the cross entropy loss in our case. The localization function $g(\mathbf{I}; \omega_g)$ is also modeled with a CNN. Both model parameters ω_f and ω_g are learnt jointly to improve the classification task. However, we do not perform a supervised optimization of this regression task, but rather follow the principles of the STN [7] to link the localization and classification. Unlike max-pooling layers that seek to achieve spatial invariance, a STN implicitly looks for the ROI that improves the outcome of the classification task. More precisely, a STN regresses the optimal warping parameters $\mathbf{p}$ driven only from the classification loss, and thus, without the need of prior knowledge from bounding box annotations. In practice, the key component of a STN is the Spatial Transformer, a module defining the geometrical warping and resampling operations in $\mathcal{W}_{\mathbf{p}}$. The fact that these transformations have an analytical expression, enables the flow of the gradient updates from the classification to the localization network during a back-propagation stage.

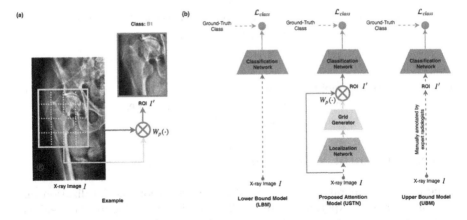

Fig. 2. Overview of the approach. **(a)** Localization of ST **(b)** Graphical representation of three models

We use the simplest form of the ST to act as our attention model, based on a similarity transformation $\mathcal{T}_{\mathbf{p}}$ and bilinear interpolation. The transformation $\mathcal{T}_{\mathbf{p}}$ defined by $\mathbf{p}$, allows for cropping, translation and isotropic scaling and is used to sample the locations of the ROI grid $\{x'_i, y'_i\}_{i=1}^{\text{gridSize}} \in \mathcal{G}$ from the original image (Fig. 2):

$$\begin{bmatrix} x_i \\ y_i \end{bmatrix} = \mathcal{T}_{\mathbf{p}} \left(\begin{bmatrix} x'_i \\ y'_i \end{bmatrix} \right) = \begin{bmatrix} s & 0 & t_r \\ 0 & s & t_c \end{bmatrix} \cdot \begin{bmatrix} x'_i \\ y'_i \end{bmatrix}$$

where x_i and y_i are the mapped locations of the grid in the input image $\mathbf{I}$. The intensity values to fill the ROI grid are finally obtained through the bilinear interpolation of the sampled locations:

$$\mathbf{I}'_i = \sum_r^H \sum_c^W \mathbf{I}_{r,c} \max(0, 1 - |x_i^s - r|) \max(0, 1 - |y_i^s - c|).$$

During training, the differentiation of these simple analytical relations allow to propagate the gradient from the classification task to a pixel of the ROI $\frac{\partial y}{\partial \mathbf{I}'_i}$, and backwards to the sampling locations $\frac{\partial \mathbf{I}'_i}{\partial x_i^s}, \frac{\partial \mathbf{I}'_i}{\partial y_i^s}$ and transformation parameters $\frac{\partial x_i^s}{\partial \mathbf{p}}, \frac{\partial y_i^s}{\partial \mathbf{p}}$, to finally reach the localization network through $\frac{\partial \mathbf{p}}{\partial \mathbf{I}_i}$.

Adapted Network Architecture. To deal with our challenging classification task, we replace the shallow localization and classification networks from [7] with the pre-trained Googlenet (inception v3) [11], which has been successfully validated for these particular tasks in medical applications [10]. For our data, training this architecture with the original ST module leads to unstable learning curves and a flat evolution of the objective function. When during the training the ROIs are pushed outside of the image, the learning is not able to recover. As for other medical applications, in our case it is sufficient to restrict the search space of the parameters to lie within the image rescaled to be inside -1 and 1, *i.e.* $-1 \leq t_r, t_c \leq 1$ and $0 \leq s \leq 1$. To this end we attach a differentiable sigmoid layer right after the localization network, such that:

$$t_r = 2 \cdot \sigma(t_r) - 1, \qquad t_c = 2 \cdot \sigma(t_c) - 1, \qquad s = \sigma(s),$$

where $\sigma(\cdot)$ is the sigmoid function. The saturation of the sigmoid for values outside the range, serves to cancel out the effect of outliers, and provides the means to improve the convergence.

3   Experimental Validation

We perform a comparative evaluation of the classification and localization task with three series of experiments. In the **first series**, we compare the results of classifying full images to manually annotated ROIs, without any attention model. The purpose is to set up the upper and lower bounds for our method. Here and for the other experiments, we evaluate three levels of discrimination: (i) fracture vs. normal detection, (ii) classification among 3 groups: normal, A and B, and (iii) classification among 6 subgroups: A1, A2, A3, B1, B2, B3. In the **second series** of experiments, we evaluate the integration of the multi-task components. In particular, we aim to show that the automatic location of the ROI places the classification performance between the upper and lower bounds of classification. Finally, our **third series** of experiments provides an independent evaluation of the localization component as well as a qualitative analysis of the proposed approach based on feature visualization. Next, we describe the details of our dataset and implementation, as well as the results for the different experiments.

Dataset collection and preparation. From the records of the trauma surgery department of the *Anonymous* clinic, we collected a total of 669 proximal femur X-ray images acquired mostly in an anterior/posterior (AP) view. The dataset includes a total of 584 patients. The images have a standard size of 2500×2048 and varying dynamic range and resolution.

AP images showing both femurs are tiled equally into two images each with one femur and part of pelvis adding one normal class to the dataset. After dividing the images, there is a total of 1221 images, from which we rejected 48 images with implants and artefacts. The resultant dataset was annotated by our clinical experts, who provided along with the image class also a bounding box of the femur head. We pre-process the images with histogram normalization. Furthermore, as the frequency of the cases remitted to the department, the class distribution for 6 classes is highly unbalanced, with as little as 15 cases for class A3, and as many as 187 and 193 for A2 and B2 respectively. For our experiments we balance the dataset through data augmentation based on rotation, flipping and scaling, leading to 195 images per class. To ensure the clinical value of our results, we train our models on 900 images and report performances on a completely separate test set of 270 images.

Implementation. The networks are implemented using MatConvNet [12]. For all the models the learning rate was set to decay logarithmically from 10^{-4} to

Table 1. Quantitative evaluation of the different set-ups, including 3 methods and different levels of hierarchical discrimination (2,3, and 6 classes).

LBM	2 Classes	3 Classes				6 Classes						
	Fract.	A	B	N	Avg.	A1	A2	A3	B1	B2	B3	Avg.
Accuracy	0.81	0.82	0.87	0.80	0.83	0.82	0.86	0.94	0.88	0.78	0.88	0.86
Precision	0.76	0.68	0.79	0.77	0.75	0.46	0.71	0.93	0.66	0.26	0.53	0.59
Recall	0.84	0.76	0.82	0.68	0.75	0.48	0.58	0.77	0.66	0.31	0.68	0.58
F1-score	0.80	0.72	0.81	0.72	0.75	0.47	0.64	0.84	0.66	0.28	0.60	0.58
USTN	**2 Classes**	**3 Classes**				**6 Classes**						
	Fract.	A	B	N	Avg.	A1	A2	A3	B1	B2	B3	Avg.
Accuracy	0.84	0.84	0.86	0.79	0.83	0.75	0.77	0.94	0.88	0.77	0.8	0.82
Precision	0.74	0.65	0.82	0.77	0.75	0.36	0.13	0.89	0.64	0.20	0.49	0.45
Recall	**0.93**	0.83	0.78	0.66	0.76	0.29	0.21	0.78	0.63	0.26	0.42	0.43
F1-score	0.82	0.73	0.80	0.71	0.75	0.32	0.16	0.83	0.64	0.23	0.45	0.44
UBM	**2 Classes**	**3 Classes**				**6 Classes**						
	Fract.	A	B	N	Avg.	A1	A2	A3	B1	B2	B3	Avg.
Accuracy	**0.88**	0.88	0.86	0.83	**0.86**	0.90	0.88	0.92	0.89	0.83	0.93	**0.89**
Precision	**0.91**	0.71	0.81	0.84	**0.79**	0.73	0.53	0.93	0.93	0.26	0.73	**0.68**
Recall	0.85	0.90	0.78	0.71	**0.80**	0.68	0.72	0.71	0.61	0.52	0.84	**0.68**
F1-score	**0.88**	0.80	0.79	0.77	**0.79**	0.70	0.61	0.80	0.74	0.35	0.78	**0.66**

10^{-5} during 60 epochs and then kept unchanged until epoch 80. The momentum was set to 0.9 and the batch size to 10. The training of our USTN network with backpropagation and stochastic gradient descent requires 3.5 h.

Quantitative evaluation. Here we compare the performance of three models. The lower bound (LBM) is given by the classification network fine-tuned to our dataset on full-images down-sampled to match the input size of the network 224×224. The upper bound (UBM), on the other hand, corresponds to the same network fine-tuned to perform classification directly on ROIs provided by the experts. The USTN corresponds to our adaption of the spatial transformer. The results are reported in the top and bottom rows of Table 1. As expected for the pure classification networks, the manual ROI localization of the UBM improves the accuracy of binary classification in 7%, and that of the 3- and 6-classes problems in 3%. There is also a significant improvement in precision and recall, reflected in increases of the F1-scores of 8% for the 2 and 6 classes and of 4% in the 3 classes. The mean accuracy values of at least 81% for the full-image and of 86% for the ROI-based approaches are meaningful in the light of the measured inter-expert correlation reported in [4] for the classes A1, A2 and A3 with Cohen's Kappa correlation values of 68% (71% for experts and 66% for residents). With the USTN, the performance scores of the binary classification

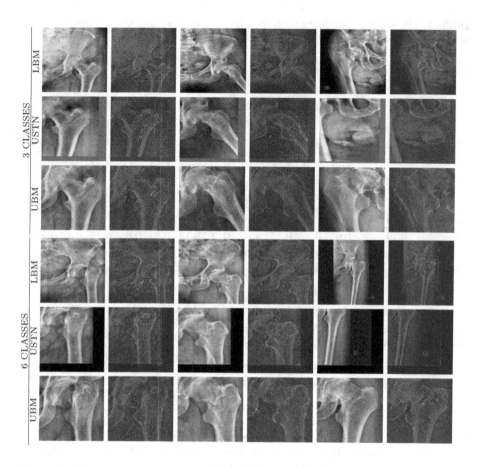

Fig. 3. Qualitative comparison with activation heatmaps for 3 and 6 class problem demonstrating the importance of implicit localization.

are close to those of UBM on ROI, and have the best recall overall. In accordance with the expert study, the performance scores decay for the more challenging discrimination among finer sub-categories (3/6 classes), approaching the LBM on full images. We also attribute that behavior to the high imbalance in the original distribution of the classes, which calls for larger amounts of preferably balanced data.

Localization results. We evaluated the performance of the localization block of our USTN, which has been trained unsupervised manner from the propagation of the classification loss, to the same localization block trained with the supervision of the ROIs provided by the experts. For 3 classes, the supervised localization has an RMSE error of 7.6 ± 4.8 pixels and a DICE coefficient of 0.4982 ± 0.0864, these values reflect the difficulty of the task, in particular for predicting the right scale. It is to be noted that the expert annotations for the femur head are difficult to standardise and therefore introduce additional variability to the regression target values. The scores drop respectively to 33.2 ± 14.16 and 0.4262 ± 0.0690 for end-to-end training of our USTN, as the lack of supervision makes the task even harder. Despite the lack of average precision, successful localization cases improve as expected the classification prediction.

Qualitative evaluation. Finally, we illustrate the performance of the three evaluated methods in Fig. 3. We have selected example images that are misclassified by the LBM on full images but correctly classified by the UBM applied to the expert provided ROIs. In the center row we have added the performance of the USTN, for cases where both classification and localization are correct (left column), cases where only the predictions for the localizations are correct (center column), and cases where both task fail. We use the visualization library in [5], which generates a heat-map of activations, by deconvolving activations back to the input space, to highlight the importance of good localization to the classification task.

4   Conclusion

We have presented a method to automatically classify fracture X-ray images of proximal femur from clinical records. The problem is formalized in a multitask manner, where localization and classification tasks are cascaded and trained end-to-end by means of a spatial transformer (ST). Our work sets the guidelines to use such attention models in order to solve complex medical image analysis to train in an end-to-end fashion. Performance values are good in the light of the known inter-expert correlation. Our proof-of-concept solution will be extended to the remaining long-bones of the body within an interactive setup that visualizes the activations and probabilities, and which allows to correct for possible errors in the localization step. Further the approach will be compared to method having localization and classification trained separately.

References

1. Bayram, F., Çakıroğlu, M.: Diffract: diaphyseal femur fracture classifier system. Biocybern. Biomed. Eng. **36**(1), 157–171 (2016)
2. Burns, J.E., Yao, J., Muñoz, H., Summers, R.M.: Automated detection, localization, and classification of traumatic vertebral body fractures in the thoracic and lumbar spine at CT. Radiology **278**(1), 64–73 (2016)
3. Ebsim, R., Naqvi, J., Cootes, T.: Detection of wrist fractures in X-ray images. In: Shekhar, R., Wesarg, S., González Ballester, M.Á., Drechsler, K., Sato, Y., Erdt, M., Linguraru, M.G., Oyarzun Laura, C. (eds.) CLIP 2016. LNCS, vol. 9958, pp. 1–8. Springer, Cham (2016). doi:10.1007/978-3-319-46472-5_1
4. van Embden, D., Rhemrev, S., Meylaerts, S., Roukema, G.: The comparison of two classifications for trochanteric femur fractures: the AO/ASIF classification and the jensen classification. Injury **41**(4), 377–381 (2010)

5. Grün, F., Christian Rupprecht, N.: A taxonomy and library for visualizing learned features in convolutional neural networks. In: ICML Visualization for Deep Learning Workshop (2016)
6. Girshick, R., Donahue, J., Darrell, T., Malik, J.: Rich feature hierarchies for accurate object detection and semantic segmentation. In: IEEE Computer Vision and Pattern Recognition (CVPR), pp. 580–587 (2014)
7. Jaderberg, M., Simonyan, K., Zisserman, A., Kavukcuoglu, K.: Spatial transformer networks. In: Neural Information Processig Systems (NIPS), pp. 2017–2025 (2015)
8. Jin, W.J., Dai, L.Y., Cui, Y.M., Zhou, Q., Jiang, L.S., Lu, H.: Reliability of classification systems for intertrochanteric fractures of the proximal femur in experienced orthopaedic surgeons. Injury **36**(7), 858–861 (2017)
9. Lindner, C., Thiagarajah, S., Wilkinson, J.M., arcOGEN Consortium, T., Wallis, G.A., Cootes, T.F.: Fully automatic segmentation of the proximal femur using random forest regression voting. IEEE TMI 32(8), 1462–1472 (2013)
10. Shin, H.C., Roth, H.R., Gao, M., Lu, L., Xu, Z., Nogues, I., Yao, J., Mollura, D., Summers, R.M.: Deep convolutional neural networks for computer-aided detection. IEEE TMI **35**(5), 1285–1298 (2016)
11. Szegedy, C., Liu, W., Jia, Y., Sermanet, P., Reed, S., Anguelov, D., Erhan, D., Vanhoucke, V., Rabinovich, A.: Going deeper with convolutions. In: IEEE Computer Vision and Pattern Recognition (CVPR) (2015)
12. Vedaldi, A., Lenc, K.: MatConvNet: Convolutional neural networks for matlab. In: Proceedings of the International Conference on Multimedia, pp. 689–692. ACM (2015)
13. Wu, J., Davuluri, P., Ward, K.R., Cockrell, C., Hobson, R., Najarian, K.: Fracture detection in traumatic pelvic CT images. J. Biomed. Imaging (2012)

Joint Supervoxel Classification Forest
for Weakly-Supervised Organ Segmentation

Fahdi Kanavati[1]([✉]), Kazunari Misawa[2], Michitaka Fujiwara[3], Kensaku Mori[4],
Daniel Rueckert[1], and Ben Glocker[1]

[1] Biomedical Image Analysis Group, Department of Computing,
Imperial College London, 180 Queen's Gate, London SW7 2AZ, UK
fk412@imperial.ac.uk
[2] Aichi Cancer Center, Nagoya 464-8681, Japan
[3] Nagoya University Hospital, Nagoya 466-0065, Japan
[4] Information and Communications, Nagoya University,
Furo-cho, Chikusa-ku, Nagoya 464-8603, Japan

Abstract. This article presents an efficient method for weakly-supervised organ segmentation. It consists in over-segmenting the images into object-like supervoxels. A single joint forest classifier is then trained on all the images, where (a) the supervoxel indices are used as labels for the voxels, (b) a joint node optimisation is done using training samples from all the images, and (c) in each leaf node, a distinct posterior distribution is stored per image. The result is a forest with a shared structure that efficiently encodes all the images in the dataset. The forest can be applied once on a given source image to obtain supervoxel label predictions for its voxels from all the other target images in the dataset by simply looking up the target's distribution in the leaf nodes. The output is then regularised using majority voting within the boundaries of the source's supervoxels. This yields sparse correspondences on an over-segmentation-based level in an unsupervised, efficient, and robust manner. Weak annotations can then be propagated to other images, extending the labelled set and allowing an organ label classification forest to be trained. We demonstrate the effectiveness of our approach on a dataset of 150 abdominal CT images where, starting from a small set of 10 images with scribbles, we perform weakly-supervised image segmentation of the kidneys, liver and spleen. Promising results are obtained.

1 Introduction

Large datasets of medical images are increasingly becoming available; however, only a small subset of images tend to be fully labelled due to the time-consuming task of providing manual segmentations. This is one of the main hurdles for conducting large scale medical image analysis. Recently, a method [3,11] using random classification forests to estimate correspondences between pairs of images

Electronic supplementary material The online version of this chapter (doi:10.
1007/978-3-319-67389-9_10) contains supplementary material, which is available to
authorized users.

© Springer International Publishing AG 2017
Q. Wang et al. (Eds.): MLMI 2017, LNCS 10541, pp. 79–87, 2017.
DOI: 10.1007/978-3-319-67389-9_10

at the level of compact supervoxels has been proposed. Given a pair of images, the method [11] consists in training a forest per image, applying it on the other image, and then extracting mutual correspondences. While the method is efficient if the application is restricted to a pair of images, it does not scale well when applied to a large dataset of images: obtaining correspondences between images in a dataset of n images would entail training n distinct forests and testing $n(n-1)$ forests. In this paper we similarly use random forests to estimate correspondences; however, we make modifications to make it applicable to a large dataset: (a) we use object-sized supervoxels instead of small compact supervoxels, (b) we train *one* shared forest for *all* the images instead of one forest per image. We do this by allowing the trees to share the same structure by performing joint optimisation at the nodes. All the images are thus encoded by the same forest structure, where each leaf node stores a distinct supervoxel label distribution per image. This method makes it possible to compute correspondences efficiently between all the image in a large dataset on a supervoxel-level by a simple look up process in the leaf nodes. The obtained correspondences can then be used to propagate semantic labels. We investigate using the proposed method in a weakly-supervised medical image segmentation setting on an abdominal CT dataset consisting of 150 images, starting only from 10 weakly-labelled images.

Related Work: In the computer vision community, there has been considerable research done in the domain of weakly supervised image segmentation [2,6,10], segmentation propagation [7,13], and co-segmentation [17], where the minimal assumption is that a common object is present in all of the images. Other form of weak annotations could be included such as bounding boxes, scribbles or tags indicating the presence of some object of interest. The main motivation behind these methods is the idea that a large dataset containing similar objects is bound to have repeating patterns and shapes, so they could potentially be exploited to discover and jointly segment the common objects. One issue when attempting to apply some of the methods to medical images is scalability, where the main bottleneck is obtaining correspondences between the images. Some state-of-the-art methods [13] rely on dense pixel-wise correspondences, which is infeasible to apply to a large dataset of 3D medical images. In an attempt to overcome such issues, other methods advocate using superpixels in an image as a building block in unsupervised and weakly supervised segmentation [7,14, 18], where feature descriptors are typically computed on a pixel-level and then aggregated within superpixels; however, descriptor choice is non-trivial and can still be computationally costly for 3D images depending on the type of features.

To investigate whether weak supervised segmentation can be performed efficiently on a large 3D medical dataset, we make use of random forests, which are one of the most popular supervised machine learning algorithms that have been used in medical image analysis [4,5,12,20]. Their popularity comes from their flexibility, efficiency, and scalability. The random forest framework makes it possible to do feature selection from a large pool of features. Additionally, random forest can scale up efficiently to large data, like 3D images, especially when simple cuboid feature, coupled with integral images, are used. Due to the nature of medical images, where anatomical structures follow certain patterns, context around voxels plays a role in improving classification [19]. Random forest with offset cuboid features can efficiently exploit context in an image to improve the prediction accuracy.

2 Method

The problem is similar to one in [11], except that instead of pairs of images, we extend it to multiple images. Given a set of images $\mathcal{I} = \{I_i\}_1^N$ and their set of associated supervoxels $\mathcal{R} = \{R_{ik}\}$, $k = 1\ldots|C^i|$, the aim is to establish correspondences between supervoxels across all images. We note $C^i = 1, \ldots, |C^i|$ as the index set of the supervoxels of image I_i.

2.1 Object-Sized Supervoxels

We over-segment each image into a set of supervoxels using a 3D extension of the efficient graph-based segmentation algorithm [8]; it takes in three parameters: k, min_size, and σ (Gaussian smoothing). For more details about the parameters, please refer to [8]. The number of supervoxels generated depends on the image. This algorithm allows obtaining segments that potentially represent different anatomical structures and organs; it has been used as a component of region proposal algorithms [16]. However, it is not possible to accurately segment each organ such that each organ is contained in one supervoxel. Over-segmentation and under-segmentation still occurs. Given two neighbouring voxels p ad q, we modify the weighting term used in the algorithm to

$$w(p, q) = \frac{|I(p) - I(q)|}{\max(10, S_\beta(p))} \times \sqrt{G(p) \times G(q)}, \qquad (1)$$

where $G(p)$ is the gradient magnitude obtained using the Sobel filter and helps in reducing the sensitivity to noise. $S_\beta(p)$ is a Gaussian filtered image, with smoothing parameter β, of the average of the absolute value of the gradient in the 3 directions; this term provides adaptive contrast normalisation. The proposed modification results in better looking supervoxels and reduces the impact of noise in CT images. In addition, during the post-processing step, we add an additional constraint where we only merge a pair of supervoxels if any of their sizes is less than min_size and their edge weight is less than m. Any remaining supervoxels that are smaller than min_size are excluded from the final output. Examples are shown in the Fig. 1 as well as in the supplementary material.

2.2 Joint Supervoxel Random Classification Forest

Due to lack of space, we directly describe the random forest framework as applied to our problem. A more extensive overview can be found at [4].

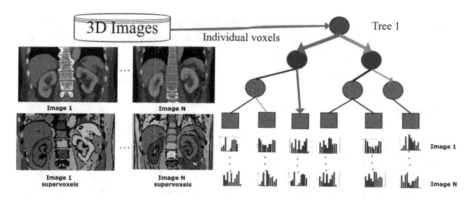

Fig. 1. An overview of the joint supervoxel forest. For illustration, only one tree is shown. Voxels from all the images in the dataset are used to train each tree. Each voxel has its supervoxel index as a label. At the nodes, we perform joint optimisation by maximising the sum of the information gain from all the images. At the leaf nodes, we store a distribution per image of the supervoxel indices, such that there could be up to N distributions stored at each leaf node. During testing, a voxel starts at the root node, and depending on its response to the binary split function at each node (circle), it is sent left or right until it reaches a leaf node (square). Once a voxel from a given image reaches a leaf node, it is possible to look up simultaneously its correspondences to all the other images.

We train a single forest on all images simultaneously such that all the images are encoded in that single forest. Figure 1 shows an overview of the proposed method, where only one tree is shown.

Node Optimisation: At each node, we perform joint optimisation of the feature selection, where the feature selected at each node is the one that maximises the sum of the total information gain from all the images.

$$IG(S) = \sum_i IG(S^i) \tag{2}$$

where $IG(S^i)$ is the information gain of the ith image with samples S^i, and

$$IG(S^i) = H(S^i) - \sum_{j=\{L,R\}} \frac{|S_j^i|}{|S^i|} H(S_j^i) \,, \tag{3}$$

where $H(S) = - \sum_{c \in C} p(c) \log p(c)$ is the Shannon entropy and $p(c)$ is the normalised empirical histogram of the labels of the training samples in S^i.

In addition, we randomly select, with ratio r_s, at each node, a subset of the images to perform node optimisation on. This allows speeding up the training process and increasing the randomisation between the trees.

Leaf Nodes: At each leaf node, we store the posterior distributions $p_i(c = l|\mathbf{v}), l \in C^i, i = 1 \dots n$ of the supervoxel labels for each one of the n images.

After training is done, the distributions for the *ith* image in the leaf nodes are computed by re-passing down *all* the image's voxels. We have found that this increases the accuracy of the correspondences, as the initial low sampling rate used during training is not enough to create an accurate distribution.

Appearance Features: Similarly to other methods, we use a set of context appearance features as they have been found to be quite effective and efficient [4, 9, 20] The features consist of local mean intensities and mean intensity differences between two different cuboid regions at different offsets, which are efficient to compute via the use of 3D integral images. The feature generation function $\psi(\mathbf{x}) : \mathbb{R}^3 \rightarrow \mathbb{R}$ takes as input the position $\mathbf{x}$ of the voxel and computes a feature value based on: a pair of offsets $(\Delta\mathbf{x}_0, \Delta\mathbf{x}_1) \in \mathbb{R}^3 \times \mathbb{R}^3$; a pair of size parameters $(\mathbf{s}_0, \mathbf{s}_1) \in \mathbb{R}^3 \times \mathbb{R}^3$, where a given $\mathbf{s}$ characterises the dimensions of a cuboid centred at position $\mathbf{u}$; $B_s(\mathbf{u})$ is the mean intensity of the voxels within the cuboid centred at $\mathbf{u}$ and of size $\mathbf{s}$; and $b \in \{0, 1\}$ is a binary value that indicates whether to take the intensity difference between two cuboids or only the value from a single cuboid. Let $\kappa = \{\mathbf{s}_0, \mathbf{s}_1, \Delta\mathbf{x}_0, \Delta\mathbf{x}_1, b\}$ denote the set of parameters. Given some choice of values for κ, the feature response for a voxel at $\mathbf{x}$ in image I is: $\psi_\kappa(\mathbf{x}) = B_{s_0}(\mathbf{x} + \Delta\mathbf{x}_0) + b \times B_{s_1}(\mathbf{x} + \Delta\mathbf{x}_1)$.

Once the feature response $\psi_\kappa(\mathbf{x})$ has been evaluated for all samples at a given node m, the optimal value for the threshold τ_m is obtained via a grid search.

Establishing Correspondences: Once the forest has been trained, correspondences between all the n images in the dataset can be obtained by applying the forest once on each image. Once a voxel $\mathbf{v}_i$ from image I_i reaches a leaf node of a tree t, it gets assigned a set of probabilities $\{p_j^t(c = l|\mathbf{v}_i) \mid l \in C^j\}_{j=1...n}$ for each one of the other images I_j in the dataset.

Correspondences on the supervoxel level are then obtained via majority voting, by aggregating all the probabilities of a supervoxel's voxels from all the trees and finding the labels that have maximum probabilities. So, given a supervoxel sv_k^i from image I_i, it gets assigned n labels $c_k^{ij}, j = 1 \ldots n$ obtained as follows:

$$c_k^{ij} = \arg\max_{c \in C^j} \sum_{t=1...T} \sum_{v \in sv_k^i} p_j^t(c|\mathbf{v}), \tag{4}$$

Mutual Correspondences: The correspondences are pruned such that a match $A \rightarrow B$ is considered valid only if there is also a match from $B \rightarrow A$. This helps in pruning out false correspondences. For each supervoxel A, we get a correspondence set M_A consisting of all the supervoxels from the other images that match with it. We expand the set of correspondences to neighbouring ones such that if we have a mutual correspondence between $A \leftrightarrow B$, and $B \leftrightarrow C$, then a correspondence between $A \leftrightarrow C$ is created. In addition, in each set M_A, we prune out the elements that do not mutually match with at least 50% of the other elements in M_A.

2.3   Weakly-Supervised Segmentation

Given a dataset where a subset has scribbles on organs, each object-sized super-voxel gets assigned the label of its organ scribble. We then use the obtained correspondences to propagate the organ labels, resulting in a larger subset of labelled images. Some images remain unlabelled, however, if they did not receive any correspondences. We therefore train another set of forests, one per organ; however, this time using the organs as labels and using the subset of images that have obtained a given organ label. Applying each organ label forest on *all* the images results in a probabilistic output as to whether a voxel is of a given organ or background. It is applied on all the images so as to potentially correct the initial over-segmentation errors and to segment the remaining unlabelled images. The probabilistic outputs (only probabilities larger than 0.85 are used) are fed in as the unary cost to graph-cut [1] so as to obtain regularised binary segmentation outputs. For each image, we then fuse the binary organ segmentations into a single image. The result is a fully-segmented dataset.

3   Experiments and Results

Dataset: We use an abdominal CT dataset consisting of 150 distinct subjects, which mostly contains pathological cases. The 3D scans have an in-plane resolution of 512×512; the number of slices is between 238 and 1061. Voxel sizes vary from 0.55 to 0.82; slice spacing ranges from 0.4 to 0.8 mm. Manual organ segmentations of the liver, spleen, kidneys, and pancreas are available.

Experimental Set-up: We generate dot scribbles on 10 randomly selected images, where each image receives 4 dot scribbles, representing the 4 organs. We repeat the experiment 10 times. Supervoxels are computed on images re-sampled to 2 mm, with $k = 80$, minimum size $3000 \, \text{mm}^3$, $\sigma = 0.5 \, \text{mm}$, $\beta = 5 \, \text{mm}$, and $m = 50$ (all set empirically). For the joint forest, images are re-sampled to 6 mm; we train 20 trees, with a max depth of 14, max offset (in native resolution) of 200 mm, cuboid sizes up to 32 mm, 15 features/node, a grid search with 10 bins, min number of samples 5, $r_s = 50\%$ and a sampling rate of 1%. Node growing during training stops when the maximum depth is reached, the number of samples is less than 5, or there is no entropy improvement. For the organ forest, we use similar parameters, except that we increase the re-sampling to 3 mm, the features/node to 100, and the sampling rate to 5%. Graph-cut is applied using the pairwise Potts model on images of 2 mm spacing, with $\lambda = 4$.

Results: From an initial set of 10 weakly organ labelled images (with dot scribbles), the number of images that received an organ supervoxel label via the correspondences were on average: 101, 110, 144, and 121 for the right kidney, left kidney, liver, and spleen, respectively. We report the dice overlap of the final segmentation output with graph-cut applied on all the 150 images. For each image, the dice overlap was averaged from the 10 random runs; box plots of those averages are reported in Fig. 2, where we see that apart from the pancreas

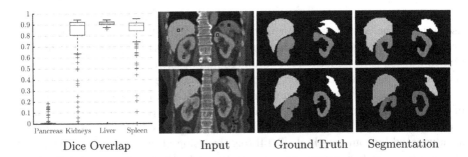

Dice Overlap   Input   Ground Truth   Segmentation

Fig. 2. Left: Final dice overlap score computed for the 150 images in the dataset at a 2 mm spacing. We see that apart from a few outliers cases for the kidneys, liver and spleen, we get an overall median dice of 0.9 for all three organs. Poor results were obtained for the pancreas. Right: Image on the top left had organ scribbles (square dots), which were then assigned to its supervoxels (coloured overlay correspond to the supervoxels that were assigned an organ label. Full supervoxels are shown in Fig. 1). The bottom left image was unlabelled and did not have any organ scribbles; however, it received a liver and spleen label for its supervoxels via the joint forest correspondences. The right column shows the segmentation output after applying the organ forest and graph-cut. We see that the bottom image gets segmentations for the kidneys. (Color figure online)

and a few outlier cases for the kidneys, liver, and spleen, we get good segmentation accuracy with extremely minimal user input. The reader is advised to refer to the supplementary material for more visual results from each step of the pipeline.

4   Discussion and Conclusion

In this paper, we have presented an efficient method for weakly-supervised organ segmentation. The method consisted in over-segmenting the images into object-sized supervoxels and training a single shared forest using all the images via joint node optimisation. The joint forest was then used to efficiently estimate correspondences between supervoxels in an abdominal CT dataset. These correspondences were used to propagate weak organ labels from a small set of 10 images to 140 unlabelled images. A second forest was then trained using organ labels on a supervoxel level. The organ forest was applied on all the images so as to correct potential inaccuracies in the over-segmentation and to segment any remaining unlabelled image. The probabilistic output from the forest was then used as the unary cost for graph-cut to regularise the output. Apart from poor results for the pancreas, which is difficult to segment due to its extremely deformable nature, the liver, kidney and spleen obtain good segmentation results, excluding a few outlier cases (a fully-supervised method [15] applied on the same dataset obtains a dice overlap of 94.9%, 93.6%, and 92.5% for liver, kidneys, and spleen, respectively). Our method could potentially be used to provide coarse segmentation or mine a large dataset of medical images, with extremely minimal user input. The advantage of our method is that it is efficient, as images can be greatly down-sampled and the random forest framework is easily parallelisable. One limitation is that method is not able to handle extremely deformable organs, such as the pancreas. Another limitation is that the initial supervoxel over-segmentation parameters were determined empirically; however, the availability of a small subset of fully-labelled images could help in determining the parameters. An alternative would be generating multiple over-segmentations per image, as advocated by some methods [7,14] (e.g. by using object proposals). We could then train a joint forest per over-segmentation set. The output from the multiple joint forests could then be used as an ensemble. Future work would involve investigating this, as well as investigating the use of alternative supervised algorithm (e.g. convolutional network), alternative image features to attempt to segment the pancreas and a more integrated interactive user input, which could help in correcting outliers and speeding up the interactive segmentation process.

References

1. Boykov, Y.Y., Jolly, M.M.P.: Interactive graph cuts for optimal boundary & region segmentation of objects in ND images. In: ICCV 2001, vol. 1, pp. 105–112 (2001)
2. Chen, X., Shrivastava, A., Gupta, A.: Enriching visual knowledge bases via object discovery and segmentation. In: Proceedings of the IEEE conference on CVPR, pp. 2027–2034 (2014)
3. Conze, P.H., Tilquin, F., Noblet, V., Rousseau, F., Heitz, F., Pessaux, P.: Hierarchical multi-scale supervoxel matching using random forests for automatic semi-dense abdominal image registration. In: IEEE ISBI (2017)
4. Criminisi, A., Shotton, J.: Decision Forests for Computer Vision and Medical Image Analysis. Springer, London (2013). doi:10.1007/978-1-4471-4929-3
5. Criminisi, A., Shotton, J., Robertson, D., Konukoglu, E.: Regression forests for efficient anatomy detection and localization in CT studies. In: Menze, B., Langs, G., Tu, Z., Criminisi, A. (eds.) MCV 2010. LNCS, vol. 6533, pp. 106–117. Springer, Heidelberg (2011). doi:10.1007/978-3-642-18421-5_11
6. Deselaers, T., Alexe, B., Ferrari, V.: Weakly supervised localization and learning with generic knowledge. IJCV 100(3), 275–293 (2012)
7. Dutt Jain, S., Grauman, K.: Active image segmentation propagation. In: Proceedings of the IEEE Conference on CVPR, pp. 2864–2873 (2016)
8. Felzenszwalb, P., Huttenlocher, D.: Efficient graph-based image segmentation. IJCV 59, 167–181 (2004)
9. Glocker, B., Zikic, D., Haynor, D.R.: Robust registration of longitudinal spine CT. In: Golland, P., Hata, N., Barillot, C., Hornegger, J., Howe, R. (eds.) MICCAI 2014. LNCS, vol. 8673, pp. 251–258. Springer, Cham (2014). doi:10.1007/978-3-319-10404-1_32
10. Grauman, K., Darrell, T.: Unsupervised learning of categories from sets of partially matching image features. In: 2006 IEEE Computer Society Conference on CVPR, vol. 1, pp. 19–25. IEEE (2006)
11. Kanavati, F., Tong, T., Misawa, K., Fujiwara, M., Mori, K., Rueckert, D., Glocker, B.: Supervoxel classification forests for estimating pairwise image correspondences. Pattern Recogn. 63, 561–569 (2017)

12. Montillo, A., Shotton, J., Winn, J., Iglesias, J.E., Metaxas, D., Criminisi, A.: Entangled decision forests and their application for semantic segmentation of CT images. In: Székely, G., Hahn, H.K. (eds.) IPMI 2011. LNCS, vol. 6801, pp. 184–196. Springer, Heidelberg (2011). doi:10.1007/978-3-642-22092-0_16

13. Rubinstein, M., Liu, C., Freeman, W.T.: Joint inference in weakly-annotated image datasets via dense correspondence. IJCV 119(1), 23–45 (2016)

14. Russell, B.C., Efros, A.A., Sivic, J., Freeman, W.T., Zisserman, A.: Using multiple segmentations to discover objects and their extent in image collections. In: Proceedings of the IEEE Computer Society Conference on CVPR, vol. 2, pp. 1605–1612 (2006)

15. Tong, T., Wolz, R., Wang, Z., Gao, Q., Misawa, K., Fujiwara, M., Mori, K., Hajnal, J.V., Rueckert, D.: Discriminative dictionary learning for abdominal multi-organ segmentation. Med. Image Anal. 23(1), 92–104 (2015)

16. Uijlings, J.R., Van De Sande, K.E., Gevers, T., Smeulders, A.W.: Selective search for object recognition. IJCV 104(2), 154–171 (2013)

17. Vicente, S., Rother, C., Kolmogorov, V.: Object cosegmentation. In: 2011 IEEE Conference on CVPR, pp. 2217–2224. IEEE (2011)

18. Xu, J., Schwing, A.G., Urtasun, R.: Learning to segment under various forms of weak supervision. In: Proceedings of the IEEE Conference on Computer Vision and Pattern Recognition, pp. 3781–3790 (2015)

19. Zhou, S.: Introduction to medical image recognition, segmentation, and parsing, Chap. 1. In: Zhou, S.K. (ed.) Medical Image Recognition, Segmentation and Parsing, pp. 1–21. Academic Press, New York (2016)

20. Zikic, D., Glocker, B., Criminisi, A.: Encoding atlases by randomized classification forests for efficient multi-atlas label propagation. Med. Image Anal. 18, 1262–1273 (2014)

Accurate and Consistent Hippocampus Segmentation Through Convolutional LSTM and View Ensemble

Yani Chen[1], Bibo Shi[2], Zhewei Wang[1], Tao Sun[1], Charles D. Smith[3], and Jundong Liu[1(✉)]

[1] School of Electrical Engineering and Computer Science,
Ohio University, Athens, USA
`liuj1@ohio.edu`
[2] Department of Radiology, Duke University, Durham, USA
[3] Department of Neurology, University of Kentucky, Lexington, USA

Abstract. In this work, a novel deep neural network is developed to automatically segment human hippocampi from MR images. To take advantage of the efficiency of 2D convolutional operations, as well the inter-slice dependence within 3D volumes, our model stacks fully convolutional neural networks (CNN) through convolutional long short-term memory (CLSTM) to extract voxel labels. Enhanced slice-wise label consistency is ensured, leading to improved segmentation stability and accuracy. We apply our model on ADNI dataset, and demonstrate that our proposed model outperforms the state-of-the-art solutions.

Keywords: Hippocampus segmentation · Brain · MRI · CNN · LSTM

1 Introduction

The human hippocampus plays a crucial role in memory formation, and it is also one of the first brain structures to suffer tissue damage in Alzheimer's Disease [6]. Accurate segmentation of hippocampus from MR images provides a quantitative foundation for many other analyses, and therefore has long been an important task in neuro-image research. Traditional solutions for automatic hippocampus segmentation include atlas-based [8] and patch-based methods [5,11,13,14], where the common practice is to identify certain similarity between the target image and anatomical atlases, at the entire structure or certain patch level, to infer the labels for individual voxels.

In recent years, deep learning models, especially convolutional neural networks (CNNs), have emerged as a new and more powerful paradigm for automatic segmentation of brain structures, including the hippocampus. The most well-known CNN architecture, in medical image analysis, is arguably the U-Net [10], designed to segment two-dimensional (2D) microscopy images. Following the similar idea of fully convolutional networks (FCN) [7], U-Net uses skip connections to concatenate features from the contracting (convolution) and expanding (deconvolution) paths.

© Springer International Publishing AG 2017
Q. Wang et al. (Eds.): MLMI 2017, LNCS 10541, pp. 88–96, 2017.
DOI: 10.1007/978-3-319-67389-9_11

Segmentation of three-dimensional (3D) structures such as hippocampi can be performed on sequences of 2D slices or directly on 3D volumes. The former is carried out by repeatedly applying a 2D model, e.g., a U-Net-like-NN, on individual slices and later stacking the obtained segmentations together. Such approaches omit the contextual information along the perpendicular axis, easily resulting in inconsistent and non-smooth segmentation surfaces. In this regard, 3D models would be more desired as they can capture all the spatial contexts naturally. However, this benefit comes with a cost, especially for CNNs. Comparing with 2D convolutions on planar patches, 3D convolutions on volumes, as in 3D U-Net [4], are computationally more expensive. 3D CNNs also commonly have more parameters to tune, but with much fewer training samples. As an alternative, combining 2D slice-based decisions from multiple views would make a compromise solution that can well incorporate 3D information while keep the system as a light 2D NN. Within each individual view, however, the inconsistency issue remains and cannot be directly resolved by view ensemble. Recurrent Neural Networks (RNN) for image segmentation models [2,9,12,15], while not originally designed for reducing inter-slice inconsistency, can actually be utilized to provide a remedy for this issue.

In this paper, we propose a long short-term memory (LSTM) + CNN + multiview solution to improve both the accuracy and slice-wise consistency in hippocampus segmentation. We use a modified U-Net, which we call U-Seg-Net, to accommodate to our data and application, and use LSTM to propagate the features generated from the middle-layers of U-Seg-Net. This setup allows the most essential features of each slice to be shared and spread along the slice sequence. At the end, we use three-view ensemble to supplement the individual segmentations with 3D neighborhood information.

2 Method

Our proposed segmentation model, as shown in Fig. 1, is based on the hardwiring of two major components, a 2D slice based segmentation network – U-Seg-Net, and a sequence learning network – convolutional long short-term memory (CLSTM).

U-Seg-Net. Similar to the original U-Net, our U-Seg-Net also utilizes the encoding, decoding and bridge architecture, as shown in Fig. 2. Several modifications were made on U-Net to better suit our data and task. First, we use padded convolution to maintain the spatial dimension of the feature maps, which is different from the unpadded convolutions in U-Net. Second, for the two convolution layers prior to each pooling/deconvolutional layer in U-Net, we remove one of them to reduce the number of parameters. Third, dropout operations are added in several places of the decoding path to prevent overfitting and enhance the system robustness. In addition, as our segmentation outputs are binary masks, we use only one 3×3 filter in the last convolution layer to generate a single channel of feature map. This feature map is later fed into a logistic function to produce the segmentation probability map for the current 2D slice. Detailed setting of each

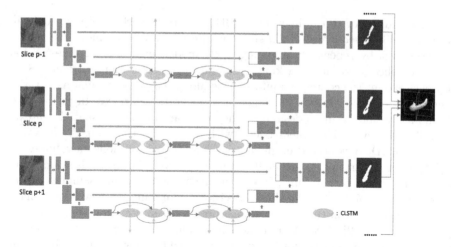

Fig. 1. The overall architecture of our proposed model: U-Seg-Net + CLSTM.

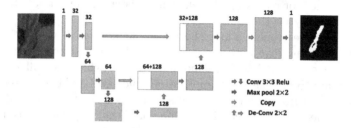

Fig. 2. The architecture of our slice-wise CNN model: U-Seg-Net

layer is shown in Fig. 2. There are totally $1,141,825$ parameters in the U-Seg-Net model.

2.1   U-Seg-Net + CLSTM

With U-Seg-Net in place for 2D slice segmentation, the next task is to capture the 3D contextual information among neighboring slices via sequence learning. To this end, we utilize LSTM to process sequential feature maps $x_1, x_2, ..., x_n$, generated from our 2D U-Seg-Net.

The original LSTMs use full connections in input-to-state and state-to-state transitions, which makes spatial locations irrelevant. Convolutional LSTM (CLSTM) [16] extends the conventional LSTM by replacing the multiplication operations in LSTM with convolutions, as in CNN. This modification enables CLSTM to maintain and propagate spatial information along the recurrent structure. Being able to encode spatial contexts makes CLSTM suitable to handle 2D or high dimensional spatio-temporal data. The replacement of full connection with convolutional operations also reduces the number of model parameters in LSTM. Detailed formulation of CLSTM can be found in [16].

Combining CLSTM with U-Seg-Net can be rather straightforward. In practice, the recurrent connections can be inserted at different positions of the U-Seg-Net. More specifically, it can be applied on the sequence of feature maps (a) in the beginning of encoding path of the U-Seg-Net, (b) in the end of decoding path, or (c) between the encoding and decoding paths. In this work, we choose (c), and take the middle layer feature maps as the most essential semantic information to share and spread among 2D slices. In some experiments we conducted, we also found this approach outperformed the setups in (a) and (b).

The combined U-Seg-Net + CLSTM architecture is shown in Fig. 1. For a 3D volume of n slices along certain axis, n weight-sharing U-Seg-Nets are applied to process the 2D slices independently, following the encoding pathway, to extract high level latent features. At the bottom of encoding part, the inter-slice information residing

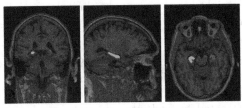

Fig. 3. Sagittal, coronal and axial views of hippocampi in an MRI scan.

in the extracted n feature maps is processed by two layers of bi-directional CLSTMs. As shown in Fig. 1, the sequence of feature maps from the encoding path of n U-Seg-Nets are fed into the first layer bi-directional CLSTM (two CLSTMs in opposite directions). The outputs of these two CLSTMs at the corresponding neurons are concatenated as the input to the second layer bi-directional CLSTM. This two-layer design is intended to construct a deep structure for bi-directional CLSTMs to better catch the 3D contextual information. With the spatial neighborhood information integrated and conveyed along the two CLSTMs, the decoding paths of n U-Seg-Nets will be carried on independently to reconstruct the final segmentations following the "deconvolution/upsampling" layers. There are totally $2,912,321$ parameters in the U-Seg-Net + CLSTM model.

View Ensemble. The proposed U-Seg-Net + CLSTM model can be trained and applied to perform 3D segmentation along different anatomical planes. As demonstrated by several studies [3], aggregating 3D probability maps generated independently from different views indeed can produce a combined segmentation that is more accurate than all individual contributors. Some structure boundaries that are very vague in one view may be much clearly separable in other view(s). In this work, we train three proposed models for sagittal, coronal, and axial views respectively, and then combine their segmentation probability maps through majority voting to generate an overall segmentation. Figure 3 illustrates the orientations and geometries of the left and right hippocampi in an MRI scan, viewing from sagittal, coronal and axial planes.

3   Implementation Details

The data used in this work were obtained from the ADNI database. We utilized 110 normal control subjects, and downloaded their baseline T1-weighted whole brain MRI images along with their hippocampus masks. To facilitate our analysis, instead of using the whole brain area as the input, we roughly cropped the left and right hippocampus of each subject for segmentation. The size of the cropping box for the left hippocampus is $24 \times 48 \times 40$, and $24 \times 56 \times 48$ for the right hippocampus. In clinical practice, this manual step can and should be replaced by an automatic atlas-based segmentation, rather easily.

Training and Testing. We evaluated our proposed model with 10-fold cross validation, specifically, with 99 subjects used for training and 11 subjects for testing in each fold. For each cropped hippocampus 3D array of training subjects, three sets of 2D image slices along sagittal, coronal, and axial view were firstly extracted to feed into and train our U-Seg-Net + CLSTM model, respectively. Then, the outputs of three sets of 3D probability maps were combined using majority voting. Note that we conducted the training and testing procedure independently for left and right hippocampus.

Optimization. The whole network, U-Seg-Net + CLSTM are trained end-to-end using a two-step fine-tuning method [1]. We first trained 2D U-Seg-Net alone separately for each view. This will not only provide a good starting point for training the combined U-Seg-Net + CLSTM model, but also serve as a baseline competing method in experiments. For 2D U-Seg-Net, we ran 50 training epochs on an Nvidia GTX 1080 GPU, which took approximately 1 h for each view. We set momentum as 0.99, weight decay as 10^{-9} and learning rate as 10^{-3} for the SGD optimizer. The batch size was set to 2, and we reduced the learning rate after 40 epochs by a factor 0.1. For the U-Seg-Net+ CLSTM model, we first fixed the parameters for U-Seg-Net part initialized by the previous step, and only updated the parameters for CLSTM part. We ran this step for 500 epochs with the same setting for optimization hyper parameters. Then, all weights of the whole network were jointly trained for another 500 epochs with learning rate decreased to 10^{-5}. The sequence length is set to the 3-rd dimension of subjects from each view.

4   Experimental Results

In this section, we present and evaluate the experimental results for the proposed model. Three different performance metrics, 3D Dice ratio, Hausdorff distance and 2D slice-wise Dice ratio, were used to measure the performance (accuracy and consistency) of the segmentation models. The 3D Dice ratio and Hausdorff distance were calculated subject-wise for each view and their combinations. Mean and standard deviation averaged from 10 folds are reported. The 2D slice based Dice ratio was calculated slice by slice, and the mean and standard deviation were averaged from all test subjects' slices along three views.

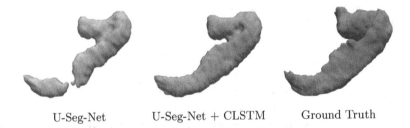

U-Seg-Net   U-Seg-Net + CLSTM   Ground Truth

Fig. 4. Surface rendering of segmentation results of U-Seg-Net, U-Seg-Net + CLSTM and ground truth of one case from the axial view. (The Dice ratio for the obtained segmentations are 72.26% and 80.87%). Please refer to text for details.

Table 1. Means and standard deviations of subject Dice ratios (%) for the hippocampus segmentation results using U-Seg-Net and U-Seg-Net + CLSTM.

		Sagittal	Coronal	Axial	Ensemble
Left	U-Seg-Net	87.44 ± 1.76	88.15 ± 1.72	85.87 ± 2.55	89.10 ± 1.59
	U-Seg-Net + CLSTM	**87.69 ± 1.76**	**88.30 ± 1.73**	**86.84 ± 2.84**	**89.21 ± 1.68**
Right	U-Seg-Net	**87.69 ± 1.42**	87.93 ± 1.92	86.23 ± 2.19	89.21 ± 1.40
	U-Seg-Net + CLSTM	87.59 ± 1.43	**88.05 ± 1.85**	**87.48 ± 1.99**	**89.37 ± 1.46**

First, we analyze the effect of utilizing CLSTM to catch inter-slice contextual information. We compared the segmentation results of the proposed U-Seg-Net + CLSTM model with U-Seg-Net based on 3D Dice ratios, and the results are shown in Table 1. For 2D U-Seg-Nets, the segmentation results on axial views are least accurate, and the results along the sagittal and coronal views are significantly better. Combing 3 views via majority voting generates the most accurate results, which confirms that multi-view combination does compensate the information lost in single view segmentation. Utilizing the two CLSTMs, the proposed U-Seg-Net + CLSTM produced better segmentations for coronal and axial views, and also led to an improvement in the overall combination. For the axial view in particular, the improvements are significant. To visualize the effect of the added CLSTM, we plotted the segmentation of axial view for one of the subjects, and show the results of U-Seg-Net, U-Seg-Net + CLSTM, together with the ground truth, in Fig. 4. It can be observed that the breakage in the middle of hippocampus segmentation using U-Seg-Net no longer exists in that of the U-Seg-Net + CLSTM model, indicating our goal of utilizing CLSTM to convey inter-slice information for better coherence is achieved. Meanwhile, we also noticed that the improvements for the sagittal, coronal views and the final combination are not as significant as for the axial view. We believe this is in great part due to the noise existing in the ground truth segmentations, and there may be very little room for improvement along these two views.

Second, we look into details to inspect if hardwiring U-Seg-Net and CLSTM would indeed lead to smoother and more consistent segmentations. We utilized

Table 2. Means and standard deviations of Hausdorff distances for the hippocampus segmentation results by U-Seg-Net and U-Seg-Net + CLSTM.

		Sagittal	Coronal	Axial	Ensemble
Left	U-Seg-Net	3.08 ± 0.78	3.05 ± 0.60	3.10 ± 0.48	2.32 ± 0.26
	U-Seg-Net + CLSTM	$\mathbf{2.71 \pm 0.54}$	$\mathbf{2.72 \pm 0.59}$	$\mathbf{2.41 \pm 0.30}$	$\mathbf{2.24 \pm 0.28}$
Right	U-Seg-Net	2.69 ± 0.30	3.35 ± 1.36	3.39 ± 0.89	2.26 ± 0.17
	U-Seg-Net + CLSTM	$\mathbf{2.56 \pm 0.30}$	$\mathbf{2.81 \pm 0.96}$	$\mathbf{2.72 \pm 0.73}$	$\mathbf{2.19 \pm 0.22}$

two other measurements, Hausdorff distance and 2D Dice ratio, to compare the segmentation results. The Hausdorff distances between produced segmentations and the ground truth are presented in Table 2. Compared with U-Seg-Net, the proposed U-Seg-Net + CLSTM model achieves smaller average and variances, in all 3 single views. Small Hausdorff distances indicate the obtained segmentations have no major deviation from the ground truth, which can be regarded as an indirect indicator of good stability and consistency of our model. To further investigate the smoothness property, we calculated 2D slice-wise Dice ratios between slice segmentations and the ground truth, with the consideration that segmentation smoothness can be reflected by the variance of 2D Dice ratios. The results are summarized in Table 3. As expected, our model yields higher means (more accurate) and smaller standard deviations (more stable) of slice-wise Dice ratios than U-Seg-Net.

Table 3. Means and standard deviations of slice-wise Dice ratios (%) in three views U-Seg-Net and U-Seg-Net + CLSTM.

		Sagittal	Coronal	Axial
Left	U-Seg-Net	81.36 ± 16.01	87.34 ± 10.56	83.71 ± 12.91
	U-Seg-Net + CLSTM	$\mathbf{81.88 \pm 15.62}$	$\mathbf{87.48 \pm 10.32}$	$\mathbf{84.54 \pm 12.11}$
Right	U-Seg-Net	81.62 ± 15.54	87.19 ± 10.23	83.89 ± 13.39
	U-Seg-Net + CLSTM	$\mathbf{81.64 \pm 15.36}$	$\mathbf{87.23 \pm 10.18}$	$\mathbf{84.96 \pm 12.25}$

In the end, we compared the performance of our proposed model with several recent works [5,8,11,13,14] that have also focused on hippocampus segmentation. As the studies were conducted and reported based on different datasets, subjects, ground truth setup and evaluation metrics, we do not intend to make a direct head-to-head quantitative comparison among these methods. The best overall (average) performance from Table 4 still could be used as a side evidence for the effectiveness of our proposed model.

Table 4. Comparison of the proposed method with other state-of-the-art methods on hippocampus segmentation (in 3D Dice ratios (%)).

.....	Method	Left	Right	Average
Morra *et al.* [8]	Ada-SVM	81.40	82.20	81.80
Coupe *et al.* [5]	Nonlocal patch-based	——	——	88.40
Tong *et al.* [13]	DDLS	87.20 (median)	87.20 (median)	87.20
Wu *et al.* [14]	Hierarchical multi-atlas	——	——	88.50
Song *et al.* [11]	Progressive SPBL	88.20	88.50	88.35
Our method	U-Seg-Net + CLSTM	**89.21**	**89.37**	**89.29**

5 Conclusion

In this work, we proposed an end-to-end trainable automatic hippocampus segmentation network based on the hardwiring of CNN and RNN models. More specifically, we integrate U-Seg-Net and CLSTM together to restore 3D contextual information back to the 2D CNN model. Our experimental results show that, without significant increase in the complexity (trainable parameters), the proposed model indeed achieves our design goals. With very high accuracy and consistency, our model provides a new and very competitive solution for hippocampus segmentation.

References

1. Branson, S., et al.: Bird species categorization using pose normalized deep convolutional nets. arXiv preprint arXiv:1406.2952 (2014)
2. Chen, J., et al.: Combining fully convolutional and recurrent neural networks for 3d biomedical image segmentation. In: NIPS 2016, pp. 3036–3044 (2016)
3. Chen, Y., et al.: Hippocampus segmentation through multi-view ensemble ConvNets. In: ISBI 2017, pp. 192–196 (2017)
4. Çiçek, Ö., Abdulkadir, A., Lienkamp, S.S., Brox, T., Ronneberger, O.: 3D U-Net: learning dense volumetric segmentation from sparse annotation. In: Ourselin, S., Joskowicz, L., Sabuncu, M.R., Unal, G., Wells, W. (eds.) MICCAI 2016. LNCS, vol. 9901, pp. 424–432. Springer, Cham (2016). doi:10.1007/978-3-319-46723-8_49
5. Coupé, P., et al.: Patch-based segmentation using expert priors: application to hippocampus and ventricle segmentation. NeuroImage **54**(2), 940–954 (2011)
6. Hobbs, K.H., et al.: Quad-mesh based radial distance biomarkers for Alzheimer's disease. In: ISBI 2016, pp. 19–23. IEEE (2016)
7. Long, J., et al.: Fully convolutional networks for semantic segmentation. In: CVPR 2015, pp. 3431–3440 (2015)
8. Morra, J.H., et al.: Comparison of AdaBoost and support vector machines for detecting Alzheimer's disease through automated hippocampal segmentation. IEEE TMI **29**(1), 30 (2010)
9. Poudel, R.P., et al.: Recurrent fully convolutional neural networks for multi-slice MRI cardiac segmentation. arXiv preprint arXiv:1608.03974 (2016)

10. Ronneberger, O., Fischer, P., Brox, T.: U-Net: convolutional networks for biomedical image segmentation. In: Navab, N., Hornegger, J., Wells, W.M., Frangi, A.F. (eds.) MICCAI 2015. LNCS, vol. 9351, pp. 234–241. Springer, Cham (2015). doi:10.1007/978-3-319-24574-4_28

11. Song, Y., Wu, G., Sun, Q., Bahrami, K., Li, C., Shen, D.: Progressive label fusion framework for multi-atlas segmentation by dictionary evolution. In: Navab, N., Hornegger, J., Wells, W.M., Frangi, A.F. (eds.) MICCAI 2015. LNCS, vol. 9351, pp. 190–197. Springer, Cham (2015). doi:10.1007/978-3-319-24574-4_23

12. Stollenga, M.F., et al.: Parallel multi-dimensional LSTM, with application to fast biomedical volumetric image segmentation. In: NIPS 2015, pp. 2998–3006 (2015)

13. Tong, T., et al.: Segmentation of MR images via discriminative dictionary learning and sparse coding: application to hippocampus labeling. NeuroImage **76**, 11–23 (2013)

14. Wu, G., et al.: Hierarchical multi-atlas label fusion with multi-scale feature representation and label-specific patch partition. NeuroImage **106**, 34–46 (2015)

15. Xie, Y., Zhang, Z., Sapkota, M., Yang, L.: Spatial clockwork recurrent neural network for muscle perimysium segmentation. In: Ourselin, S., Joskowicz, L., Sabuncu, M.R., Unal, G., Wells, W. (eds.) MICCAI 2016. LNCS, vol. 9901, pp. 185–193. Springer, Cham (2016). doi:10.1007/978-3-319-46723-8_22

16. Xingjian, S., et al.: Convolutional LSTM network: a machine learning approach for precipitation nowcasting. In: NIPS 2015, pp. 802–810 (2015)

STAR: Spatio-Temporal Architecture for Super-Resolution in Low-Dose CT Perfusion

Yao Xiao[1], Ajay Gupta[2], Pina C. Sanelli[3], and Ruogu Fang[1(✉)]

[1] University of Florida, Gainesville, FL, USA
Ruogu.Fang@bme.ufl.edu
[2] Weill Cornell Medical College, New York, NY, USA
[3] Northwell Health, Manhasset, NY, USA

Abstract. Computed tomography perfusion (CTP) is one of the most widely used imaging modality for cerebrovascular disease diagnosis and treatment, especially in emergency situations. While cerebral CTP is capable of quantifying the blood flow dynamics by continuous scanning at a focused region of the brain, the associated excessive radiation increases the patients' risk levels of developing cancer. To reduce the necessary radiation dose in CTP, decreasing the temporal sampling frequency is one promising direction. In this paper, we propose STAR, an end-to-end Spatio-Temporal Architecture for super-Resolution to significantly reduce the necessary scanning time and subsequent radiation exposure. The inputs into STAR are multi-directional 2D low-resolution spatio-temporal patches at different cross sections over space and time. Via training multiple direction networks followed by a conjoint reconstruction network, our approach can produce high-resolution spatio-temporal volumes. The experiment results demonstrate the capability of STAR to maintain the image quality and accuracy of cerebral hemodynamic parameters at only one-third of the original scanning time.

1 Introduction

Computed tomography perfusion (CTP) is one of the most widely used imaging modality for disease diagnosis and therapeutics planning such as stroke and oncology [3,11], especially in emergency situations. Cerebral CTP scans a focused brain region for a prolonged amount of time to quantify the blood flow dynamics in the brain. However, a single 40-second cerebral CTP scan can subject the human body to as much as a year's worth of radiation exposure from natural surroundings [7]. In contrast, a chest x-ray would be on par with about ten days worth of exposure. Also, by repetitively scanning a particular region of the brain, there is always a chance the patient may experience the effects of excessive exposure to radiation. Effects such as hair loss (epilation) and skin reddening (erythema) have been reported in a CT brain perfusion over-exposure incident [13]. Risks such as cancer and congenital disabilities are also within public concern [2]. Solutions such as lowering the radiation dose will increase image noise [8] and optimizing a CT scan system will increase the cost. Significant research continues with the goal of reducing radiation exposure from CTP scans.

© Springer International Publishing AG 2017
Q. Wang et al. (Eds.): MLMI 2017, LNCS 10541, pp. 97–105, 2017.
DOI: 10.1007/978-3-319-67389-9_12

In recent years deep learning has achieved significant performance improvement in super-resolution (SR) and image reconstruction [1,5,9,10]. Deep learning models, especially convolutional neural network (CNN) structure, allows the use of learning from low-resolution (LR) image input to reconstruct a high-resolution (HR) output, thus providing a practical solution for image reconstruction. However, most of the super-resolution frameworks using deep learning techniques favor to focus on the 2D natural image SR, since adding the temporal dimension is more challenging, especially with medical images. In this work, we aim to address the challenges in temporal SR and demonstrate the feasibility of our CNN based framework in cerebral CTP for the purpose of increasing scanning intervals and thus reducing the overall scanning time, such that reducing the radiation amount to the patients.

Contributions: This paper proposes STAR an end-to-end Spatio-Temporal Architecture for super-Resolution, and we validate this framework on the clinical cerebral CTP dataset. The proposed STAR architecture consists of two main components: single-directional networks (SDN) and a multi-directional conjoint CNN. SDNs can capture both spatial and temporal features from CTP slices simultaneously by different cross-section patch representations, and the multi-directional conjoint CNN can integrate various single-directional information to reconstruct the final HR spatio-temporal cerebral CTP sequences. Specifically, the contributions are three-fold: (1) Our patch representation layer extracts CTP features from both spatial and temporal dimension. With the cross-section information, the STAR model can represent both spatial and temporal details for CTP image SR, especially for improving CTP sequence temporal resolution. (2) We integrate multiple SDNs with a conjoined multi-directional network to boost the performance for 3D spatio-temporal CTP data. (3) STAR can reduce the scanning time to only one-third of the current method with comparable image quality and accuracy, regarding peak signal-to-noise ratio (PSNR) and structural similarity index measure (SSIM) of the hemodynamic maps for disease diagnosis.

2   Methodology

In this section, we first introduce our patch representation schema for generating 2D spatio-temporal LR inputs. Then, we explain how to improve the spatial and temporal resolution simultaneously for each cross-section by the SDNs. Last but not least, we describe our conjoint model to synthesize multi-directional inputs into a spatio-temporal HR image sequence.

Patch Representation. The input 2D LR patches for image SR are generated from 3D cerebral CTP slices ($X \times Y \times T$). X and Y represent the 2D spatial dimensions and T indicates the temporal dimension of the sequence. We also consider the diagonal (D) direction from $X \times Y$ as one spatial dimension, where X and Y are equal in our data. We extract 2D patches on the $X \times Y$ direction as well as on one of the spatial directions with T dimension: $X \times T$, $Y \times T$, and $D \times T$. With these cross-section data, we can re-scale them on spatial direction,

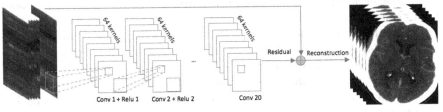

Fig. 1. Single directional network. This model learns the difference between the LR inputs and the HR ground truth image from each cross-section from the high-dimensional medical images. By adding a skip connection between with the input image to the reconstruction layer, the model learns the reside between the LR and HR images. The convolution and ReLU layer occur in pairs and we set 64 filters with size 3×3 for each convolutional layer.

temporal direction, or both spatial and temporal directions to create 2D LR patches. For instance, a 2D spatio-temporal patch represents a single spatial vector change through time, re-scale on temporal dimension allows the change of CTP scanning time in a particular ratio. After feeding these LR patches into the convolution layers for learning the spatio-temporal details, HR output will be generated in the testing stage based on the captured features.

Single Directional Network. The Single Directional Network takes the input patches from one of the four combinations of spatial and temporal dimensions: $X \times Y$, $X \times T$, $Y \times T$, and $D \times T$. Selecting a proper CNN model is a critical component for learning spatio-temporal features for SR problems. We adapt the very deep network for super-resolution (VDSR) [5] with optimized network structure to the SDN (See Fig. 1) due to its high performance in 2D natural image SR. With numerous small filters of size 3×3 in the convolution layers the deep net architecture not only captures the detailed image information but also reduces the computational complexity [12].

The convolution layers of SDN exploit the spatio-temporal information over large cross-section regions by cascading small filters many times. A filter is an integral component of the layered architecture. It refers to an operator applied to the entire image which transforms the information encoded in the pixels. We set 64 filters of size 3×3 in the convolutional layers where a filter operates on the 3×3 region of the 2D input patches. The first layer of convolution operates on the spatio-temporal patches directly to obtain the feature maps, while the kernels in middle layers are convolved with the results from the previous layer. The computed intermediate j^{th} feature map $f_j^{(l)}$ for the middle layer l are calculated by convolving kernels w_{kj}^l with the output feature maps $f_k^{(l-1)}$ from the previous layer $l-1$, that is $f_j^{(l)} = \frac{1}{K} \sum_{k=1}^{K} f_k^{(l-1)} \otimes w_{kj}^l$, where $\otimes$ is the convolution operator. By padding zeros for every convolutional layer during training, we ensure our output size is the same as the input. The ReLU activation layer is used after each convolutional layer; it ensures only certain features are most relevant and will be passed to the next convolution layer. It's activation function $max(0, x)$ defines the output of a node given an input or set of inputs x.

The last layer of SDN is for CTP image reconstruction. A reconstruction function $y = \phi(p, f^{(L)})$ is responsible for constructing HR outputs. In this function, p denotes the 2D patches result from the middle convolution layers, and ϕ is the reconstruction function that sums up the predicted residuals and LR inputs to generate the HR outputs. We also set a high learning rate and apply residual learning to accelerate the convergence and ensure a less training time.

STAR Architecture. The Single Directional Network only extracts features from one of the directions: $Y \times T$, $X \times T$, $D \times T$ or $X \times Y$. By simply stacking the output from various cross-sections into a spatio-temporal volume, the subvoxel information and the contextual cues from different planes are missed. Thus we enhance the SDN by integrating different cross-sections together into spatio-temporal volume through a conjoint layer and another CNN architecture, with the goal of preserving the complementary inter-directional information.

Figure 2 visualizes the proposed STAR model. In this model, the left side shows the extraction of 2D patches through the four directions: $Y \times T$, $X \times T$, $D \times T$ and $X \times Y$. Followed by the arrows, we feed those patches into a single dimensional network $S_i^{(L)}$ respectively, where $i = 1, 2, 3, 4$ is the index of different directional inputs and L indicates the number of convolution layers. After the reconstruction of the perfusion slices P_i through a single directional network $S_i^{(L)}$, we calculate the mean $M = mean(\phi(P_i, S_i^{(L)}))$ of all directions' output in the conjoint layer. In the end, we supply another deep neural network for the conjoint learning, and the result from that is the final HR CTP slices. The advantage of combining different direction spatial-temporal features can be seen from two aspects. On one hand, the sub-voxel information and contextual cues from different planes of brain CTP volume can be learned to alleviate the bias

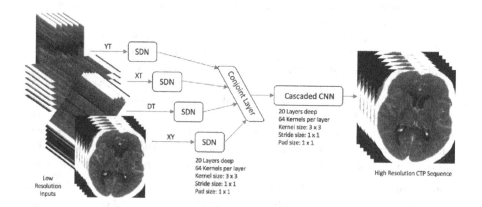

Fig. 2. STAR Architecture.

that is caused by only learning from one direction. On the other hand, the central anatomical structure of the brain can always be captured from different directions. This ensures the pixels in the same area of the brain will be reinforced after the conjunction; providing complementary details to overcome the blurring caused by the bicubic interpolation for LR patches generation.

3   Experiments and Results

Our models are built on top of Caffe, a deep learning framework by the BVLC [4], and trained with a GPU server that contains NVIDIA K40 GPU with 64 GB of RAM. The models are evaluated on 22 patients' 10,472 CTP slices scanned at four 5 mm thickness brain regions with the spatial resolution of 0.43 mm. The slices within one sequence are intensity normalized and co-registered over time. We randomly split these slices into two subsets: 7,140 for training (15 patients), 1,428 for validation (3 patients) and 1,904 for testing (4 patients). The size for each sequence is $512 \times 512 \times 119$ ($X \times Y \times T$). In order to create more input images to brew a robust model, we clip patches with size 41×41 pixel and a stride of 21 from four directions, which yields 36,800, 36,800, 73,600, and 62,951 patches in the directions of XY, YT, DT, and XY. We create the LR patches by using bicubic method re-size to $1/3$ on the original 2D HR patches.

Experiment on SDNs. We test on two different CNN structures, and the result shows that the basic single directional network outperforms the shallow network in SRCNN (3 layers) [1] at all four cross-sections. This confirms that for both spatial and temporal SR, deeper is better than the shallow net. In Fig. 3, three single directional SDNs that have temporal SR are compared with the bicubic interpolation and SRCNN method, and it shows that the 20 layer model achieves better PSNR on average. Among these three types of single directional networks, YT direction gives the best PSNR by the 20 layer structure. The XY spatial direction has a lower PSNR value (39.899 dB) compared to the temporal cross-sections which yield to about 2.690 dB and 1.733 dB higher than bicubic

Table 1. PSNR comparison for perfusion maps that are generated by different methods.

	CBF		CBV	
sSVD	PSNR	SSIM	PSNR	SSIM
Bicubic	19.271	0.901	18.909	0.880
Spat-SDN	22.311	0.946	21.203	0.925
Temp-SDN	24.919	0.974	21.730	0.945
STAR	**26.131**	**0.978**	**23.003**	**0.955**

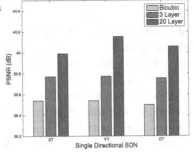

Fig. 3. PSNR comparison between 3 layer CNN and 20 layer CNN in SDNs.

and SRCNN. Therefore, we choose this 20 layer deep CNN structure for our SDN model. To maintain the output image is the same size of the input, the kernel size, stride size, and pad size of our deep directional CNN is set to be 3, 1, 1 respectively. Except the last layer outputs one feature map, other convolution layers have 64 outputs. With residual learning, the loss function is determined by the sum of estimated residuals between the HR ground truth image and the LR input. The basic learning rate is set to be 0.1, and the weight decay is set to be 0.0001 for faster convergence.

Furthermore, we also compare the performance based on the different patch representations in the basic model. The result of down-sampling on temporal direction only can be seen in Fig. 3. We also evaluate on SDNs with YT, XT and DT LR inputs that are scaled down on both spatial and temporal directions, they bring about 2.13 dB, 2.98 dB and 4.01 dB lower PSNR than temporal direction only. However, these SNDs outperform much better results where they achieved a greater improvement on image SR - on average of 0.9 dB higher than the differences between the improvement of temporal only SDNs. This experiment indicates that the temporal pattern can be predicted more precisely than the spatial features through the proposed approach. In other words, there is an extensive potential of our basic networks to combine the spatial and temporal learning to produce better performance in an appropriate way, for which the high performance will be explained in our STAR cross-section learning approach.

Experiment on STAR. The proposed STAR network is a combination of multiple SDNs from different cross-sections together and is cascaded with another deep convolution network where the convolution occurs in pairs with the ReLU layer. The cascaded layers have the same parameter settings of SDN. In the first convolution layer, filters are convolved on top of the mean outputs from the previous spatial SDN and the three temporal SDNs. Thus the sub-voxel information and the contextual cues can be learned through different directions.

As can be seen in Fig. 4, the resolution of images from left to right of the columns have been improved gradually. The first row of the figure is the grayscale CTP slice. The following two rows are the cerebral hemodynamic parameters: Cerebral Blood Flow (CBF) and Cerebral Blood Volume (CBV); which are calculated by Perfusion Mismatch Analyzer (PMA, [6]) from the corresponding CTP sequences in the first row. The first row LR images in column (a) are downscaled with a ratio of 3 from the ground truth gray-scale images in column (e). Column (b) and (c) are the intermediate results from spatial SR SDN where we only perform spatial SR on the XY direction, and temporal SR SDN where we only perform temporal cross-section SR. The superior outcomes of the proposed STAR method are shown in the column (d). As the areas that the arrows are pointing at, the images with LR are missing the details and the rough sketch is blurry. The spatial SR images can show more details than the LR images, but still, the boundaries are not clear enough; and the temporal SR images are similar to the spatial SR images, which with drawbacks in different areas. By combining the spatial and temporal details, we can get a much better SR result: the images present more clearly and with extra details.

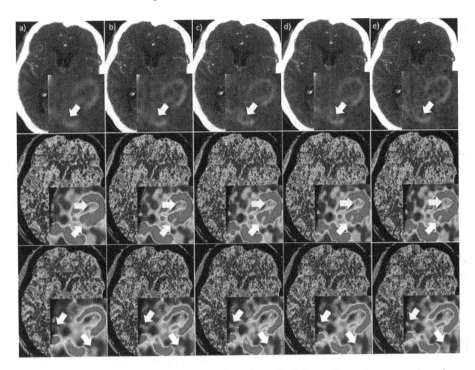

Fig. 4. The gray-scale images (first row) and cerebral hemodynamic parameters (second row: CBF, third row: CBV) have achieved a higher resolution through different stages: column (*a*): LR input, column (*b*): SDN spatial, column (*c*): SDN temporal, column (*d*): STAR spatio-temporal, column (*e*): the ground truth image.

We also measure the PSNR and SSIM for the perfusion images. The highlighted row in Table 1 shows the best values for our method. The basic models no matter the spatial-only SDN (Spat-SDN) or the temporal-only SDN provides better image quality than the bicubic method in different degrees. Our final STAR model gives the highest PSNR of 26.131 dB on CBF which is 6.86 dB higher than the baseline and in CBV calculation, the STAR improves bicubic about 4.094 dB. Other than that, in the SSIM comparison, STAR still achieves the best results of 0.978 and 0.955 respectively. These experiments show the perfusion maps at only 1/3 of the original scanning time with comparable perfusion map quality and accuracy through the STAR framework. Our model allows the input with 1/3 of CTP scanning time and provides high-resolution outputs which potentially reduce the possibility of radiation over-exposure.

4   Conclusion

In this paper, we have presented STAR, an end-to-end spatio-temporal super-resolution framework. The experimental results show that the proposed basic model of single directional network improves both spatial and temporal resolution, while the multi-directional conjoint network further enhances the SR results - comparing favorably with only temporal or only spatial SR. By learning the spatial-temporal features, our approach ensures the ability to maintain the quality of brain CTP slices within one-third of the original scanning time. In the future, we believe that by reducing the scanning time, our approach will provide an applicable solution for improving spatial and temporal resolution and help to lower the possibility of excessive patient radiation exposure, while increasing the potential of assisted clinical diagnosis of cerebrovascular disease with high-quality perfusion images. Our plans include applying our pipeline to a variety of imaging modalities, including functional MRI, PET/CT for functionality super-resolution and investigating the correlation between the temporal and spatial upscale ratios with super-resolution quality.

Acknowledgements. This work is partially supported by the National Key Research and Development Program of China (No: 2016YFC1300302), National Science Foundation under Grant No. IIS-1564892, National Center for Advancing Translational Sciences of the National Institute of Health under Award No. UL1TR000457 and by National Natural Science Foundation of China (No: 61525106).

References

1. Dong, C., Loy, C.C., He, K., Tang, X.: Learning a Deep Convolutional Network for Image Super-Resolution. In: Fleet, D., Pajdla, T., Schiele, B., Tuytelaars, T. (eds.) ECCV 2014. LNCS, vol. 8692, pp. 184–199. Springer, Cham (2014). doi:10. 1007/978-3-319-10593-2_13
2. de González, A.B., Mahesh, M., Kim, K.P., Bhargavan, M., Lewis, R., Mettler, F., Land, C.: Projected cancer risks from computed tomographic scans performed in the united states in 2007. Archives Intern. Med. **169**(22), 2071–2077 (2009)
3. Hoeffner, E.G., Case, I., Jain, R., Gujar, S.K., Shah, G.V., et al.: Cerebral perfusion CT: technique and clinical applications 1. Radiology **231**(3), 632–644 (2004)
4. Jia, Y., Shelhamer, E., Donahue, J., et al.: Caffe: Convolutional architecture for fast feature embedding. arXiv preprint. (2014). arXiv:1408.5093
5. Kim, J., Lee, J.K., Lee, K.M.: Accurate image super-resolution using very deep convolutional networks. In: IEEE Conference on Computer Vision and Pattern Recognition (CVPR Oral)., June 2016
6. Kudo, K.: Perfusion mismatch analyzer, version 3.4.06. asist-japan web site. http:// asist.umin.jp/index-e.htm Accessed 15 Dec 2016
7. Mettler Jr., F.A., Bhargavan, M., et al.: Radiologic and nuclear medicine studies in the united states and worldwide: Frequency, radiation dose, and comparison with other radiation sources 1950–2007 1. Radiology **253**(2), 520–531 (2009)
8. Nelson, T.R.: Practical strategies to reduce pediatric ct radiation dose. J. Am. Coll. Radiol. **11**(3), 292–299 (2014)
9. Oktay, O., Bai, W., Lee, M., Guerrero, R., Kamnitsas, K., Caballero, J., Marvao, A., Cook, S., O'Regan, D., Rueckert, D.: Multi-input Cardiac Image Super-Resolution Using Convolutional Neural Networks. In: Ourselin, S., Joskowicz, L., Sabuncu, M.R., Unal, G., Wells, W. (eds.) MICCAI 2016. LNCS, vol. 9902, pp. 246–254. Springer, Cham (2016). doi:10.1007/978-3-319-46726-9_29

10. Shi, W., et al.: Real-time single image and video super-resolution using an efficient sub-pixel convolutional neural network. In: Proceedings of the IEEE Conference on Computer Vision and Pattern Recognition. pp. 1874–1883 (2016)
11. Shrier, D.A., Tanaka, H., Numaguchi, Y., Konno, S., Patel, U., Shibata, D.: CT angiography in the evaluation of acute stroke. Am. J. Neuroradiol. **18**(6), 1011–1020 (1997)
12. Szymanski, L., McCane, B.: Deep networks are effective encoders of periodicity. IEEE Trans. Neural Netw. Learn. Syst. **25**(10), 1816–1827 (2014)
13. Wintermark, M., Lev, M.: FDA investigates the safety of brain perfusion ct. Am. J. Neuroradiol. **31**(1), 2–3 (2010)

Classification of Alzheimer's Disease by Cascaded Convolutional Neural Networks Using PET Images

Danni Cheng and Manhua Liu[(✉)]

Department of Instrument Science and Engineering,
School of EIEE, Shanghai Jiao Tong University, Shanghai 200240, China
mhliu@sjtu.edu.cn

Abstract. Accurate and early diagnosis of Alzheimer's disease (AD) plays important role for the patient care and development of future treatment. Positron Emission Tomography (PET) is a functional imaging modality which can help physicians to predict AD. In recent years, machine learning methods have been widely studied on analysis of PET brain images for quantitative evaluation and computer-aided-diagnosis (CAD) of AD. Most existing methods extract the hand-craft imaging features from images, and then train a classifier to distinguish AD from other groups. This paper proposes to construct cascaded 3D convolutional neural networks (3D-CNNs) to hierarchically learn the multi-level imaging features which are ensembled for classification of AD using PET brain images. First, multiple deep 3D-CNNs are constructed on different local image patches to transform the local image into more compact high-level features. Then, a deep 3D CNNs is learned to ensemble the high-level features for final classification. The proposed method can automatically learn the generic features from PET imaging data for classification. No image segmentation and rigid registration are required in preprocessing the PET images. Our method is evaluated on the PET images from 193 subjects including 93 AD patients and 100 normal controls (NC) from Alzheimer's Disease Neuroimaging Initiative (ADNI) database. Experimental results show that the proposed method achieves an accuracy of 92.2% for classification of AD vs. NC, demonstrating the promising classification performance.

Keywords: Alzheimer's disease diagnosis · Convolutional neural network (CNN) · Cascaded CNN · PET image · Image classification

1 Introduction

Alzheimer's disease (AD) is an irreversible brain degenerative disorder with progressive impairment of the memory and cognitive functions [1]. Currently there is no effective cure for AD, but it is a great interest to develop treatments that can delay its progression, especially if diagnosis is provided at an early stage [2]. Accurate and early diagnosis of AD is not only challenging but also important for patient care and developing future treatments.

Positrons Emission Tomography (PET) is a functional medical imaging modality which can help physicians to diagnose AD. A positron-emitting radionuclide (tracer)

© Springer International Publishing AG 2017
Q. Wang et al. (Eds.): MLMI 2017, LNCS 10541, pp. 106–113, 2017.
DOI: 10.1007/978-3-319-67389-9_13

with a biologically active molecule, such as (18)F-fluorodeoxy-glucose, is introduced in the body. Concentrations of this tracer are imaged using a camera and indicate tissue metabolic activity by virtue of the regional glucose uptake [3]. Fluorodeoxiglucose positron emission tomography (FDG-PET) provides a powerful functional imaging biomarker to help understand the anatomical and neural changes and assist AD diagnosis. In recent years, various pattern recognition methods have been investigated in analysis of PET brain images to identify the patterns related to AD and decode the disease states for computer-aided-diagnosis (CAD). A region based method was proposed to extract features for classification of AD with PET images [3]. In this method, brain images are mapped into 116 anatomical regions of interest (ROIs) and the first four moments and the entropy of the histograms of these regions are computed as the regional features. Receiver Operating Characteristics curves are used to rank the discriminability of ROIs to distinguish PET brain images and the features from top 21 regions are input to both support vector machine (SVM) and random forest classifiers for AD classification. In [4], 286 features were extracted from 116 cerebral anatomical volumes of interest (VOIs) based on the automated anatomical labeling (AAL) cortical parcellation map, and a semi-supervised method was proposed to integrate the labelled and unlabeled data by random manifold learning with affinity regularization for AD classification.

To capture the rich image information, the voxel-wise intensity features were extracted after preprocessing of the PET images including co-registration to their baseline PET scan, reorientation into a standard space, voxel intensity normalization and smoothing with a 8 mm FWHM Gaussian filter for AD classification. In [2, 5], a boosting classification method was proposed for classification of PET images based on a mixture of simple classifiers, which performs feature selection concurrently with the classification to solve high dimensional problem. A favorite class ensemble of classifiers was proposed with each base classifier in the ensemble using a different feature subset which is optimized for a given class.

Recently, deep learning methods were also explored to extract the latent features from measurements of ROIs for AD classification [6, 7]. Suk et al. [6] used a stacked autoencoder to learn the latent high-level features separately from 93 ROIs of the MRI and PET images and a multi-kernel SVM was used to combine these features to improve the classification performance. Liu et al. [7] extracted a set of latent features from 83 ROIs of the MRI and PET scans and trained a multi-layered neural network consisting of several auto-encoders to combine multimodal features for classification. Azmi et al. [8] proposed an AD classification method based on segmented brain features use neural network. A deep learning based framework was proposed for estimating the missing PET imaging data for multimodal classification of AD in [9].

Convolutional neural networks (CNNs) have been widely explored for MR brain image analysis [10, 11]. Hosseini-Asl et al. [10] proposed to predict AD with a deep 3D-CNNs, which is built upon a 3D convolutional autoencoder and pre-trained to capture anatomical shape variations in structural MRI scans. The deep CNNs were studied for AD classification using MRI and fMRI [11]. Vu et al. [12] combined sparse autoencoder (SAE) and convolution neural network (CNN) for multimodality learning. The above methods focused on the AD diagnosis from MRI or multimodality images. In the case of PET images, further investigation is needed to determine their ability to diagnose AD.

This paper proposes a novel classification method based on cascaded 3D-CNNs to learn the multi-level imaging features and ensemble these features for classifications of AD *vs.* NC using PET brain images. First, a number of local 3D patches are extracted from the whole brain image. Second, a deep 3D CNN is built to hierarchically and gradually transform the image patch into more compact discriminative features. Third, a high-level 3D CNN is cascaded to ensemble the features learned from multi-local CNNs for image classification. The proposed method works well to extract the generic features from the high dimensional imaging data for classification. The rest of this paper is organized as follows. Section 2 presents the proposed classification method. Experiments are provided in Sect. 3. Section 4 concludes this paper.

2   Materials and Proposed Method

In this section, we will present the proposed AD classification method using PET brain images in detail. PET image is a functional imaging modality which is often used as a biomarker to help physicians for AD diagnosis. For analysis of high dimensional PET brain images, the cascaded CNNs are constructed to hierarchically learn the multi-level generic features and ensemble for classification of AD. There are three main advantages to apply deep CNNs for our task. First, their deep complex architecture of CNNs can extract the low-, mid- to high-level features from a high volume of training images. Second, they can explicitly make use of the spatial structure of brain images and learn local spatial filters useful to the classification task. Finally, cascading multiple CNNs can construct a hierarchy of more complex features representing larger spatial regions, finally providing a global label. Figure 1 shows the flow chart of the proposed classification method based on cascaded CNNs, which consists of three main steps: image preprocessing, feature extraction with multi-CNNs, and ensemble classification by cascading CNNs, as detailed below.

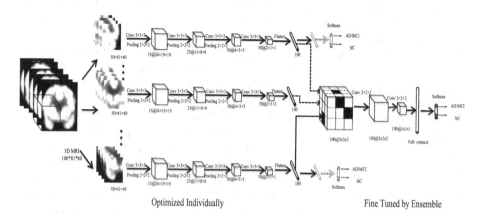

Fig. 1. The flow chart of the proposed classification method and the structures of deep CNNs denoted with the sizes of input, convolution, max pooling and output layers and the numbers and sizes of generated feature maps.

2.1   Image Acquisition and Processing

The data used in this work were obtained from 193 participants in the Alzheimer's Disease Neuroimaging Initiative (ADNI) database (www.loni.ucla.edu/ADNI). The 193 baseline FDG-PET brain images were taken from 93 AD subjects and 100 NC subjects. Detailed information about FDG-PET acquisition procedures is available at the ADNI website. The PET images were processed to make the images from different systems more similar. The image processing included co-registration to their baseline PET scans and reorientation into a standard space. In addition, we also perform intensity normalization and conversion of the image to a uniform isotropic resolution of 8 mm FWHM as in [2]. The voxels outside the brain are removed from the image analysis and the final PET images used for test are of size $100 \times 81 \times 80$ voxels. The voxel intensities of each PET image are used for classification.

2.2   Feature Extraction with Multiple 3D CNNs

If all voxel intensities of each image are directly used for classification, there are 648,000 features input to the classifier. The voxel intensity features are of huge dimensionality, far more features than training samples, which may lead to low classification performance due to the 'curse of dimensionality'. Motivated by the success of CNNs in computer vision, this paper proposes to build the deep CNNs to learn image features for AD classification. To capture the subtle local variations of the high-dimensional PET images, a number of local 3D patches are extracted from the whole brain image and a deep CNN is constructed to hierarchically and gradually transform each image patch into more compact high-level features. In this work, 27 local 3D patches of $54 \times 41 \times 40$ voxels are uniformly extracted from each PET image at a fixed step with 50% overlapping.

Convolutional neural networks (CNNs) have been successfully studied for various applications such as image classification and object detection. However, most of the CNNs architectures are used in 2D image area. In this work, we adopt the fundamental structure just like LeNet [13] for each CNNs and extend it to 3D formation to learn the features of each 3D image patch, which can capture the 3D image structures. For simplicity, the same network structure is used to build the deep CNNs for all 3D patches. Each deep CNNs consists of the following types of layers, as illustrated in Fig. 1.

The first one is the input layer which accepts a 3D image patch of fixed size ($50 \times 41 \times 40$ voxels in this work). The second type is the convolutional layers which convolve the learned filters with the input image patch and produce a feature map for each filter. Through convolution, the features can capture the discriminatory information of the image. The layer following the convolutional layer is the max pooling layers which down-sample the input feature map along the spatial dimensions by replacing each non-overlapping block with their maximum. Max pooling can help to reduce feature dimension and achieve the invariance to shift, scale and rotation at a certain level. The forth type of layer is the fully connected layers which consist of a number of output neurons. Each neuron outputs the learned linear combination of all inputs from the previous layer and passed through nonlinearity. The last layer is a prediction layer which uses a softmax function to generate a prediction score for each class label. The softmax function is a derivation of logistic function that highlights the largest values in a vector while suppressing those that are significantly below the maximum.

In this work, each deep CNNs is built with 4 convolutional layers, 3 max pooling layers, and one fully connected layer. The sizes of all convolution filters are $3 \times 3 \times 3$ and the numbers of filters are set to 15, 25, 50, and 50 for 4 convolution layers, respectively. Max pooling is applied for each $2 \times 2 \times 2$ region, and *Tanh* is adopted as the activation function in these layers because of its good performance for CNNs. During the pre-training period, each deep CNNs is optimized individually to output the class prediction score by the softmax layer. The image patch is transformed into high-level features by building deep CNNs.

2.3   Cascaded Ensemble Classification for AD Diagnosis

While the lower layers of the predictive 3D-CNNs extract discriminative features of local image patches, the upper layers have to facilitate task-specific classification by ensemble with these features. Different from the conventional ensemble methods by averaging the class prediction scores, this paper proposes a cascaded CNNs to combine the features learned by local 3D CNNs for ensemble classification. The features of the low-level CNNs are piled up to form feature maps of a 3D-structure and a deep 3D CNNs is further built at high level to learn the global features followed by full connection and softmax layer for ensemble classification. The cascaded CNNs have the advantages on making full use of the spatial information and learning high-level global features when compared with concatenating all features of local patches for classification.

Training the proposed cascaded ensemble classification consists of pre-training of individual CNNs, and final task-specific fine-tuning for ensemble classification. Initially, we train a deep 3D CNNs for each image patch individually by directly mapping the outputs of the fully connected layer to the probabilistic scores of class labels with the softmax layer. In the ensemble learning process, we keep the initial-trained parameters of the first 3 convolution and pooling layers in the low-level CNNs, while the parameters of the last convolutional layer and upper fully connected layers are fine-tuned jointly with the high-level CNNs to ensemble the features for final classification.

3   Experimental Results

In this section, experiments are performed to test the proposed classification algorithm. There are 193 PET brain images of 93 AD subjects and 100 NC subjects from ADNI for our experiments. Ten-fold cross-validation is used to avoid random factors affecting results. Each time, one fold of the image set is used for testing, another fold used for validation while the left eight folds were used for training. The validation part is for parameter tuning. To increase training data, augmentation is performed by shift, sampling and rotation to generate additional images for the training set. The proposed algorithm is implemented with the Keras [17] library based on Theano [16] in Python. The experiment is conducted on PC with GPU NVIDIA GTX1080. In the low level, 27 deep CNNs are independently trained to extract the local features with the output of the prediction scores by softmax layer. The Adadelta gradient descent algorithm [15] is used to train the local deep CNNs. To avoid overfitting, dropout, L1 and L2 regulation are adopted in our network [14].

To evaluate the classification performance, we compute the classification accuracy (ACC), the sensitivity (SEN), the specificity (SPE), and the area under receiver operating characteristic curve (AUC) in the experiments. The first experiment is to compare the proposed cascaded CNNs to the best local 3D CNNs and the ensemble by averaging the predictions of low-level CNNs. Their results are compared in Table 1. Figure 2 compares the ROC (receiver operating characteristic) curves of different methods for classification of AD vs. NC. From the results, the proposed cascaded CNNs performs better than other methods. Since there are some patches irrelevant to AD, ensemble by averaging degrades the classification performance.

Table 1. Comparison of classification performances on AD vs. NC.

Methods	ACC (%)	SEN (%)	SPE (%)	AUC (%)
The best CNNs	88.6	90.8	86.8	92.7
Ensemble by average	86.0	89.2	83.5	94.6
Cascaded CNNs	**92.2**	**91.4**	**92.4**	**94.9**

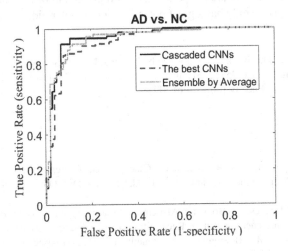

Fig. 2. Comparison of ROC curves for classification of AD vs. NC.

In addition, we compared the results of the proposed method with some results reported in the literature that also used the PET data of ADNI, as shown in Table 2. It is worth to note that the classification accuracies in Table 2 are only based on the PET images and subjects in the test are different. These results further validate the efficacy of our proposed method for classification of AD.

Table 2. Comparison of the classification performances for AD vs. NC (%) reported in the literature.

Method	ACC	SEN	SPE	AUC
Silveira et al. [2]	91.0	-	-	-
Lu et al. [4]	89.4	88.7	90.0	-
Liu et al. [7]	91.4	92.3	90.4	-
Suk et al. [6]	88.7	-	-	-
Li et al. [8]	-	-	-	89.8
Vu et al. [10]	91.1	-	-	-
Azmi et al. [9]	90.6	82.4	95.3	-
Our method	92.2	91.4	92.4	94.9

"-" mean the results were not mentioned in literature.

4   Conclusions

This paper has presented a classification method based on the cascaded 3D-CNNs to classify AD vs. NC using PET brain images. Multiple deep CNNs have been built on different local image patches to learn the discriminative features. Then a high-level 3D CNN is cascaded to ensemble the features learned from local CNNs and generate the high-level features for image classification. Our experimental results and comparison on ADNI database demonstrate the performance improvement of the proposed method for AD diagnosis. This study has a great potential for computer-aided diagnosis in other biomedical fields.

Acknowledgement. This work was supported by National Natural Science Foundation of China (NSFC) under grants No. 61375112, Shanghai Medical Guidance Project No. 134119a9700, and SMC Excellent Young Faculty program of SJTU.

References

1. Minati, L., Edginton, T., Bruzzone, M.G., Giaccone, G.: Current concepts in Alzheimer's disease: a multidisciplinary review. Am. J. Alzheimer's Dis. Other Dement. **24**, 95–121 (2008)
2. Silveira, M., Marques, J.: Boosting Alzheimer disease diagnosis using PET images. In: International Conference on Pattern Recognition, pp. 2556–2559 (2010)
3. Garali, I., Adel, M., Bourennane, S., Guedj, E.: Region-based brain selection and classification on pet images for Alzheimer's disease computer aided diagnosis. In: IEEE International Conference on Image Processing, pp. 1473–1477 (2015)
4. Shen, L., Xia, Y., Cai, T.W., Feng, D.D.: Semi-supervised manifold learning with affinity regularization for Alzheimer's disease identification. In: International Conference of the IEEE EMBS, p. 2251 (2015)
5. Cabral, C., Silveira, M.: Classification of Alzheimer's disease from FDG-PET images using favourite class ensembles. In: Engineering in Medicine and Biology Society, pp. 2477–2480. IEEE (2013)

6. Suk, H.I., Lee, S.W., Shen, D.: Latent feature representation with stacked auto-encoder for AD/MCI diagnosis. Brain Struct. Funct. **220**(2), 841–859 (2015)
7. Liu, S., Cai, W., Che, H., Pujol, S., Kikinis, R., Feng, D., Fulham, M.J.: Multimodal neuroimaging feature learning for multiclass diagnosis of Alzheimer's disease. IEEE Trans. Biomed. Eng. **62**(4), 1132–1140 (2015)
8. Azmi, M.H., et al.: 18F-FDG PET brain images as features for Alzheimer classification. Radiat. Phys. Chem. **137**, 135–143 (2016)
9. Li, R., Zhang, W., Suk, H.-I., Wang, L., Li, J., Shen, D., Ji, S.: Deep learning based imaging data completion for improved brain disease diagnosis. Med. Image Comput. Comput. Assist. Interv. **17**(03), 305–312 (2014)
10. Hosseiniasl, E., Keynto, R., Elbaz, A.: Alzheimer's disease diagnostics by adaptation of 3D convolutional network. In: IEEE International Conference on Image Processing, Phoenix, Arizona, USA, 25–28 September 2016
11. Sarraf, S., Tofighi, G.: DeepAD: Alzheimer's disease classification via deep convolutional neural networks using MRI and fMRI. biorxiv.org
12. Vu, T.D., et al.: Multimodal learning using convolution neural network and Sparse Autoencoder. In: IEEE International Conference on Big Data and Smart Computing, Jeju, South Korea, 13–16 February 2017
13. LeCun, Y., Bottou, L., Bengio, Y., Haffner, P.: Gradient-based learning applied to document recognition. Proc. IEEE **86**(11), 2278–2324 (1998)
14. Srivastava, N., Hinton, G., Krizhevsky, A., Sutskever, I., Salakhutdinov, R.: Dropout: a simple way to prevent neural networks from overfitting. J. Mach. Learn. Res. **15**(1), 1929–1958 (2014)
15. Zeiler, M.D.: ADADELTA: an adaptive learning rate method. arXiv:1212.5701 (2012)
16. Chollet, F.: Keras: Theano-based deep learning library (2015). https://github.com/fchollet/keras
17. Bastien, F., Lamblin, P., Pascanu, R., Bergstra, J., Goodfellow, I., Bergeron, A.: Theano: new features and speed improvements. Computer Science (2012)

Finding Dense Supervoxel Correspondence of Cone-Beam Computed Tomography Images

Yuru Pei[1($\boxtimes$)], Yunai Yi[1], Gengyu Ma[2], Yuke Guo[3], Gui Chen[4], Tianmin Xu[4], and Hongbin Zha[1]

[1] Key Laboratory of Machine Perception (MOE),
Department of Machine Intelligence, Peking University, Beijing, China
Peiyuru@cis.pku.edu.cn
[2] uSens Inc., San Jose, USA
[3] Luoyang Institute of Science and Technology, Luoyang, China
[4] School of Stomatology, Peking University, Beijing, China

Abstract. Dense correspondence establishment of cone-beam computed tomography (CBCT) images is a crucial step for attribute transfers and morphological variation assessments in clinical orthodontics. However, the registration by the traditional large-scale nonlinear optimization is time-consuming for the craniofacial CBCT images. The supervised random forest is known for its fast online performance, thought the limited training data impair the generalization capacity. In this paper, we propose an unsupervised random-forest-based approach for the supervoxel-wise correspondence of CBCT images. In particular, we present a theoretical complexity analysis with a data-dependent learning guarantee for the clustering hypotheses of the unsupervised random forest. A novel tree-pruning algorithm is proposed to refine the forest by removing the local trivial and inconsistent leaf nodes, where the learning bound serves as guidance for an optimal selection of tree structures. The proposed method has been tested on the label propagation of clinically-captured CBCT images. Experiments demonstrate the proposed method yields performance improvements over variants of both supervised and unsupervised random-forest-based methods.

1 Introduction

Malocclusions, giving rise to the functional and esthetic problems, is viewed as a worldwide health issue. The CBCT images are widely used in clinical orthodontics to provide patient-specific morphological information for treatment planning and evaluation. Dense voxel-wise correspondence, equivalent to image registration, is a crucial step to establish the mapping between CBCT images, and in turn the label propagation [8]. 3D image registration has been thoroughly studied in medical image processing for decades. However, it is not a trivial task to

---

Electronic supplementary material The online version of this chapter (doi:10.1007/978-3-319-67389-9_14) contains supplementary material, which is available to authorized users.

Q. Wang et al. (Eds.): MLMI 2017, LNCS 10541, pp. 114–122, 2017.
DOI: 10.1007/978-3-319-67389-9_14

realize a fast online CBCT image registration by the traditional intensity-based registration technique using conventional metrics, such as the mutual information (MI) and the normalized correlations (NC), under the large-scale nonlinear optimization framework. The image registration often costumes several minutes due to hundreds of millions of voxels in the head CBCT images.

The random forest is known for its robustness, scalability, and the fast online performance. The random-forest-based label propagation has reported promising efficiency and accuracy [5]. However, the supervised random forest needs a large set of annotated data for training. The manual labeling of volumetric data is known to be laborious and subjective. The pseudo-labeling by supervoxel decomposition of one image relieve the manual annotation [8]. However, the limited annotation impairs the generalization capacity of the random forest. A variety of unsupervised clustering random forests, such as those learned by the GINI impurity [2] and the multi-variate Gaussian distribution [4], have been employed for affinity estimation and correspondence establishment [9]. However, unlike the supervised forest and the similar multi-label boosting [6,7], there is no theoretical analysis of the convergence rate and the complexity of hypothesis function family for the unsupervised clustering forest. Moreover, the forest size is often too large for the volumetric images. Even for the random forest built upon supervoxels, the local aggregation of voxels with similar appearances, there are nearly ten thousand leaf nodes in one randomized tree with a dozen layers.

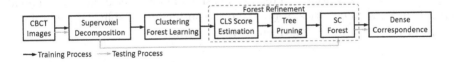

Fig. 1. Flowchart of our system.

To address the above problems, we propose an unsupervised clustering random-forest-based framework for affinity estimation and correspondence establishment of supervoxels in CBCT images. Specifically, (1) we derive the data-dependent learning guarantee of the unsupervised randomized clustering tree based on the Rademacher complexity. (2) Given the dimension-free learning bound, we propose a tree-pruning algorithm to minimize the expected clustering errors of supervoxels. In particular, we define a confident score according to contextual leaf assignments (CLS score), which favors the supervoxel with similar contexts to others belonging to the same leaf node. The tree pruning penalizes the supervoxels with small CLS scores, and results to a spatially-consistent tree. The main point of this work is to provide the theoretical analysis to randomized clustering trees. Furthermore, the derived theory guides a tree-pruning algorithm for a compact and spatially-consistent clustering random forest (SC forest), where experimental results demonstrate improvements over variants of both supervised and unsupervised random-forest-based methods.

2   Methods

The proposed unsupervised forest-based correspondence establishment framework (see Fig. 1) consists of two main steps, (1) clustering forest learning from decomposed supervoxels of the training CBCT images (Sect. 2.1), (2) tree pruning based forest refinement for an SC forest (Sect. 2.2). Instead of the empirical evaluation of the clustering random forest, we derive the learning bound of the clustering loss, a product of leaf assignment and compactness evaluation weighted by the CLS scores, by the Rademacher complexity.

2.1   Clustering Forest

We build the clustering forest for the affinity estimation and correspondence establishments, which avoid the annotation of the training data [5] and the limitation of pseudo labels from the supervoxel decomposition of just one volume image [8]. We follow the density forest [4] to find the optimal node splitting under an assumption of the Gaussian distribution in tree nodes. Furthermore, we replace the determinant operator in the information gain estimation by the trace operator [9] to avoid the rank deficiency in the covariance matrix of the high dimensional feature vectors of the supervoxels. The feature channels of the supervoxels are defined as an intensity histogram of inside voxels and an average intensity histogram of one-ring neighboring supervoxels similar to [11]. Similar to the supervised classification and regression random forest, the clustering random forest is built in an empirical way, where the optimal node splitting is obtained independently by maximizing the information gain.

2.2   Tree Pruning

Considering the large number of supervoxels, each tree in the forest has dozens of layers, and results to more than ten thousand leaf nodes. Some leaf nodes contribute trivially or even negatively to the final clustering. Moreover, in the clustering forest, the consistent supervoxel correspondence in the contextual sense is only addressed by feature channels. A tree-pruning algorithm is proposed to handle the trivial and inconsistent leaf nodes based on a theoretical learning bound of the randomized clustering tree. We start by introducing the notations of the clustering random forest, and reformulating the clustering loss function in a compact way for our further formulation.

Leaf assignment function $s(x, l)$. When given binary questions stored in tree nodes, the tree maps a data point x to a leaf node. $s(x, l) = 1$ when x is assigned to the l-th leaf node.

Leaf compactness evaluation $f_l(x)$. The leaf nodes provide a partition of given data. Each leaf node is viewed as a cluster. The compactness evaluation gives a clue of the clustering performance, and $f_l(x) = (1 - \tau)\|x - \mu_l\|^2$. τ denotes the CLS score of the supervoxel x estimated based on the leaf assignment of its context, when given the leaf assignment of suerpvoxels from CBCT image set $\mathcal{V}$ by the random forest. For a supervoxel $x \in V \cap L_l$, and $V \in \mathcal{V}$,

$$\tau(x) = \frac{1}{Z} \sum_{i=1}^{n_R} \sum_{x' \in \mathcal{B}(x)} \max_{x^{r'} \in \mathcal{B}(x^r)} d(x', x^{r'}). \tag{1}$$

Given the training volume image set $\mathcal{V}$, $V_{ref} \in \mathcal{V} - V$. Supervoxel $x^r \in V_{ref}$, belonging to the same leaf node L_l as x, and $s(x, l) = s(x^r, l)$. We assess the affinity of supervoxels in a contextual cube $\mathcal{B}(x)$ centered at x and their counterpart in the contextual cube $\mathcal{B}(x^r)$ of x^r. Function d is defined based on the common traversal path $\mathcal{P}(x', x^{r'})$ of x' and $x^{r'}$, and $d(x', x^{r'}) = |\mathcal{P}(x', x^{r'})|/\nu$, where ν denotes the maximum length of traversal paths of x' and $x^{r'}$. Z is a normalization constant determined by supervoxel number n_B of $\mathcal{B}(x)$ and number n_R of reference images V_{ref} with supervoxels in L_l, and $Z = n_R \cdot n_B$. For all points belonging to leaf node L_l, the CLS scores are normalized, and $\frac{\tau_i}{\sum_{i=1}^{n_l} \tau_i} \to \tau_i$.

The clustering center of leaf node L_l is defined as $\mu_l = \sum_{i=1}^{n_l} \tau_i x_i$, which favors the supervoxels bearing consistent contexts with their counterparts in the same leaf node. The clustering loss function of leaf node L_l is rewritten as $f_l(x) = (1 - \tau)\|x - X_l T_l \mathbf{e}\|^2$. X_l is a k by n_l dimensional matrix, where the i-th column of X_l is the feature vector $x_i \in \mathbb{R}^k$. T_l is a n_l by n_l dimensional diagonal matrix with the diagonal entry set as τ. $\mathbf{e}$ denotes a n_l-dimensional vector with all entries set at one. Thus, the clustering loss function of one randomized clustering tree

$$g(x) = \sum_{l=1}^{n_v} s(x, l) f_l(x) = \sum_{l=1}^{n_v} (1 - \tau) s(x, l)\|x - X_l T_l \mathbf{e}\|^2, \tag{2}$$

where n_v is the number of leaf nodes. Let's denote the data domain as $\mathcal{D}$. The training data set $X \in \mathcal{D}$. The hypothesis of the randomized clustering tree is determined by a vector of leaf nodes centers $(\mu_1, \mu_2, \ldots, \mu_{n_v})$.

Definition 1 (*Rademacher Complexity of Clustering tree*). *For an independent distributed sample set* $X = \{x_1, x_2, \ldots, x_n\}$, *and* $X \in \mathcal{D}$, *if* $\mathcal{G}$ *is a class of clustering hypothesis on* $\mathcal{D}$, *the Rademacher complexity of* $\mathcal{G}$ *is defined as*

$$\mathfrak{R}(\mathcal{G}) = E_\sigma \sup_{g \in \mathcal{G}} \frac{1}{n} \sum_{i=1}^{n} \sigma_i g(x_i) = E_\sigma \sup_{g \in \mathcal{G}} \frac{1}{n} \sum_{i=1}^{n} \sigma_i \sum_{l=1}^{n_v} s(x_i, l) f_l(x_i),$$

where σ *is i.i.d. random variable equal to 1 or* -1 *with the probability* $p \in [0, 1/2]$, *and 0 with the probability of* $1 - 2p$.

Since the clustering loss g is defined as a product of the leaf assignment s and the clustering compactness function f (Eq. 2), $\sum_{l=1}^{n_v} \mathfrak{R}(\mathcal{G}_l) \leq \sum_{l=1}^{n_v} \mathfrak{R}(\mathcal{S}_l) + \sum_{l=1}^{n_v} \mathfrak{R}(\mathcal{F}_l)$ (Lemma by DeSalvo et al. [7]), where $\mathcal{S}_l$ and $\mathcal{F}_l$ denote the hypothesis class of leaf assignment and clustering compactness in leaf nodes L_l. Moreover, the complexity of the leaf assignment hypothesis $\mathfrak{R}(\mathcal{S}_l)$ is determined by sequential binary questions stored in the branched nodes,

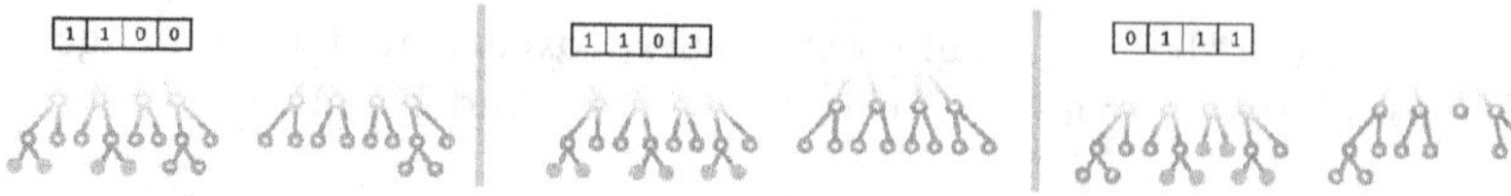

Fig. 2. Three leaf pruning examples on a tree with five layers and eleven leaf nodes. The pruning indicator vectors are shown, where one means pruning. The leaf nodes to be pruned are orange colored, and the remained leaf nodes are green colored. (Color figure online)

and $\mathfrak{R}(\mathcal{S}_l) \leq \sqrt{\frac{2\nu_l(r\log\frac{e}{\eta}+\log 2nr)}{n}}$, similar to the supervised classification forest [7]. ν_l is the depth of the l-th leaf. r is the number of feature channels used in node spitting. $\eta = r/\alpha$, where α is the cardinality of a feature family.

Theorem 1. *For a randomized clustering tree, any independently distributed instance $x_1, x_2, \ldots, x_n \in X$, $X \in \mathcal{D}$, and $\delta > 0$, with probability of at least $1 - \delta$, the following holds*

$$
\begin{aligned}
E_x g(x) \leq &\frac{1}{n}\sum_{i=1}^{n} g(x_i) \\
&+ \sum_{l=1}^{n_v}\left(\frac{\sqrt{\pi/2}a_l^2(2+\sqrt{n_l})}{n_l}\sqrt{\sum_{i=1}^{n_l}(1-\tau_i)^2 + \sqrt{\frac{2\nu_l(r\log\frac{e}{\eta}+\log 2nr)}{n}}}\right).
\end{aligned}
\tag{3}
$$

The learning bound is given considering the sequential tree traversals determined by questions stored in branch nodes, as well as the clustering compactness. a_l denotes the data radius of leaf node L_l, and $\forall x \in L_l, \|x\| \leq a_l$. The proof of Theorem 1 is given in the supplemental material.

Given the learning bound in Theorem 1 and the randomized clustering forest (Sect. 2.1), we propose a tree-pruning algorithm to remove the trivial and inconsistent leaf nodes. (1) For each tree in the randomized clustering forest, locate the paired leaf nodes with brothers as pruning candidates (Fig. 2). For a clustering tree with q paired leaf nodes, there are 2^q possibilities for tree pruning. (2) Randomly sample n_q possibilities, and find the one minimizing the learning bound (Eq. 3). The procedure is repeated for each tree in the forest. Since the clustering loss favors the supervoxels with high CLS scores, the resulted SC forest is spatially consistent in the sense that corresponding supervoxels bear similar contextual leaf assignments.

Given the SC forest, it is straightforward to get the pairwise affinity matrix A. For the k-th tree, $A_{k,ij} = d(x_i, x_j)$, determined by the common traversal path as in Eq. 1. The affinity estimated by the forest with n_t trees is $A = 1/n_t \sum_{k=1}^{n_t} A_k$.

3   Experiments

The experimental dataset consists of 150 clinically-captured CBCT images of orthodontic patients. All CBCT images are of the same size ($500 \times 500 \times 476$)

and resolution ($0.4 \times 0.4 \times 0.4$ mm^3). The histogram matching is applied in the preprocessing. The supervoxels are extracted by the SLIC algorithm [1]. It is intuitive that the small supervoxel produces accurate correspondence because the fine structure boundary can be captured. The supervoxel number extracted from each CBCT image is set at 5000 for a tradeoff between the forest complexity and the correspondence accuracy. The comparably large context is helpful to discriminate supervoxels regarding the contextual leaf assignments, though it introduces additional computational costs. In our experiments, the cube size is set at 40 mm considering the discriminative capacity and the computational complexity.

It is not a trivial task to label the supervoxel-wise correspondence between CBCT images manually. The benchmark supervoxel correspondence is established by the non-rigid B-spline based registration, where the supervoxel labels of the reference CBCT image are transferred to others. Due to independent supervoxel decompositions of CBCT images, the supervoxel boundaries are variable. The supervoxel is labeled by its counterpart of the reference image with the largest overlapping volume in our experiments.

The supervoxel correspondence by the proposed method is evaluated by the accurate label ratio (ALR) $e_l = n_a/n_s$, where n_a is the number of supervoxel with accurate labels by the correspondence establishment. n_s is a total number of tested supervoxels. We also qualitatively assess the correspondence performance by two metrics, the Dice Similarity coefficients (DSC) and the average Hausdorff distance (AHD), under the label propagation scenarios. The labeling accuracies of four structures, i.e. the mandible, the maxilla, the zygoma arch, and the teeth, are reported. The four-fold cross-validation is performed. In the training step, the supervoxels from 75% CBCT images of the training set are used to train the clustering random forest. We compare with other random-forest-based methods, including the classification forest (CLA-forest), the regression forest (REG-forest) [8], and the clustering forest (CLU-forest) [9]. All forests are composed of ten trees with a minimum leaf size set at five.

Table 1. The label propagation accuracies assessed by the DSC and AHD on the clinically-captured CBCT images by the proposed method (SC-forest), the classification forest (CLA-forest), the regression forest (REG-forest) [8], and the clustering forest (CLU-forest) [9].

	Mandible		Maxilla		Zygoma Arch		Teeth	
	DSC	AHD	DSC	AHD	DSC	AHD	DSC	AHD
CLA-forest	0.88 ± 0.02	0.3 ± 0.03	0.81 ± 0.03	0.31 ± 0.03	0.9 ± 0.02	0.29 ± 0.03	0.87 ± 0.02	0.32 ± 0.03
REG-forest	0.81 ± 0.03	0.32 ± 0.03	0.76 ± 0.03	0.35 ± 0.03	0.88 ± 0.03	0.3 ± 0.03	0.83 ± 0.02	0.34 ± 0.03
CLU-forest	0.89 ± 0.02	0.31 ± 0.03	0.86 ± 0.03	0.32 ± 0.03	0.92 ± 0.02	0.28 ± 0.03	0.9 ± 0.03	0.31 ± 0.03
SC-forest	0.92 ± 0.02	0.29 ± 0.02	0.89 ± 0.02	0.29 ± 0.03	0.94 ± 0.02	0.27 ± 0.03	0.93 ± 0.02	0.29 ± 0.02

3.1   Correspondence Results

Table 1 illustrates the mean and standard deviation of DSC and AHD of four structures, including the mandible, the maxilla, the zygoma arch, and the teeth, by the supervised CLA and REG forests, and the unsupervised CLU forest with and without tree-pruning. Figure 3(a-d) illustrate the DSC boxplots of four types of structures on the clinically-captured CBCT images. The ALR by the CLA, REG, CLU-forests are 0.83, 0.79, 0.85 vs. 0.89 by the proposed SC-forest as shown in Fig. 3(e). The label propagation of all structures by the proposed method outperforms other supervised and unsupervised random-forest-based methods. The unsupervised forest built upon a large image set, including approx. 110 CBCT images in our experiments, outperforms the supervised random forests trained by limited data from just one volumetric image. Moreover, the SC forest with tree pruning under the guidance of the learning bound produces an improvement to the original clustering forest (CLU-forest). Experiments demonstrate that the leaf node pruning facilitates affinity estimation and correspondence establishment. The average DSC of label propagation of the maxilla by the conventional patch fusion (PF) [3] and the convex optimization (CO) [10] based methods are 0.81 and 0.87 vs. 0.89 by the proposed SC forest. It turns out the proposed method also yields improvements to PF and CO based methods. Moreover, the testing costs by the SC forest-based method, depending

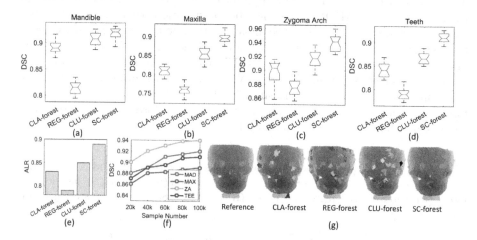

Fig. 3. The DSC boxplots of the label propagation accuracies on clinically-captured CBCT images of the proposed method (SC-forest), the classification forest (CLA-forest), the regression forest (REG-forest) [8], and the clustering forest (CLU-forest) [9] on four craniofacial structures, including (a) the mandible, (b) the maxilla, (c) the zygoma arches, and (d) the teeth. (e) The ALR of the proposed SC-forest, as well as the CLA, REG, and CLU forests. (f)The labeling accuracies with different sample numbers. (g) One supervoxel labeling case by forest-based methods. From left to right are the reference image, labeling results based on the CLA-forest, the REG-forest, the CLU-forest, and the SC-forest.

on fast tree traversals, are lower than registration-based PF [3] and nonlinear CO-based method [10].

The SC forest is built with tree pruning to minimize the learning bound. In our experiments, n_q of 2^q pruning possibilities are randomly selected to find the optimal tree pruning. Figure 3(f) illustrates the labeling accuracy with variable n_q. We observe that the more samples, the better labeling performances. The brute searching of all possibilities will result to the globally-optimal tree pruning, though it is time-consuming. n_q is set at 100k in all tree pruning experiments.

4   Conclusion

In this paper, we present a theoretical analysis of the clustering hypothesis complexity for the unsupervised random forest. Under the guidance of the learning bound, we propose a tree-pruning algorithm to refine the randomized clustering forest by removing the trivial and inconsistent paired leaf nodes. The proposed method has been applied to the affinity estimation and correspondence establishment of supervoxels extracted from CBCT images. The experiments demonstrate the proposed method has better performances in the correspondence-based label propagation than the compared conventional approaches.

Acknowledgments. This work was supported by National Natural Science Foundation of China under Grant 61272342.

References

1. Achanta, R., Shaji, A., Smith, K., Lucchi, A., Fua, P., Süsstrunk, S.: Slic superpixels compared to state-of-the-art superpixel methods. IEEE Trans. Pattern Anal. Mach. Intell. **34**(11), 2274–2282 (2012)
2. Breiman, L.: Random forests. Mach. Learn. **45**(1), 5–32 (2001)
3. Coupé, P., Manjón, J.V., Fonov, V., Pruessner, J., Robles, M., Collins, D.L.: Patch-based segmentation using expert priors: Application to hippocampus and ventricle segmentation. NeuroImage **54**(2), 940–954 (2011)
4. Criminisi, A., Shotton, J., Konukoglu, E.: Decision forests for classification, regression, density estimation, manifold learning and semi-supervised learning. Microsoft Research Cambridge, Technical report MSRTR-2011-114, vol. 5, no. 6, p. 12 (2011)
5. Criminisi, A., Shotton, J., Robertson, D., Konukoglu, E.: Regression forests for efficient anatomy detection and localization in CT studies. In: Menze, B., Langs, G., Tu, Z., Criminisi, A. (eds.) MCV 2010. LNCS, vol. 6533, pp. 106–117. Springer, Heidelberg (2011). doi:10.1007/978-3-642-18421-5_11
6. Denil, M., Matheson, D., De Freitas, N.: Narrowing the gap: random forests in theory and in practice. In: ICML, pp. 665–673 (2014)
7. DeSalvo, G., Mohri, M.: Random composite forests. In: AAAI, pp. 1540–1546 (2016)
8. Kanavati, F., Tong, T., Misawa, K., Fujiwara, M., Mori, K., Rueckert, D., Glocker, B.: Supervoxel classification forests for estimating pairwise image correspondences. Pattern Recogn. **63**, 561–569 (2017)

9. Pei, Y., Kim, T.K., Zha, H.: Unsupervised random forest manifold alignment for lipreading. In: Proceedings of the IEEE International Conference on Computer Vision, pp. 129–136 (2013)
10. Wang, L., et al.: Automated segmentation of CBCT image using spiral CT atlases and convex optimization. In: Mori, K., Sakuma, I., Sato, Y., Barillot, C., Navab, N. (eds.) MICCAI 2013. LNCS, vol. 8151, pp. 251–258. Springer, Heidelberg (2013). doi:10.1007/978-3-642-40760-4_32
11. Zikic, D., Glocker, B., Criminisi, A.: Encoding atlases by randomized classification forests for efficient multi-atlas label propagation. Med. Image Anal. **18**(8), 1262–1273 (2014)

Multi-scale Volumetric ConvNet with Nested Residual Connections for Segmentation of Anterior Cranial Base

Yuru Pei[1(✉)], Haifang Qin[1], Gengyu Ma[2], Yuke Guo[3], Gui Chen[4], Tianmin Xu[4], and Hongbin Zha[1]

[1] Key Laboratory of Machine Perception (MOE),
Department of Machine Intelligence, Peking University, Beijing, China
Peiyuru@cis.pku.edu.cn
[2] uSens Inc., San Jose, USA
[3] Luoyang Institute of Science and Technology, Luoyang, China
[4] School of Stomatology, Peking University, Beijing, China

Abstract. Anterior cranial base (ACB) is known as the growth-stable structure. Automatic segmentation of the ACB is a prerequisite to superimpose orthodontic inter-treatment cone-beam computed tomography (CBCT) images. The automatic ACB segmentation is still a challenging task because of the ambiguous intensity distributions around fine-grained structures and artifacts due to the limited radiation dose. We propose a fully automatic segmentation of the ACB from CBCT images by a volumetric convolutional network with nested residual connections (NRN). The multi-scale feature fusion in the NRN not only promotes the information flows, but also introduces the supervision to multiple intermediate layers to speed up the convergence. The multi-level shortcut connections augment the feature maps in the decompression pathway and the end-to-end voxel-wise label prediction. The proposed NRN has been applied to the ACB segmentation from clinically-captured CBCT images. The quantitative assessment over the practitioner-annotated ground truths demonstrates the proposed method produces improvements to the state-of-the-arts.

1 Introduction

In clinical orthodontics, the anterior cranial base (ACB) is recognized as one stable structure, reaching a full growth at a very early age [1]. Automatic segmentation of the ACB is crucial for the superimposition of inter-treatment cone-beam computed tomography (CBCT) images [4], and in turn for the treatment planning and evaluation in clinical orthodontics. The manual annotation is extremely tedious and prone to inter- and intra-observer variations. Given the blurry CBCT images with artifacts due to the limited radiation dose, it is not a trivial job to obtain complete and reliable contours even by the level-set method using interactively-defined shape priors. Faced with the blurry images of fine-grained

© Springer International Publishing AG 2017
Q. Wang et al. (Eds.): MLMI 2017, LNCS 10541, pp. 123–131, 2017.
DOI: 10.1007/978-3-319-67389-9_15

structures compared with surrounding tissues, the automatic and reliable segmentation of the ACB from CBCT images is much needed yet challenging.

The automatic structure segmentation is a well-defined problem and has been addressed in medical image processing for several decades. The statistical shape model [16] was efficient for solving in a reduced parameter space but subjected to limited capacities to accommodate shape variations of fine-grained bony structures. Segmentation based on non-rigid registration or template-warping [6] involved high online computational costs. The level-set-based (LS) method [9] relied on a variety of deliberately-designed shape priors and suffered from inheritable error accumulations in the label propagation process. Nowadays the ConvNet is one of the mainstream machine learning techniques. The end-to-end pixel-wise prediction networks for image segmentation [12] have been extended for 3D volumetric medical image segmentation [2,3,5,10,13,15]. The voxel-wise label prediction network generally includes two parts: an image compression pathway and a decompression pathway for label images. Shortcut connections are added to the ConvNet [2,3,5,13] using the multi-scale abstracted feature maps for label prediction, which can be seen as variants of the residual network [8]. A mixture of long-jump and local residual connections has been used for 3D volumetric image segmentation [10,15]. The above networks just fused feature maps of the same scale. Furthermore, a set of variations have been introduced to the fully convolutional network to take advantage of multi-scale features, such as zooming out features [11], hypercolumns descriptors [7], and deep supervision network (DSN) [14]. Although existed variants of ConvNet do not explicitly discuss the integration of multi-scale feature fusion and multi-level deep supervision in end-to-end 3D image segmentations, they have shown a great potential to further volumetric medical image processing of fine-grained structures.

In this paper, we propose a novel 3D ConvNet with nested residual connections (NRN) (see Fig. 1) by an integration of the multi-scale feature fusion and multi-level deep supervision for the ACB segmentation from CBCT images. The NRN, built upon the deconvolutional U-net [5], utilizes cross-level shortcut connections to exploit a full potential of multi-scale abstracted image features. The NRN is effective to enforce the information propagation and to speed up the convergence rate. Moreover, the multiple connections from image feature maps to the final label map introduce labeling supervisions to the intermediate feature map learning. In the NRN, the deconvolutional upsampling with fractional strides is used for the cross-level feature map fusion. Given the cross-level shortcut connections, the NRN can be seen as a nested residual network, where a large residual block encloses a small one. In our system, a four-ring nested residual network is built as shown in Fig. 1. The long-jump cross-level shortcut connections, as well as residual connection inside convolutional and deconvolutional blocks, augment feature maps in the decompression pathway, especially for the fine-grained structures such as the ACB.

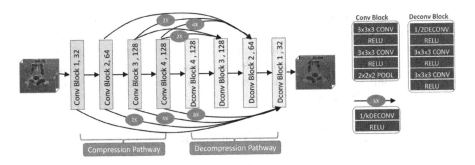

Fig. 1. Architecture of the proposed NRN.

2 Methods

We investigate the integration of the multi-scale feature fusion and the multi-level deep supervision for reliable segmentation of the ACB, where the nested residual connections are introduced to promote information propagation and further reinforce the final binary label prediction.

2.1 Network Architecture

As shown in Fig. 1, the network is built upon the deconvolution network [5,12] with symmetric compression and decompression pathways. The compression pathway is composed of four convolutional blocks (Conv-block) and four deconvolutional blocks (Deconv-block). Each Conv-block consists of two duplicated $3 \times 3 \times 3$ convolution layers with a stride of one and a $2 \times 2 \times 2$ pooling layer. The Rectified Linear Unit layer (RELU) follows each convolutional layer. Thus, the abstracted feature maps in the compression pathway are of four resolution levels. The decompression pathway is composed of four Deconv-blocks. The Deconv-block consists of one convolutional layer with a stride of $1/2$ for upsampling feature maps, and duplicated convolutional layers with a stride of 1 and a receptive field of $3 \times 3 \times 3$.

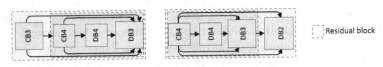

Fig. 2. Examples of nested residual blocks in the proposed NRN. (CB-Conv block, DB-Deconv block)

The shortcut connections are appended between four levels of Conv-blocks and the Deconv-blocks of the same or higher resolutions. Aside from the shortcut connections between blocks of the same resolution, the proposed NRN also has the cross-level connections, e.g. Conv block 2 → Deconv block 1. For the cross-level connections illustrated as side arrows (Fig. 1), the deconvolution with fractional strides are utilized to up-sample the feature maps to be of the same resolution as the counterparts in the decompression pathway. Let's denote the output label map as X_o. The sigmoid function is used to convert the continuous feature map to a label map.

$$X_o = sigm\left(X_d^{(1)} + \sum_{i=1}^{L} g(X_c^{(i)}, W_r^{(i)}, b_r^{(i)})\right),\tag{1}$$

where function $g(\cdot)$ is the convolution followed by ReLU. W_r and b_r are the weight and bias parameters of cross-level connections. L is the number of Conv-blocks, and set at four in our network. The final output X_o is affected by both the mainstream convolution $X_d^{(1)}$ and the accumulated deconvolved feature maps $g(X_c^{(i)}, W_r^{(i)}, b_r^{(i)})$ from the compression pathway. That is, the supervision is introduced to intermediate multi-scale layers in the compression pathway. X_c and X_d denote feature maps in the compression and decompression pathways respectively. Given the multi-level shortcut connections, the fused l-th level feature map $\tilde{X}_d^{(l)} = X_c^{(l)} + H^{(l)}$. The residual function

$$H^{(l)} = g(\tilde{X}_d^{(l+1)}, W_d^{(l)}, b_d^{(l)}) + \sum_{i=l+1}^{L} g(X_c^{(i)}, W_r^{(i)}, b_r^{(i)}).\tag{2}$$

W_d and b_d are the weight and bias parameters of the convolution layer in the decompression pathway. The shortcut connections introduce a residual network as described in [8]. It's interesting to note that the NRN is nested since there are connections between feature maps of different scales. We rewrite Eq. 2 as

$$H^{(l)} = g(H^{(l+1)}, W_d^{(l)}, b_d^{(l)}) + K,\tag{3}$$

where $K = g(X_c^{(l+1)}, W_d^{(l)}, b_d^{(l)}) + \sum_{i=l+1}^{L} g(X_c^{(i)}, W_r^{(i)}, b_r^{(i)})$. We explicitly address the integration of the multi-scale feature fusion and multi-level deep supervision in the end-to-end 3D image segmentations. The deconvolutional connections between multi-scale feature maps in the compression and decompression pathways strengthen feature maps for the segmentation map prediction. The proposed method is different from the deep residual network (DRN) [8], which is a concatenation of local residual blocks. The shortcut connections across multi-scale feature maps result in a nested residual network (see Fig. 2). At the same time, the supervision is introduced to the intermediate feature maps by the shortcut connections to the final segmentation maps, which looks similar to the DSN [14] and MRN [15]. However, the proposed work is different from the DSN [14] and MRN [15] in that the nested multi-scale shortcut connections also contribute to the intermediate feature maps aside from the final label map.

2.2 Training

The proposed NRN is utilized to perform the ene-to-end segmentation map inference, where per-voxel labels of the whole input volume are obtained simultaneously without subvolume sliding and cropping. The stochastic gradient descent solver of the Keras toolkit is used to train the network. The voxel-wise cross entropy loss function $\mathcal{L} = -\sum (x_o \ln y + (1 - x_o) \ln (1 - y)) + \sum_{i=\{d,c,r\}} \alpha_i \|W_i\|^2$, where y denotes the ground truth segmentation label. The constant α_c, α_d, and α_r are set at 1, 1, and 0.5 for the regularization of the compression, decompression, and long-jump connection parameters. The training is performed on a PC with a NVIDIA TITAN X GPU, and took 10 h after 300 epochs. The batch size is set at two considering the GPU memory. The momentum is set at 0.9. The learning rate is set at 1e-4, and divided by 10 after every 100 epochs. The weight decay is set at 5e-4. The batch normalization is imposed on each layer to handle the internal covariance shift problem by making the input data of each layer to be of zero mean and unit variance.

3 Experiments

Data Set. The training data set includes 120 clinically captured CBCT images. The CBCT images are captured by a NewTom scanner with a 12-in field of view. The volume block of the ACB is of a resolution of $160 \times 160 \times 64$. The ground truth label maps are interactively defined using the software ITKSnap. The isotropic voxel size is 0.4 mm $\times$ 0.4 mm $\times$ 0.4 mm.

3D medical image segmentation tasks are often faced with limited training data in contrast to large amounts of annotation data in natural image processing. We use the non-rigid data augmentation to improve shape variations in limited clinically-captured data, where the randomly sampled B-spline deformations are utilized to generate a training data set of 4 k volumetric images.

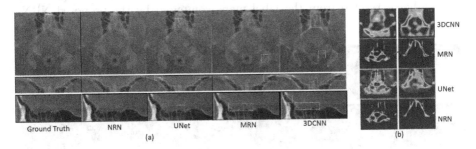

Fig. 3. (a) Comparison of ACB segmentations by the proposed NRN, U-Net [5], MRN [15], and 3DCNN [12] (with failed cases yellow outlined). (b) Comparisons of feature maps of Deconv block 2 by the proposed NRN, U-Net [5], MRN [15], and 3DCNN [12]. (Color figure online)

Qualitative Assessment. We perform the ablation experiments to evaluate the effectiveness of the cross-level residual connections. The four-fold cross-validation scheme is employed. The proposed NRN is compared with three variants of the CNN, including the U-Net with long jump connections [13], the mixed residual network (MRN) with both local and long residual connections [15], and the 3D-CNN without residual connections [12] as shown in Fig. 3(a). In our experiments, except for the shortcut connections, all network have the same mainstream architectures. That is, all networks have four Conv-blocks and four Deconv-blocks in the mainstream architectures. The segmentation accuracy is evaluated using three metrics: the Dice similarity coefficient (DSC), the average Hausdorff distance (AHD), and the mean surface deviation (MSD) of ACB surface meshes as shown in Table 1. We also compare the proposed NRN with traditional segmentation methods, including the level set (LS) [9] and the registration-based (REG) methods [6] as shown in Table 1. The segmentation accuracies in term of the DSC, AHD, and MSD of thirty images in the test set are shown in Fig. 5(a–c). The DSC, AHD, and MSD of the ACB segmentation by the proposed NRN are $0.81, 0.33$ mm, and 0.50 mm, which outperform compared approaches.

Table 1. Segmentation accuracies of the proposed NRN, U-Net [5], MRN [15], 3DCNN [12], LS [9], and REG [6] methods.

	NRN	U-Net [5]	MRN [15]	3DCNN [12]	REG [6]	LS [9]
DSC	**0.81 ± 0.003**	0.78 ± 0.003	0.76 ± 0.002	0.63 ± 0.002	0.42 ± 0.006	0.12 ± 0.004
AHD	**0.33 ± 0.02**	0.49 ± 0.03	0.44 ± 0.02	0.64 ± 0.01	0.96 ± 0.08	1.43 ± 0.15
MSD	**0.50 ± 0.002**	0.56 ± 0.002	0.72 ± 0.002	1.16 ± 0.005	1.77 ± 0.02	0.85 ± 0.03

We measure the surface mesh deviation (MSD) between the surfaces extracted from the volumetric label maps of the ground truth annotations as shown in Table 1. The iso-surfaces are extracted by ITKSnap. The sampled surface meshes extracted from the label maps computed by the proposed NRN,

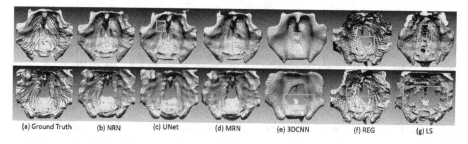

(a) Ground Truth   (b) NRN   (c) UNet   (d) MRN   (e) 3DCNN   (f) REG   (g) LS

Fig. 4. Comparisons of surface meshes extracted from the label maps of (a) the ground truth, (b) the proposed NRN, (c) U-Net [5], (d) MRN [15], (e) 3DCNN [12], (f) REG [6], and (g) LS [9] methods (with failed cases blue outlined). (Color figure online)

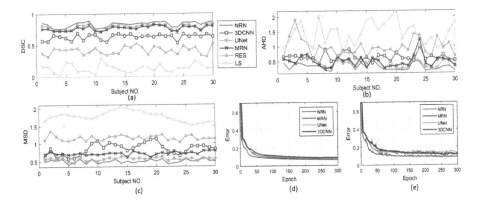

Fig. 5. Comparisons of the ACB segmentations by the proposed NRN, U-Net [5], MRN [15], 3DCNN [12], REG [6], and LS [9] methods in terms of (a) the DSC, (b) the AHD, and (c) the MSD of thirty images in the test set. (d) The training and (e) validation errors of the NRN, 3DU-Net [5], MRN [15], and 3DCNN [12].

3DU-Net [5], MRN [15], and 3DCNN [12] are shown in Fig. 4. The surfaces defined by the NRN coincide with the ground truth in terms of surface completeness and reliability. The ACB bony surfaces obtained by our method are better than the traditional LS [9] and REG [6] methods, where our method does not need any shape priors as shown in Fig. 4.

We compare the learning behavior of the proposed NRN with 3D U-Net [5], MRN [15], and 3DCNN [12]. The validation errors decrease along with the training errors and show no apparent overfitting and no sign of gradient vanishing by the proposed NRN as shown in Fig. 5(d, e). We also compare the feature maps of Deconv block 2 as shown in Fig. 3(b). The feature maps obtained by the proposed NRN have clear contour features of the foreground ACB compared with other CNN variants. The proposed NRN has been demonstrated to be efficient in the learning process with a relatively fast convergence rate.

4   Discussion and Conclusion

We present a novel 3D ConvNet with the multi-scale feature fusion as well as the multi-level deep supervision to handle the segmentation of bony structures of the ACB. The long-jump residual connections across multi-level feature maps augment the information propagation, and introduce the supervision into intermediate layers. In the ablation experiments, the proposed NRN shows faster convergence than other CNN variants with or without residual connections. Moreover, the NRN shows obvious improvements to traditional segmentation methods, including the LS [9] and the registration-based [6] methods. The ACB surfaces extracted from the resulted label maps are complete and consistent with the manually-extracted ACB surfaces, and effectively avoid surface missing and false leaking to surrounding soft tissues. The DSC, AHD, and MSD are

0.81, 0.33 mm, and 0.50 mm for the ACB segmentation by the proposed method, and outperforms the state-of-the-arts in terms of the segmentation accuracy and surface consistency. The proposed NRN is a general framework and can be applied to other volume image processing tasks. In future work, we will investigate the potential of the NRN for the challenging structure segmentation with a noisy background such as occluded dentitions.

Acknowledgments. This work was supported by National Natural Science Foundation of China under Grant 61272342.

References

1. Afrand, M., Ling, C.P., Khosrotehrani, S., Flores-Mir, C., Lagravère-Vich, M.O.: Anterior cranial-base time-related changes: a systematic review. Am. J. Orthod. Dentofac. Orthop. **146**(1), 21–32 (2014)
2. Kayalibay, B., Jensen, G., van der Smagt, P.: Cnn-based segmentation of medical imaging data. arXiv:1701.03056 [cs.CV] (2017)
3. Brosch, T., Tang, L.Y., Yoo, Y., Li, D.K., Traboulsee, A., Tam, R.: Deep 3d convolutional encoder networks with shortcuts for multiscale feature integration applied to multiple sclerosis lesion segmentation. IEEE TMI **35**(5), 1229–1239 (2016)
4. Cevidanes, L.H., Motta, A., Proffit, W.R., Ackerman, J.L., Styner, M.: Cranial base superimposition for 3-dimensional evaluation of soft-tissue changes. Am. J. Orthod. Dentofac. Orthop. **137**(4), S120–S129 (2010)
5. Çiçek, Ö., Abdulkadir, A., Lienkamp, S.S., Brox, T., Ronneberger, O.: 3D U-Net: learning dense volumetric segmentation from sparse annotation. In: Ourselin, S., Joskowicz, L., Sabuncu, M.R., Unal, G., Wells, W. (eds.) MICCAI 2016. LNCS, vol. 9901, pp. 424–432. Springer, Cham (2016). doi:10.1007/978-3-319-46723-8_49
6. Coup, P., Tong, T., Misawa, K., Fujiwara, M., Mori, K., Rueckert, D., Glocker, B., Manjn, J.V., Fonov, V., Pruessner, J., Robles, M., Collins, D.L.: Patch-based segmentation using expert priors: application to hippocampus and ventricle segmentation. NeuroImage **54**(2), 940–954 (2011)
7. Hariharan, B., Arbeláez, P., Girshick, R., Malik, J.: Hypercolumns for object segmentation and fine-grained localization. In: CVPR, pp. 447–456 (2015)
8. He, K., Zhang, X., Ren, S., Sun, J.: Deep residual learning for image recognition. In: CVPR, pp. 770–778 (2016)
9. Li, C., Xu, C., Gui, C., Fox, M.D.: Level set evolution without re-initialization: a new variational formulation. In: CVPR, vol. 1, pp. 430–436 (2005)
10. Milletari, F., Navab, N., Ahmadi, S.A.: V-net: fully convolutional neural networks for volumetric medical image segmentation. In: 3DV, pp. 565–571
11. Mostajabi, M., Yadollahpour, P., Shakhnarovich, G.: Feedforward semantic segmentation with zoom-out features. In: CVPR, pp. 3376–3385 (2015)
12. Noh, H., Hong, S., Han, B.: Learning deconvolution network for semantic segmentation. In: ICCV, pp. 1520–1528 (2015)
13. Ronneberger, O., Fischer, P., Brox, T.: U-Net: convolutional networks for biomedical image segmentation. In: Navab, N., Hornegger, J., Wells, W.M., Frangi, A.F. (eds.) MICCAI 2015. LNCS, vol. 9351, pp. 234–241. Springer, Cham (2015). doi:10.1007/978-3-319-24574-4_28
14. Xie, S., Tu, Z.: Holistically-nested edge detection. In: ICCV, pp. 1395–1403 (2015)

15. Yu, L., Yang, X., Chen, H., Qin, J., Heng, P.A.: Volumetric convnets with mixed residual connections for automated prostate segmentation from 3d mr images. In: AAAI (2017)
16. Zhang, S., Zhan, Y., Dewan, M., Huang, J., Metaxas, D.N., Zhou, X.S.: Deformable segmentation via sparse shape representation. In: Fichtinger, G., Martel, A., Peters, T. (eds.) MICCAI 2011. LNCS, vol. 6892, pp. 451–458. Springer, Heidelberg (2011). doi:10.1007/978-3-642-23629-7_55

Feature Learning and Fusion of Multimodality Neuroimaging and Genetic Data for Multi-status Dementia Diagnosis

Tao Zhou, Kim-Han Thung, Xiaofeng Zhu, and Dinggang Shen[✉]

Department of Radiology, BRIC, University of North Carolina, Chapel Hill, USA
dgshen@med.unc.edu

Abstract. In this paper, we aim to maximally utilize multimodality neuroimaging and genetic data to predict Alzheimer's disease (AD) and its prodromal status, i.e., a multi-status dementia diagnosis problem. Multimodality neuroimaging data such as MRI and PET provide valuable insights to abnormalities, and genetic data such as Single Nucleotide Polymorphism (SNP) provide information about a patient's AD risk factors. When used in conjunction, AD diagnosis may be improved. However, these data are heterogeneous (e.g., having different data distributions), and have different number of samples (e.g., PET data is having far less number of samples than the numbers of MRI or SNPs). Thus, learning an effective model using these data is challenging. To this end, we present a novel *three-stage deep feature learning and fusion framework*, where the deep neural network is trained stage-wise. Each stage of the network learns feature representations for different combination of modalities, via effective training using *maximum number of available samples*. Specifically, in the first stage, we learn latent representations (i.e., high-level features) for each modality independently, so that the heterogeneity between modalities can be better addressed and then combined in the next stage. In the second stage, we learn the joint latent features for each pair of modality combination by using the high-level features learned from the first stage. In the third stage, we learn the diagnostic labels by fusing the learned joint latent features from the second stage. We have tested our framework on Alzheimer's Disease Neuroimaging Initiative (ADNI) dataset for multi-status AD diagnosis, and the experimental results show that the proposed framework outperforms other methods.

1 Introduction

Alzheimer's disease (AD) is the most common form of dementia that often affect individuals over 65 years old. According to a recent report from Alzheimer's Association, the total estimated prevalence of AD is expected to be 60 million worldwide over the next 50 years. As there is no cure for AD, the accurate diagnosis of AD and especially its prodromal stage, i.e., mild cognitive impairment (MCI), which can be further categorized into progressive MCI (p-MCI) and stable MCI (s-MCI), is highly desirable in clinical application.

© Springer International Publishing AG 2017
Q. Wang et al. (Eds.): MLMI 2017, LNCS 10541, pp. 132–140, 2017.
DOI: 10.1007/978-3-319-67389-9_16

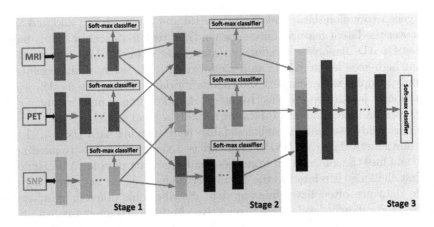

Fig. 1. Proposed diagnostic framework for AD diagnosis by deep feature learning.

In search of an accurate biomarker for AD, data from different types of modalities have been collected and investigated [6,14,17]. Among these modalities, neuroimaging techniques such as Magnetic Resonance Imaging (MRI) and Positron Emission Topography (PET), are able to provide anatomical and functional information about the brain, respectively. Many studies in recent years have shown that fusing the information from multiple neuroimaging modalities will enhance the performance of AD diagnosis [3]. On the other hand, genome-wide association studies have identified a series of genetic variations (e.g., Single Nucleotide Polymorphism (SNP)) that are associated with AD. In addition, the association between the SNP genotype data and the neuroimaging phenotype features has also been studied [1,9]. Through the genetic information from SNPs, we can asses the risk factor of an individual likely to get AD, while through the brain structural and functional information gathered from neuroimaging data, we can assess the current brain abnormality of an individual. Both types of information are complementary to each other, and, when used together, may able to improve the AD diagnosis.

Machine learning approaches have been widely used in neuroimaging-based AD diagnosis. Their performances generally depend on how well they can transform the neuroimages into representations that can be effectively used for AD identification. This transformation is commonly called feature learning or representation, which involves techniques like feature extraction and selection. For example, works in [8,15] uses sparse learning to select discriminative features for AD diagnosis. On the other hand, deep learning, which has been proven effective in many classification applications, has the ability to learn high-level abstraction (or latent patterns) from the data. Because of this, deep learning has been widely applied in biomedical research, achieving promising results. For example, Xiao et al. [16] used stacked deep polynomial networks to learn multimodal neuroimaging features for AD diagnosis. Fakoor et al. [4] used unsupervised deep learning methods such as Stack Auto-Encoder (SAE) to enhance cancer diagnosis using gene expression data, and Suk et al. [13] and Liu et al. [11] adopted SAE to discover the latent feature representation from region-of-interest (ROI) based features for AD diagnosis. In addition, some related works [11–13] focused on learning high-level features from multimodality data. However, all these methods used only samples with complete multimodality data to train the model, which may seriously jeopardize the effectiveness of deep learning, a process which generally relies on large amount of data for training a good model.

In this study, we will use multimodality neuroimaging data (i.e., MRI and PET) and genetic data (i.e., SNP). There are two challenges on how to maximally utilize and fuse the information from these multimodality data for AD diagnosis. The first challenge is related to the data heterogeneity, as the neuroimaging and genetic data are often have different data distributions, different numbers of features, and different levels of discriminative ability to AD diagnosis (e.g., SNP data in its raw form are less effective in AD diagnosis). Thus, using these data directly by simple concatenation will result in an inaccurate prediction model. The second challenge is the small sample size issue caused by incomplete data, i.e., not all samples have all the three modalities. As deep learning performs better when it is trained using a large number of samples, the small sample size issue may severely affect its performance.

In this paper, we propose a novel three-stage deep feature learning and fusion framework to address the above challenges, as shown in Fig. 1. Specifically, we train our networks stage-wise, where, at each stage, we learn the latent data representations (high-level features) for different combination of modalities by using the maximum number of available samples. Specifically, in the first stage, we learn high-level features for each modality independently, so that the heterogeneity between modalities can be better addressed and different modality data can be more comparable in the latent representation space. For instance, for SNPs with high dimensionality, we use more hidden layers (compared to MRI and PET data), but with gradually decreased number of neurons for subsequent layers, to reduce its dimensionality while capturing its latent features, so that it is more comparable with the latent features learned from the neuroimaging data. In other words, we address the data heterogeneity issue by learning latent features through progressive mapping via multiple hidden layers. In the second stage, we learn joint features for each modality combination by using the high-level latent features learned from the first stage. In the third stage, we learn the diagnostic labels by fusing the learned joint features from the second stage. It is worth noting that to effectively train each stage of the network, one must use the maximum number of available samples. For example, in the first stage, to learn the high-level latent features from MRI data, we use all the available MRI data; in the second stage, to learn the joint high-level features from MRI and PET data, we use all samples with both MRI and PET data. By this way, the small-sample-size and incomplete dataset issues are partially addressed.

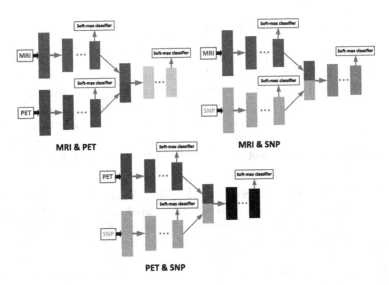

Fig. 2. Stage 2 includes training three DNN architectures for joint latent representation learning of any pair of modalities (i.e., MRI and PET, MRI and SNP, PET and SNP). Note that for each DNN architecture, there are three (soft-max) outputs which are used simultaneously to train the network.

2   Methodology

Our goal is to learn a multi-status AD diagnostic model that can identify different statuses of AD, i.e., Normal Control (NC – no dementia), MCI (prodromal status of AD, which can be further categorized to p-MCI and s-MCI), and AD. We achieve this by training a three-stage Deep Neural Network (DNN) as shown in Fig. 1, using MRI, PET and SNP data. We train our networks stage-wise, since we want to learn the latent features from different combinations of modalities by best using all the available samples for each combination. The details of this framework are discussed below.

Stage 1: Independent single-modality deep feature learning. As described earlier, three modalities have different number of samples, e.g., the PET data has far less number of samples than numbers of MRI and SNPs. Our aim in this stage is to learn discriminative high-level features from each modality by using all its available training samples. We first employ DNN architecture on each independent modality, with the respective network architecture depicted as **Stage 1** in Fig. 1. In each DNN architecture, there are multiple fully-connected layers and one output layer (e.g., soft-max classifier). The output layer consists of three neurons for the case of three-class classification (i.e., AD/MCI/NC classification task), or four neurons for the case of four-class classification (i.e., AD/p-MCI/s-MCI/AD classification task). The label information from the training data at the output layer is also used to guide the learning of the network weights. After training, the outputs of hidden layers can be regarded as the high-level features for each of different modalities. Note that we use the maximum number of available samples for each modality in this stage, for effective training. For example, assume that we have N subjects, where only N_1 subjects contain MRI data, N_2 subjects contain PET data, and N_3 subjects contain SNP data. The conventional multimodality model uses only the subjects with all three modality data, which is much less than $min(N_1, N_2, N_3)$. On the other hand, by using our proposed framework, we can use all the N_1, N_2 and N_3 samples to train three separate deep learning models for three modalities, respectively. It is expected that, by using more samples in training, our model can have better ability for feature representation.

Stage 2: Joint two-modality deep feature learning. As mentioned, different combinations of two modalities (i.e., MRI and PET, MRI and SNP, PET and SNP) are used to learn their joint or shared representations. The aim of this stage is to fuse complementary information from different modalities to further improve the performance of the model. The architecture used in this study is depicted in Fig. 2. There are a total of three DNN architectures, one for each pair of modalities. Specifically, the outputs from hidden layers in **Stage 1** are regarded as intermediate inputs in **Stage 2**, and the weights from **Stage 1** can be regarded as initial weights to initialize the DNN architecture for **Stage 2**. In addition, use three outputs to train each DNN architecture. Two of the outputs are used to guide the learning of high-level features from two different modalities, while the other is used to guide the learning of joint high-level features for the two modalities. Using three outputs simultaneously during the network training can balancing the high-level features learning at different level of modality combinations.

Stage 3: Joint three-modality deep feature learning and fusion. After training the networks in **Stage 2**, we can obtain joint representations between any pair of modalities, which can then be used to get a final prediction. The architecture used in this stage is depicted as **Stage 3** in Fig. 1. In **Stage 3**, we use the learned joint high-level features from **Stage 2** as input and the target labels as output. Obviously, in **Stage 3**, we can use only the samples with complete MRI, PET and SNP data to train the remaining network, and fine-tune the whole network. Afterward, we obtain the diagnostic label for each new sample, based on the output of the last classification layer (i.e., soft-max classifier in **Stage 3**).

3 Experimental Results and Analysis

3.1 Dataset

We use MRI, PET and SNP data from the ADNI dataset[1] for multi-status AD diagnosis. We use the baseline data from a total of 805 subjects, including 190 AD, 389 MCI and 226 normal controls (NC) subjects. All the subjects have MRI data, while only 736 subjects have SNP data, and 360 subjects have PET data.

---

[1] http://www.loni.usc.edu/ADNI.

Table 1. Demographic information of the baseline subjects in the study.

	Female/male	Education	Age	MMSE
NC	108/118	16.0 ± 2.9	75.8 ± 5.0	29.1 ± 1.0
MCI	138/251	15.6 ± 3.0	74.9 ± 7.3	27.0 ± 1.8
AD	101/89	14.7 ± 3.1	75.2 ± 7.5	23.3 ± 2.0
Total	347/458	15.5 ± 3.0	75.2 ± 6.8	26.7 ± 2.7

The MCI subjects can be further categorized into two subclasses, i.e., p-MCI and s-MCI, which are retrospectively determined by monitoring the disease status of MCI subjects after certain period of time (e.g., 24 months). However, since some MCI subjects dropped out of the study after the baseline scans, their sublabels (p-MCI or s-MCI) can not be determined. Hence, the total number of p-MCI (i.e., 205) and s-MCI (i.e., 157) subjects does not match with the total number of baseline MCI subjects. The detailed demographic information of the baseline subjects are summarized in Table.1. After preprocessing steps (including skull stripping, cerebellum removal, intensity correction, tissue segmentation, etc.), the MRI and PET images were divided into 93 ROIs, and the gray matter volumes and the average PET intensity values of these ROIs were calculated as MRI and PET features, respectively. In addition, for SNP data, according to the AlzGene database[2], we only select SNPs that belong to the top AD gene candidates, and those selected SNP data have 3023 features.

3.2 Experimental Setup

In this section, we evaluate the effectiveness of the proposed deep feature learning and fusion framework by considering two classification tasks: (1) AD vs. MCI vs. NC (i.e., three-class classification task) and (2) AD vs. p-MCI vs. s-MCI vs. NC (i.e., four-class classification task). For each classification task, a twenty-fold cross-validation technique was used for evaluation. Specifically, 5% of the subjects were randomly selected as testing samples, and the remaining subjects were used as training samples. 10% of the samples from the training set were used as validation set to select parameters of the networks. In order to reduce randomness, the process was performed 10 times. The final classification results were computed by averaging the results from all the experiments. In the first stage, we built a two-hidden-layer (i.e., 32-16) DNN for MRI and PET data, respectively, and a three-hidden-layer (i.e., 128-64-16) DNN for SNPs data. In the following stages, the outputs of the last hidden layer of the previous network were used as inputs, and a two-hidden-layer (i.e., 32-16) DNN was used for the all the modality combinations in the second and third stages. Furthermore, ℓ_1 and ℓ_2 regularizations were imposed on the weight matrices of the networks.

We compared the proposed framework with three popular dimension reduction methods, i.e., Principal Component Analysis (PCA) [7], Canonical

---

[2] www.alzgene.org.

Correlation Analysis (CCA) [5], and Lasso [10]. To fuse the three modalities, we concatenated the feature vectors of the multimodality data into a single long vector for the above three comparison methods. In addition, we also included SAE [13] as another deep feature learning method for comparison. For this method, we obtained SAE-learned features from each modality independently, and then concatenated all the learned features into a single long vector. As a baseline method, we further included the result for the experiment using just the original features without any feature selection (denoted as "Original"). We finally used SVM classifier from LIBSVM toolbox [2] to perform classification for all the above comparison methods. For each classification task, we use grid search to determine the best parameters for the feature selection algorithms and the classifier, based on their performances on the validation set. For instance, the best soft margin parameter C of SVM classifier was determined by grid searching from $\{10^{-4}, \ldots, 10^4\}$.

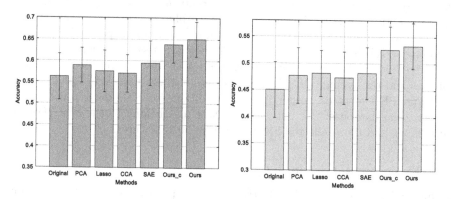

Fig. 3. Comparison of classification accuracy for the three-class classification task (left) and the four-class classification task (right).

Figure 3 shows the classification performance of all the competing methods for two multi-class classification tasks. It can be clearly seen that our proposed method outperforms all other methods, showing the advantage of deep feature learning and high-level feature fusion of our method. Comparing with another deep feature learning strategy, i.e., SAE, its learned high-level features did not perform as well as ours, probably due to the fact the SAE is an unsupervised feature learning method that did not consider label information. In addition, the good performance of our proposed framework could also be due to stage-wise feature learning strategy, which uses the maximum number of available samples for training. For fair comparison, we also include results for our proposed framework that only use samples with complete multimodality data, which are denoted as "Ours-c" in Fig. 3. From Fig. 3, we can see that our proposed framework that uses all available samples ("Ours") still performs better than its degraded version "Ours-c", which uses only complete multimodality data.

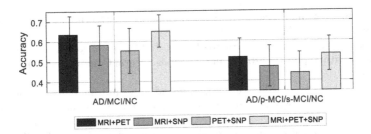

Fig. 4. Comparison of classification accuracy of the proposed framework for AD/MCI/NC and AD/p-MCI/s-MCI/NC by using with different modality combinations.

To further analyze the benefit of neuroimaging and genetic data fusion, Fig. 4 illustrates the performance of our proposed framework for different combinations of modalities. From Fig. 4, it can be seen that our proposed framework performs better when using MRI+PET data if compared with the other two data combinations (i.e., MRI+SNP, PET+SNP). However, when using all the three modalities, genetic data can further improve the classification performance.

4   Conclusion

In this paper, we present a novel three-stage deep learning framework to integrate multimodality neuroimaging and genetic data for multi-status AD diagnosis. We address the data heterogeneity issue in our framework by learning the latent feature representations for each modality before fusing them for AD diagnosis. We also use three-stage learning strategy to effectively learn the latent features for different modality combinations, using maximum number of available samples. Furthermore, small sample size issue due to incomplete dataset is addressed by using all available samples at the respective stages of the network learning. Experimental results using ADNI dataset have clearly demonstrated the effectiveness of our proposed framework in comparison with other state-of-the-art methods.

Acknowledgment. This research was supported in part by NIH grants EB006733, EB008374, EB009634, MH100217, AG041721 and AG042599.

References

1. Biffi, A., Anderson, C.D., Desikan, R.S., et al.: Genetic variation and neuroimaging measures in Alzheimer disease. Arch. Neurol. **67**(6), 677–685 (2010)
2. Chang, C.C., Lin, C.J.: LIBSVM: a library for support vector machines. ACM Trans. Intell. Syst. Tech. (TIST) **2**(3), 27 (2011)
3. Dai, Z., et al.: Discriminative analysis of early Alzheimer's disease using multimodal imaging and multi-level characterization with multi-classifier (M3). Neuroimage **59**(3), 2187–2195 (2012)

4. Fakoor, R., Ladhak, F., Nazi, A., Huber, M.: Using deep learning to enhance cancer diagnosis and classification. In: ICML (2013)
5. Hardoon, D.R., Szedmak, S., Shawe-Taylor, J.: Canonical correlation analysis: an overview with application to learning methods. Neural Comput. **16**(12), 2639–2664 (2004)
6. Hinrichs, C., et al.: Predictive markers for ad in a multi-modality framework: an analysis of MCI progression in the adni population. Neuroimage **55**(2), 574–589 (2011)
7. Jolliffe, I.: Principal Component Analysis. Wiley Online Library (2002)
8. Lei, B., Yang, P., Wang, T., Chen, S., Ni, D.: Relational-regularized discriminative sparse learning for Alzheimer's disease diagnosis. IEEE Trans. Cybern. **47**, 1102–1113 (2017)
9. Lin, D., Cao, H., Calhoun, V., Wang, Y.: Sparse models for correlative and integrative analysis of imaging and genetic data. J. Neurosci. Methods **237**, 69–78 (2014)
10. Liu, J., Chen, J., Ye, J.: Large-scale sparse logistic regression. In: Proceedings of the 15th ACM SIGKDD International Conference on Knowledge Discovery and Data Mining, pp. 547–556. ACM (2009)
11. Liu, S., Liu, S., Cai, W., Che, H., et al.: Multimodal neuroimaging feature learning for multiclass diagnosis of Alzheimer's disease. IEEE Trans. Biomed. Eng. **62**(4), 1132–1140 (2015)
12. Rastegar, S., Soleymani, M., Rabiee, H., Mohsen Shojaee, S.: MDL-CW: a multimodal deep learning framework with cross weights. In: CVPR, pp. 2601–2609 (2016)
13. Suk, H., Lee, S., Shen, D.: Latent feature representation with stacked auto-encoder for AD/MCI diagnosis. Brain Struct. Funct. **220**(2), 841–859 (2015)
14. Thung, K.H., et al.: Neurodegenerative disease diagnosis using incomplete multimodality data via matrix shrinkage and completion. NeuroImage **91**, 386–400 (2014)
15. Ye, J., Farnum, M., Yang, E., et al.: Sparse learning and stability selection for predicting MCI to AD conversion using baseline ADNI data. BMC Neurol. **12**(1), 46 (2012)
16. Zheng, X., Shi, J., Li, Y., Liu, X., Zhang, Q.: Multi-modality stacked deep polynomial network based feature learning for Alzheimer's disease diagnosis. In: 2016 IEEE 13th International Symposium on Biomedical Imaging (ISBI), pp. 851–854. IEEE (2016)
17. Zhu, X., et al.: Subspace regularized sparse multitask learning for multiclass neurodegenerative disease identification. IEEE Trans. Biomed. Eng. **63**(3), 607–618 (2016)

3D Convolutional Neural Networks with Graph Refinement for Airway Segmentation Using Incomplete Data Labels

Dakai Jin, Ziyue Xu$^{(\boxtimes)}$, Adam P. Harrison, Kevin George, and Daniel J. Mollura

National Institutes of Health, Bethesda, MD, USA
ziyue.xu@nih.gov

Abstract. Intrathoracic airway segmentation from computed tomography images is a frequent prerequisite for further quantitative lung analyses. Due to low contrast and noise, especially at peripheral branches, it is often challenging for automatic methods to strike a balance between extracting deeper airway branches and avoiding leakage to the surrounding parenchyma. Meanwhile, manual annotations are extremely time consuming for the airway tree, which inhibits automated methods requiring training data. To address this, we introduce a 3D deep learning-based workflow able to produce high-quality airway segmentation from incompletely labeled training data generated without manual intervention. We first train a 3D fully convolutional network (FCN) based on the fact that 3D spatial information is crucial for small highly anisotropic tubular structures such as airways. For training the 3D FCN, we develop a domain-specific sampling scheme that strategically uses incomplete labels from a previous highly specific segmentation method, aiming to retain similar specificity while boosting sensitivity. Finally, to address local discontinuities of the coarse 3D FCN output, we apply a graph-based refinement incorporating fuzzy connectedness segmentation and robust curve skeletonization. Evaluations on the EXACT'09 and LTRC datasets demonstrate considerable improvements in airway extraction while maintaining reasonable leakage compared with a state-of-art method and the dataset reference standard.

Keywords: Airway tree segmentation · CT · Convolutional neural network · Graph method · Incomplete label

1 Introduction

The intrathoracic airway tree is one of the major organs in the respiratory system. Its morphological changes, such as lumen shape or wall thickness, often

Z. Xu—This work is supported by the Intramural Research Program of the National Institutes of Health, Clinical Center and the National Institute of Allergy and Infectious Diseases. We also thank Nvidia for the donation of a Tesla K40 GPU.

The rights of this work are transferred to the extent transferable according to title 17 § 105 U.S.C.

Q. Wang et al. (Eds.): MLMI 2017, LNCS 10541, pp. 141–149, 2017.
DOI: 10.1007/978-3-319-67389-9_17

relate to the progression of several pulmonary diseases, e.g. asthma and chronic obstructive pulmonary disease (COPD) [1]. The development of *in vivo* computed tomography (CT)-based quantitative airway tree analysis provides valuable information for disease detection, etiologies investigation, and treatment-effects evaluation. Airway tree segmentation is also often a prerequisite for quantitative morphological analysis in image-based approaches.

Due to the structural complexity, this 3D segmentation task is extremely tedious and time consuming using manual or semi-automatic methods, taking more than 7 h or up to 2.5 h [2], respectively. In addition, annotations may be error prone. On the other hand, many automatic methods have been reported, including threshold-based [3], morphology-based [4] and 2D learning-based [5, 6]. Among these, different variations of region growing (RG) are often used. However, imaging resolution limits, airway wall thinness, and other artifacts can all harm CT contrasts, causing RG methods to struggle with leakage into the adjacent lung parenchyma. In contrast, 2D learning-based methods [5,6] potentially add more robustness; however, the extracted airway branches are limited due to the failure of exploiting 3D spatial information, which can be important for 3D airway tree delineation.

In the past decade, deep learning approaches have gained significant success within the natural image domain, due to their unparalleled performance on challenging data [7,8]. Using this powerful technique, several deep learning based-approaches have already been applied to medical image classification and segmentation tasks [6,9–11], most of which work in 2D. For airway segmentation, Charbonnier et al. [6] proposed to use 2D convolutional neural networks (CNNs) for detecting leakages, greatly increasing the extracted airway length compared to previous results. However, their framework does not directly provide a probability map for airway candidates and 3D continuity and tree structural information are not fully utilized under 2D settings. Finally, a limiting factor uniting all these learning-based methods [5,6] is the extreme cost in obtaining annotated airway segmentation as training data. Avoiding the need for fully-annotated data is a crucial quality toward wider adoption within clinical settings.

To address these gaps, we introduce a new 3D deep fully convolutional network (FCN) workflow designed for training on weakly annotated tree structures. Our method is based on the following two modules. (1) A 3D FCN is trained to perform efficient end-to-end learning and inference suitable for 3D airway trees. Crucially, instead of training on manually annotated airways, our workflow trains on incomplete and weakly labeled annotations produced by a previous, highly-specific and moderately-sensitive automated method [4]. We introduce a new domain-specific sampling scheme tailored for tree-like structures, and train our 3D FCN to learn the real airway patterns achieving a similarly high specificity, but with markedly increased sensitivity. (2) Graph-based methods are applied to refine the FCN output, by first using fuzzy-connectedness RG, which combines the 3D FCN probability map and the original CT intensity; and followed by a skeletonization guided leakages removal. We evaluate our method on the Extraction of Airways from CT 2009 (EXACT09) and Lung Tissue Research Consortium (LTRC) datasets, demonstrating high specificity while extracting on average 30 and 70 more tree branches, respectively, compared to the highly-specific baseline method [4].

2   Method

Our method's overall operation is illustrated in Fig. 1. In the following, we first provide details on our proposed 3D FCN architecture, followed by an explanation of our principled and domain-specific data sampling method that allows training with incomplete labels. Finally, we discuss our graph-based refinement methods.

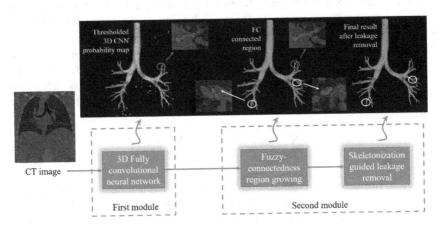

Fig. 1. Schematic illustration of the workflow of the new airway segmentation method.

2.1   3D FCN Architecture

A high quality airway probability map is crucial for a successful segmentation. Although 2D CNN-based airway segmentation may achieve improved performance compared with previous learning based methods [5], we postulate that 3D spatial information, especially the 3D branch-level continuity and junction-bifurcating patterns, is important for segmenting airway structures as well as avoiding local leakages to the neighboring lung parenchyma.

Due to high memory and computational demands, training on one entire 3D chest or whole body CT image is not possible with standard equipment. As a result, images are often broken up into relatively small 3D regions of interest (ROIs) [10,11]. One major problem with this is that the size of large organs or anatomies can exceed the ROI of the training data, therefore hampering the learning ability and robustness. In contrast, the airway is a relatively small-scale structure with tree-like topology. Thus, a relatively small 3D ROI contains sufficient spatial information to characterize the airway branch and junction-level patterns. Moreover, since conservative GR can reliably extract large airway branches, e.g. trachea and left-right main bronchi, we focus our FCN on learning the middle and small size airway branches. Thus, airways are an application highly amenable for 3D FCNs, even with current technological limitations.

We adapt and modify the 3D U-Net architecture [11]. To help preserve very small airways at peripheral sites, we trim the previously deeper 3D U-Net to contain only two pooling layers, resulting in three different spatial resolutions. Downsizing the depth of our network allowed us to increase the width of the convolutional layers at the middle and higher levels, potentially helping to learn the structure variations in 3D space. Additional upsampling path with short-cuts from the corresponding pooling layers to the upsampling layers is also incorporated aiming to better capture finer scale airways. Kernels used in all convolutional layers are $3 \times 3 \times 3$ except the last layer using a $1 \times 1 \times 1$ kernel. Apart from these modifications, we use the same architectural choices as 3D U-Net [11]. See Fig. 2 for the details of our network architecture. Cross-entropy loss is used in training. In our end-to-end training, the loss function is computed over all voxels in the ROI. Due to the sparsity of airway structures in the training data, the distribution of airway and background voxels is highly biased. Therefore, a global class-balancing weight is applied to the loss function, which is shown below:

$$loss = -\beta \sum_{j \in Y_+} \log \hat{y}_j - (1 - \beta) \sum_{j \in Y_-} \log (1 - \hat{y}_j), \tag{1}$$

where $\hat{y}_j$ is the computed value after the final convolutional layer, Y_+ and Y_- represent the set of the foreground and background airway labels, and $\beta = mean\left(|Y_-|/|Y|\right)$ is global weight precomputed over the entire training data.

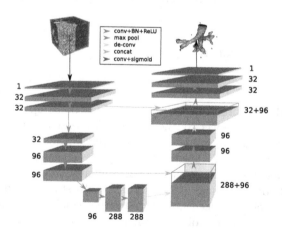

Fig. 2. 3D FCN architecture designed for small airway tubular structures. The number of channels is denoted at the side of each feature map.

2.2 Training with Incomplete Labeling

Obtaining fully-annotated medical image segmentation is always a bottleneck, but it is particularly costly, tedious, and error-prone for airways. For this reason, we investigate whether incomplete, but automatically generated, labels can serve as effective training data for our 3D FCN method. Specifically, we use labels generated from a previous conservative segmentation method that has only a small number of airway leakages, but is unable to capture all branches. In effect, this means that baseline labels are highly specific but not sufficiently sensitive. Without loss of generality, for this work we use Xu *et al.*'s method [4] as the baseline segmentation. Other methods with high specificity and moderate sensitivity are also suitable to serve as the baseline segmentation. Our aim is to retain similar specificity of the baseline segmentation, while increasing the sensitivity.

Instead of training using a sliding box across the entire volume, we use a more principled approach tailored for tree-like structures. (1) To ensure high-quality ROIs with positive examples, we extract sub-volumes along the baseline segmentation. Specifically, we generate the centerline representation of the baseline airway tree, and along each centerline we randomly sample 15% of the voxels and crop a $80 \times 80 \times 72$ voxel-size ROI centered at this centerline voxel. To augment the data, we also randomly shift within 15 voxels in each dimension. In this way, there are roughly 500 ROIs containing positive examples for one CT image. This ensures that there are sufficient examples capturing the local airway branching patterns, e.g., various locations, sizes and branch orientations, as well as the lung background parenchyma. (2) To obtain sufficient negative examples, 500 $80 \times 80 \times 72$ ROIs are also randomly sampled from each CT image.

One potential drawback of this incomplete labeling training strategy is that the baseline segmentation will contain false negatives. Fortunately, however, the use of the global weight, β, helps address this issue. Recall that with the paucity of positive examples, the loss weighting reduces the impact of each background voxel on the training process. For this reason, the detrimental effects of any false negatives will also be reduced. In contrast, foreground voxels are more highly weighted, meaning the impact of true positives will be magnified. Thus, when the labels are noisy, the weighting scheme is suited for high-specificity, moderate-sensitivity settings. This exactly describes the baseline segmentation we use.

2.3 Graph-Based Refinement

In the second module of our workflow, we propose to use graph-based refinement to address the local discontinuity, variations, and coarse spatial resolution of the probability map from the 3D FCN. First, we apply fuzzy connectedness segmentation to grow the airway region by incorporating the 3D FCN airway probability information and the CT intensity into the *fuzzy affinity* function in FC method. In this way, information from the high resolution of the original CT attenuations are used to enhance the accurate, but sometimes, coarse FCN output. The initial seeds for the FC are generated by setting a high threshold

(> 0.8) on the FCN probability map. The general form for the fuzzy affinity function incorporates adjacency, μ_α, feature homogeneity, μ_ψ, and expected object features, μ_ϕ. Let p and q denote any two voxels in 3D digital space. The adjacency component is defined as: $\mu_\alpha(p, q) = 1$, if p and q are 26-adjacent, and '0' otherwise. $\mu_\psi(p, q)$ captures the homogeneity between p and q, with a smaller value for more similar pair, whereas $\mu_\phi(p, q)$ calculates how well the pair of p and q match the expected feature distribution. We refer the reader to [4] for more details on specific forms of these affinity functions. In our context, two features are used at a given voxel p: intensity $I(p)$ and the 3D FCN probability map $FCN(p)$. Both $\mu_\psi(p, q)$ and $\mu_\phi(p, q)$ incorporate these two features into their affinity calculation. The combined affinities are given as follows:

$$\mu_k(p, q) = \gamma \mu_k(FCN(p), FCN(q)) + (1 - \gamma)\mu_k(I(p), I(q)), \quad k \in \{\psi, \phi\} \quad (2)$$

where γ is the factor to control the influence of intensity as compared with the 3D FCN features. In this paper, $\gamma = 0.75$ is used since FCN output features higher contrast in avoiding leakage.

Because of the high quality of the 3D FCN map, the segmented results after FC based refinement do not typically contain large leakages. Mostly, they are small boundary protrusions or branch like structures adjacent to airway branches as shown in Fig. 1. Therefore, post-pruning methods are applied to remove some leakages. Here, we use a robust curve skeletonization approach [12] to remove the leakages appeared as the boundary protrusions. The method generates the curve skeleton of airway tree by iteratively growing new skeletal branches computed as a minimum-cost path. The meaningfulness of a skeletal branch is defined by its global context and scales, therefore, enhancing its robustness in stopping false branches that comes from the leaked segmentation region. Based on the skeleton representation of the airway tree, we also compute the scales of terminal branches and prune those whose maximal local radius exceeds its minimal radius by three times, i.e., the extreme scale difference indicates leakage.

3   Experiments and Results

We evaluated our airway segmentation method on CT scans from the EXACT09 challenge [13] and the LTRC [14] with slice resolution 0.5 to 1.25 mm. Images from EXACT09 were acquired using different scanning protocols and reconstruction parameters. The dataset ranges from clinical dose to ultra low-dose scans, from healthy subjects to diseased patients, and from full inspiration to full expiration. In contrast, images from LTRC are those of patients with COPD and interstitial lung disease using more clinical standardized imaging protocols.

We trained our 3D FCN from scratch using 12 randomly chosen training images from the EXACT09 challenge because of its imaging diversity. This results in around 12000 training samples. For testing, we used the entire 20 volume EXACT09 test set and another randomly selected 20 volumes from LTRC. Optimization was performed using stochastic gradient descent, with initial learning rates of 1e-6, a momentum of 0.99, and a weight decay of 0.05. Training converged after 3~4 epochs. When testing, we applied overlapped sliding windows with sub-volumes sized to $80 \times 80 \times 72$ and strides of $48 \times 48 \times 40$. Afterwards, the probability maps of sub-volumes are aggregated to get the whole volume prediction. In general, it takes roughly 10 min to process one CT volume.

Here, we compared our segmentation results to the baseline results of [4]. On the other hand, because LTRC provides the airway reference segmentations, we compare our LTRC results with both baseline results of [4] and the dataset reference standard [14]. Note that the LTRC reference standard is prone to leakages. Three evaluation metrics are used: segmented branch count, tree length, and leakage count. Two experts manually examined the airway segmentations, judging if a segmented branch is a true branch or belongs to a leakage.

Table 1. Quantitative results (mean ± standard deviation) of new method compared against the baseline method Xu *et al.* [4] and LTRC reference standard [14].

	Additional branch count	Additional tree length (cm)	Additional tree length %	Additional leakage count
v.s. Xu *et al.* (EXACT09)	32.2 ± 32.1	66.8 ± 89.9	46.0 ± 49.4	5.2 ± 5.1
v.s. Xu *et al.* (LTRC)	78.8 ± 28.9	158.7 ± 59.7	82.9 ± 53.2	4.7 ± 3.2
v.s. reference (LTRC)	93.6 ± 32.6	181.4 ± 68.2	94.7 ± 60.8	1.3 ± 4.2

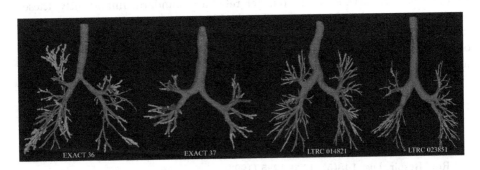

Fig. 3. 3D rendering of example airway segmentations of our method compared against Xu *et al.* [4] and the dataset reference standard [14] for EXACT09 and LTRC, respectively. Overlap regions are colored in red, and green indicates additional branches extracted by our method. Branches detected by the method of Xu *et al.* [4] or the reference standard [14], but missed by ours, are colored in blue (Color figure online).

The quantitative results are summarized in Table 1. Our method significantly increases the number of detected branches as well as the tree length in both

EXACT09 and LTRC datasets. In the EXACT09 dataset, an average of over 32 more branches and 46% tree length is obtained as compared to the baseline method [4]. In the LTRC dataset, further improvements are observed, i.e., 78 more tree branches and roughly 83% more tree length, as compared to the baseline method of [4]. Further improvements are observed when compared against the reference standard [14]. Meanwhile, the additional leakage counts are limited (< 5) in both datasets. As a result, we demonstrate markedly increased sensitivity, while retaining good specificity. Selected examples from both datasets are displayed in Fig. 3, visualizing the impact of these improvements. As shown, leakages in the new method are typically small, which will minimize the volume-based leakage metrics used in the EXACT09 challenge [13].

4   Conclusion

In this paper, we introduce a robust and accurate 3D deep learning-based workflow for airway tree segmentation, which is able to produce high-quality segmentations from incompletely labeled training data. Using a 3D fully convolutional neural network approach, we develop a training and domain-specific sampling scheme tailored for tree structure that uses incomplete labels from a previous highly specific segmentation method. Followed by the 3D FCN prediction, a graph-based refinement step is applied to address local discontinuities of the coarse 3D FCN output by incorporating fuzzy connectedness segmentation and the curve skeletonization. The airway segmentation results on the EXACT09 and LTRC dataset demonstrate considerable improvements in expanding the airway branch numbers and the tree length while maintaining limited leakage compared to a state-of-art method or the dataset reference standard. Importantly, these results are obtained without the need for highly cost manual airway annotations, increasing our method's usability and applicability going forward. Next step of our work involves more comprehensive evaluations, and full EXACT09 challenge metric will be performed to further demonstrate the effectiveness of our method.

References

1. Kuwano, K., Bosken, C.H., Paré, P.D., Bai, T.R., Wiggs, B.R., Hogg, J.C.: Small airways dimensions in asthma and in chronic obstructive pulmonary disease. Am. Rev. Respir. Dis. **148**(5), 1220–1225 (1993)
2. Tschirren, J., Yavarna, T., Reinhardt, J.M.: Airway segmentation framework for clinical environments. In: Second International Workshop on Pulmonary Image Analysis, London, UK, pp. 227–238 (2009)
3. Van Rikxoort, E.M., Baggerman, W., van Ginneken, B.: Automatic segmentation of the airway tree from thoracic CT scans using a multi-threshold approach. In: Second International Workshop on Pulmonary Image Analysis, pp. 341–349 (2009)
4. Xu, Z., Bagci, U., Foster, B., Mansoor, A., Udupa, J.K., Mollura, D.J.: A hybrid method for airway segmentation and automated measurement of bronchial wall thickness on CT. Med. Imag. Anal. **24**(1), 1–17 (2015)

5. Lo, P., Sporring, J., Ashraf, H., Pedersen, J.J., de Bruijne, M.: Vessel-guided airway tree segmentation: a voxel classification approach. Med. Imag. Anal. **14**(4), 527–538 (2010)
6. Charbonnier, J.P., van Rikxoort, E.M., Setio, A.A., Schaefer-Prokop, C.M., van Ginneken, B., Ciompi, F.: Improving airway segmentation in computed tomography using leak detection with convolutional networks. Med. Imag. Anal. **36**, 52–60 (2017)
7. Simonyan, K., Zisserman, A.: Very deep convolutional networks for large-scale image recognition. CoRR abs/1409.1556 (2014)
8. He, K., Zhang, X., Ren, S., Sun, J.: Deep residual learning for image recognition. In: IEEE Conference on Computer Vision and Pattern Recognition, June 2016
9. Ronneberger, O., Fischer, P., Brox, T.: U-Net: convolutional networks for biomedical image segmentation. In: Navab, N., Hornegger, J., Wells, W.M., Frangi, A.F. (eds.) MICCAI 2015. LNCS, vol. 9351, pp. 234–241. Springer, Cham (2015). doi:10.1007/978-3-319-24574-4_28
10. Merkow, J., Marsden, A., Kriegman, D., Tu, Z.: Dense volume-to-volume vascular boundary detection. In: Ourselin, S., Joskowicz, L., Sabuncu, M.R., Unal, G., Wells, W. (eds.) MICCAI 2016. LNCS, vol. 9902, pp. 371–379. Springer, Cham (2016). doi:10.1007/978-3-319-46726-9_43
11. Çiçek, Ö., Abdulkadir, A., Lienkamp, S.S., Brox, T., Ronneberger, O.: 3D U-Net: learning dense volumetric segmentation from sparse annotation. In: Ourselin, S., Joskowicz, L., Sabuncu, M.R., Unal, G., Wells, W. (eds.) MICCAI 2016. LNCS, vol. 9901, pp. 424–432. Springer, Cham (2016). doi:10.1007/978-3-319-46723-8_49
12. Jin, D., Iyer, K.S., Chen, C., Hoffman, E.A., Saha, P.K.: A robust and efficient curve skeletonization algorithm for tree-like objects using minimum cost paths. Pattern Recogn. Lett. **76**, 32–40 (2016)
13. Lo, P., Van Ginneken, B., Reinhardt, J.M., et al.: Extraction of airways from CT (EXACT'09). IEEE Trans. Med. Imaging **31**(11), 2093–2107 (2012)
14. Karwoski, R.A., Bartholmai, B., Zavaletta, V.A., Holmes, D., Robb, R.A.: Processing of CT images for analysis of diffuse lung disease in the lung tissue research consortium. In: Proceedings of SPIE 6916, Medical Imaging 2008: Physiology, Function, and Structure from Medical Images (2008)

Efficient Groupwise Registration for Brain MRI by Fast Initialization

Pei Dong, Xiaohuan Cao, Jun Zhang, Minjeong Kim, Guorong Wu,
and Dinggang Shen$^{(\boxtimes)}$

Department of Radiology and BRIC,
University of North Carolina at Chapel Hill, Chapel Hill, USA
dgshen@med.unc.edu

Abstract. Groupwise image registration provides an unbiased registration solution upon a population of images, which can facilitate the subsequent population analysis. However, it is generally computationally expensive for performing groupwise registration on a large set of images. To alleviate this issue, we propose to utilize a fast initialization technique for speeding up the groupwise registration. Our main idea is to generate a set of simulated brain MRI samples with known deformations to their group center. This can be achieved in the training stage by two steps. First, a set of training brain MR images is registered to their group center with a certain existing groupwise registration method. Then, in order to augment the samples, we perform PCA on the set of obtained deformation fields (to the group center) to parameterize the deformation fields. In doing so, we can generate a large number of deformation fields, as well as their respective simulated samples using different parameters for PCA. In the application stage, when given a new set of testing brain MR images, we can mix them with the augmented training samples. Then, for each testing image, we can find its closest sample in the augmented training dataset for fast estimating its deformation field to the group center of the training set. In this way, a tentative group center of the testing image set can be immediately estimated, and the deformation field of each testing image to this estimated group center can be obtained. With this fast initialization for groupwise registration of testing images, we can finally use an existing groupwise registration method to quickly refine the groupwise registration results. Experimental results on ADNI dataset show the significantly improved computational efficiency and competitive registration accuracy, compared to state-of-the-art groupwise registration methods.

1 Introduction

Groupwise registration provides an unbiased registration solution for a group of images, which is an essential process of population analysis in modern medical image analysis tasks, e.g., analyzing brain structural variations for brain developmental and neurological disorder studies [1]. Unlike conventional pairwise registration which needs to manually select a template image, groupwise registration method can simultaneously align all images to a common space, i.e., their group center. Obviously, by adopting groupwise registration, the bias of individual brain anatomy can be alleviated

© Springer International Publishing AG 2017
Q. Wang et al. (Eds.): MLMI 2017, LNCS 10541, pp. 150–158, 2017.
DOI: 10.1007/978-3-319-67389-9_18

during registration, which helps facilitate the precise population analysis, especially for the brain diseases that are only related to subtle brain structural changes.

To date, many groupwise registration methods have been developed in order to provide effective groupwise registration solutions. Joshi *et al.* [2] proposed an efficient groupwise registration method, which iteratively estimated the group center image by simply averaging all registered subject images at the tentative group mean image. Although the group center could be converged by only a few iterations in their method, it did not yield a sufficiently sharp group mean image, which indicates that the registration accuracy needs further improvement. To address this limitation, Ying *et al.* [3] proposed a hierarchical unbiased graph shrinkage (HUGS) method for groupwise registration. This approach first employed a graph model to fit the data representation on the image manifold, and then regarded groupwise registration as a dynamic graph shrinkage problem. By only connecting similar images on the graph, all images can efficiently move to the group center along the graph edge. Wu *et al.* [4] further improved this method with multi-layer graph model to address the heterogeneity issue in the imaging data. These methods can contribute to an accurate group center image with much sharper anatomical structures. However, all these methods require very long computational time because of numerous iterative optimizations, which makes these methods less practical in clinical application.

In order to tackle this limitation, we propose an efficient groupwise registration method by using a fast initialization technique, which is able to achieve comparable registration accuracy with the state-of-the-art methods, while significantly reducing the computational time. Specifically, we calculate an accurate group center image from a set of training images, as well as their deformation fields to the group center. When group-wisely registering a new group of images, we first quickly initialize all new images to a roughly estimated group center image, where all new images can be quite close to each other. Then, the final group center can be refined by adopting a conventional groupwise registration method efficiently. The main contributions of this paper can be summarized as follows:

(1) An accurate and fast groupwise registration method is proposed by fully exploiting the established deformation fields of the existing training dataset. This can help provide a fast initialization for a new image set, where the anatomical variation among the individuals can be greatly reduced. In this way, the final accurate registration results can be efficiently achieved by using a certain groupwise registration method.

(2) A novel data augmentation strategy is introduced to generate an abundantly enlarged training set from the limited number of training images and establish the respective deformation fields to a training group center. By generating the simulated data, the training images can be well distributed on the image manifold, which is essential to transfer the group center from the training set to the new testing image group to achieve an accurate initialization.

Our proposed method is evaluated on Alzheimer's Disease Neuroimaging Initiative (ADNI) dataset. The registration results show competitive registration performance with significant reduced computation time, compared to a state-of-the-art groupwise registration method [3].

2   Method

Given a set of training images, the goal of our work is to group-wisely registering all new images to their group center efficiently and accurately compared to the state-of-the-art registration method. Our proposed method composes of two stages: *training data augmentation* and efficient groupwise registration supported by *fast initialization*. To construct a training dataset with an adequate number of images, we enlarge the existing dataset by simulating MR brain samples via a wavelet-based PCA (WPCA) model [5]. In groupwise registration stage, new images in the testing set can be easily warped to the center of training dataset group by register each new image to its most similar image in training dataset. Then, the testing group center can be quickly estimated by iteratively evolving from the training group center. Finally, it is straightforward to refine all testing images to their final group center by adopting a conventional groupwise registered method in an effective way.

2.1   Training Dataset Augmentation

All training images should be well distributed in the image manifold, which requires the image samples to cover the possible variability of individual brain anatomical structures. Based on the limited training data, we propose to use the WPCA-based data augmentation to enlarge the dataset in order to simulate diversified images.

Assume we have N training images $\boldsymbol{I}^s = \{I_i^s \mid i = 1, \ldots, N\}$. The first step is to use a certain groupwise registration method to simultaneously align all training images to their group center image G^s, and obtain a set of dense deformation fields $\boldsymbol{u}^s = \{u_i^s \mid i = 1, \ldots, N\}$, which bring each training image I_i^s to its group center image G^s, respectively. Here, we employ the HUGS method [3], one of the state-of-the-art groupwise registration methods, to obtain the accurate group center image by exhaustively iterative optimization, as well as the deformation fields of all training images to the group center. In the second step, a WPCA model is employed to generate simulated deformation fields from the previous established deformation fields $\boldsymbol{u}^s$ with the warped MR brain images using the simulated deformation fields. Here, in order to accurately estimate a set of simulated deformation fields from a limited training deformation fields, we employ an wavelet-based PCA model [5] regularized by its Jacobian determinants and a Markov random field, to generate a set of simulated deformation fields $\boldsymbol{u}^{s'} = \{u_j^{s'} \mid j = 1, \ldots, M\}$ and their respective MR brain images $\boldsymbol{I}^{s'} = \{I_j^{s'} \mid j = 1, \ldots, M\}$. Therefore, we can obtain an augmented training dataset with $N + M$ brain images $\boldsymbol{I}^{\bar{s}} = \boldsymbol{I}^s \cup \boldsymbol{I}^{s'} = \{I_k^{\bar{s}} \mid k = 1, \ldots, N + M\}$ corresponding to their deformation field $\boldsymbol{u}^{\bar{s}} = \boldsymbol{u}^s \cup \boldsymbol{u}^{s'} = \{u_k^{\bar{s}} \mid k = 1, \ldots, N + M\}$, which can directly bring the images to the group center image G^s. Figure 1 shows an illustration of simulating MR brain images in the high-dimensional image manifold. The orange circle denotes the group center image G^s. The blue circle and solid curves denote the training image I_i^s and its deformation pathway u_i^s to the group center image G^s. The blue circular ring and the dashed curves denote the simulated images $I_j^{s'}$ and the simulated deformation pathway $u_j^{s'}$, respectively.

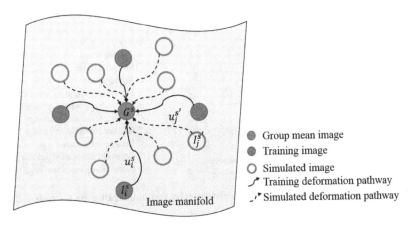

Fig. 1. Illustration of training dataset augmentation.

2.2   Efficient Groupwise Registration by Fast Initialization

Our proposed groupwise registration consists of two parts: (1) fast group center initialization and (2) efficient groupwise registration.

The group center for the testing group is fast initialized based on the group center G^s of training dataset. Given a new image group with P testing images $\mathbf{I}^t = \{I_m^t \mid m = 1, \ldots, P\}$, we first combine them with the augmented training dataset $\mathbf{I}^{\bar{s}}$. Then, the initialized group center can be obtained by two steps.

In the *first* step, each new image I_m^t finds its closest sample in the augmented training dataset $\mathbf{I}^{\bar{s}}$ by measuring the similarity between images on the image manifold. Here, for the computational efficiency, we use the sum of squared differences (SSD) as the similarity metric. Therefore, the image distance between a testing image I_m^t and a training image $I_k^{\bar{s}}$ can be defined as:

$$d = \left\| I_m^t - I_k^{\bar{s}} \right\|^2 \tag{1}$$

Then, we apply a conventional deformable registration method to obtain the deformation field $u_m^{t \to \bar{s}}$ (blue curved arrow shown in Fig. 2) between the new image I_m to its closest image in $\mathbf{I}^{\bar{s}}$ in an efficient manner. Note that, many existing deformable registration algorithms [6–9] can be used for this purpose, since the two images are already very similar and easy to register. Here, we use diffeomorphic Demons [7] to perform the deformable registration. After that, a set of deformation fields $u^{t \to G^s} = \{u_m^{t \to G^s} \mid m = 1, \ldots, P\}$, which are from each testing image to the group center of the training set (orange curved arrow shown in Fig. 2), can be obtained.

In the *second* step, we aim to iteratively estimate a tentative testing group center G' based on the testing image set, and obtain the respective deformation field of each testing image to this group center G'. Specifically, we first calculate an averaged

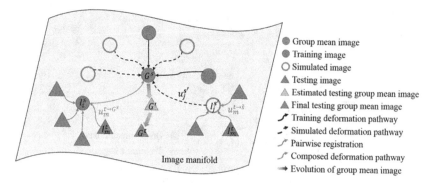

Fig. 2. Illustration of efficient groupwise registration by fast initialization on the testing dataset. (Color figure online)

deformation field $\bar{u}^{t\rightarrow G^s}$ from the previous obtained deformation fields, which can be defined as:

$$\bar{u}^{t\rightarrow G^s} = 1/P \sum_{m=1}^{P} u_m^{t\rightarrow G^s} \qquad (2)$$

Then, we compute its reverse deformation field $(\bar{u}^{t\rightarrow G^s})^{-1}$, which can bring the training group center image G^s to an initially estimated testing group center G_0'. After that, the updated the deformation fields $u^{t\rightarrow G_0'}$ from each testing image to this initial estimated testing group center can be obtained, which is calculated by:

$$u^{t\rightarrow G_0'} = \{(\bar{u}^{t\rightarrow G^s})^{-1} \circ u_m^{t\rightarrow G^s} \mid m = 1,\ldots,P\} \qquad (3)$$

where the symbol $\circ$ denotes the composition of the two deformation fields. Then, after iteratively repeating Eqs. (2) and (3), we obtain the updated testing group center G' with the respective deformation fields $u^{t\rightarrow G'}$ of each testing image to G'. By using the deformation fields $u^{t\rightarrow G'}$, we can fast initialize all testing images to the estimated testing group center, where we can obtain P warped testing images $I^{G'} = \{I_m^{G'} \mid m = 1,\ldots,P\}$. Note that, the warped testing images $I^{G'}$ will be located closely to each other in G' image space.

Based on the fast group center estimation, we further perform accurate groupwise registration by adopting an existing groupwise registration method to quickly calculate the final testing group center image G^t. It should be noted that, the reason that why using groupwise registration method can be fast at this stage is that all testing images in $I^{G'}$ image space are very similar to each other. Comparing to conventional groupwise registration methods, which align all images without initialization by using many iterations to gradually move all images to their image center, our proposed method can benefit from the fast initialization, which contributes to dramatically saving the computational time by significantly reducing the iteration numbers.

Figure 2 illustrates our proposed efficient groupwise registration. The solid blue triangle denotes the new testing images. The blue arrow is the pairwise registration between the testing image and its closest training image. The yellow triangle denotes the estimated testing group center image, and the green triangle denotes the final testing group center.

3 Experiments and Results

In the experiments, we selected 50 subjects as our training dataset and another 50 subjects as the testing image group from the dataset. All images were processed with standard pre-processing procedures. Specifically, all images were first resampled to an image size of $256 \times 256 \times 256$ with a voxel size of 1 mm $\times$ 1 mm $\times$ 1 mm. Then, we used N3 algorithm [6] to correct the inhomogeneous intensity. After that, we employed BET [7] for skull stripping. Next, each image was further segmented into gray matter (GM), white matter (WM) and cerebrospinal fluid (CSF) by using FAST software [8]. These tissue segmentations were manually corrected with visual inspection and were regarded as the ground truth for evaluating the registration performance. Figure 3 shows several typical images used in our experiment.

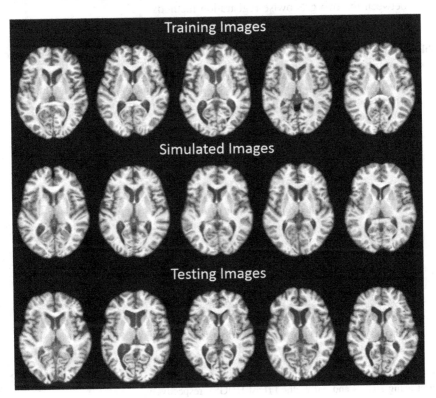

Fig. 3. Typical images from the training dataset, simulated dataset, and testing dataset.

Before performing groupwise registration, affine registration was applied to register all images to a selected image which is the closest to the geometric mean of image set using FLIRT [9]. Then, in the training stage, we employed HUGS [3] to generate the group center of the training dataset along with their deformation field to the group center. Next, we used the WPCA model to generate 250 simulated MR brain samples to enlarge our training dataset. In the application stage, we separately perform HUGS [3] registration and our proposed registration method (Fast-HUGS) on the testing dataset. For our proposed method, each new image was first registered to its closest image in the training dataset using demons [7]. At the final stage, we used HUGS method to group-wisely refine the registration result.

To quantitatively evaluate our method, the Dice ratio is used to measure the overlap degree of each tissue among the group-wisely registered images. Since no label image is available in the common space of testing images, we generate a label image in the common space by using majority voting on all aligned testing label images. The Dice ratio of different tissue types is then calculated with respect to the label image in the common space for each certain subject. The Dice ratio of each tissue type and the computational time using HUGS and Fast-HUGS are reported in Table 1. It can be observed that our method achieves a comparable Dice ratio compared to HUGS, while the number of iterations and computational time are significantly reduced. Figure 4 shows a boxplot of the Dice ratio of the three tissue types. Figure 5 illustrates the results between the two groupwise registration methods.

Table 1. Average dice ratio and standard deviation (%) by the two methods, along with iteration times and corresponding computational time.

	GM	WM	CSF	Overall	# Iteration	Time
HUGS	74.7 ± 3.0	79.1 ± 2.6	71.7 ± 3.7	75.1 ± 2.9	6	41 h
Fast-HUGS	74.2 ± 1.8	78.5 ± 1.5	73.3 ± 1.4	75.4 ± 1.4	1	7 h

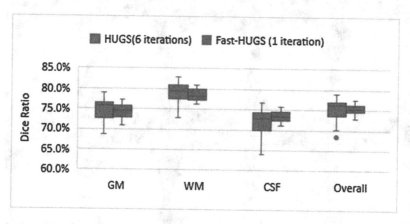

Fig. 4. Box plot of GM, WM, CSF and overall Dice ratio for the testing images from ADNI dataset using HUGS and our method (Fast-HUGS), respectively.

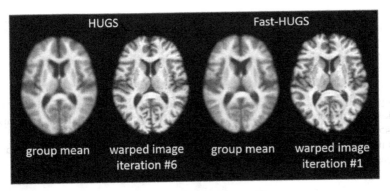

Fig. 5. Visual comparison of groupwise registration results by HUGS and our method (Fast-HUGS), respectively.

4 Conclusion

In this paper, we proposed an efficient groupwise registration method by introducing fast initialization. We first enlarge the brain anatomical variability of the training MR images with the existing deformation fields to their group center. When group-wisely registering a new set of testing images, each new testing image can find its closest image in the training dataset for fast estimating its deformation field to the group center of the training image. Then, by quickly estimating a tentative group center for the testing images, all new testing images can be fast initialized to this initialized group center, where all warped new images are close to each other. Thus, the real group center of the new testing images can be quickly refined by using an existing groupwise registration method with only a few iterations. Experimental results show our proposed registration method can dramatically reduce the computational time while maintaining competitive registration accuracy compared to the state-of-the-art groupwise registration method. Our preliminary experimental results suggest that, our groupwise registration method can be potentially extended to more applications of the large population analysis.

References

1. Viergever, M.A., Maintz, J.B.A., Klein, S., et al.: A survey of medical image registration – under review. Med. Image Anal. **33**, 140–144 (2016)
2. Joshi, S., Davis, B., Jomier, M., et al.: Unbiased diffeomorphic atlas construction for computational anatomy. NeuroImage **23**(Suppl. 1), S151–S160 (2004)
3. Ying, S., Wu, G., Wang, Q., et al.: Hierarchical unbiased graph shrinkage (HUGS): a novel groupwise registration for large data set. NeuroImage **84**, 626–638 (2014)
4. Wu, G., Peng, X., Ying, S., et al.: eHUGS: enhanced hierarchical unbiased graph shrinkage for efficient groupwise registration. PLoS ONE **11**, e0146870 (2016)

5. Xue, Z., Shen, D., Karacali, B., et al.: Simulating deformations of MR brain images for validation of atlas-based segmentation and registration algorithms. NeuroImage **33**, 855–866 (2006)
6. Sled, J.G., Zijdenbos, A.P., Evans, A.C.: A nonparametric method for automatic correction of intensity nonuniformity in MRI data. IEEE Trans. Med. Imaging **17**, 87–97 (1998)
7. Smith, S.M.: Fast robust automated brain extraction. Hum. Brain Mapp. **17**, 143–155 (2002)
8. Zhang, Y., Brady, M., Smith, S.: Segmentation of brain MR images through a hidden Markov random field model and the expectation-maximization algorithm. IEEE Trans. Med. Imaging **20**, 45–57 (2001)
9. Jenkinson, M., Smith, S.: A global optimisation method for robust affine registration of brain images. Med. Image Anal. **5**, 143–156 (2001)

Sparse Multi-view Task-Centralized Learning for ASD Diagnosis

Jun Wang[1,2] (ID), Qian Wang[3], Shitong Wang[2], and Dinggang Shen[1,4(✉)]

[1] Department of Radiology and Biomedical Research Imaging Center,
University of North Carolina at Chapel Hill, Chapel Hill, NC 27599, USA
dgshen@med.unc.edu
[2] School of Digital Media, Jiangnan University, Wuxi 214122, Jiangsu, China
[3] School of Biomedical Engineering,
Med-X Research Institute, Shanghai Jiao Tong University, Shanghai, China
[4] Department of Brain and Cognitive Engineering,
Korea University, Seoul, Korea

Abstract. It is challenging to derive early diagnosis from neuroimaging data for autism spectrum disorder (ASD). In this work, we propose a novel sparse multi-view task-centralized (Sparse-MVTC) classification method for computer-assisted diagnosis of ASD. In particular, since ASD is known to be age- and sex-related, we partition all subjects into different groups of age/sex, each of which can be treated as a classification task to learn. Meanwhile, we extract multi-view features from functional magnetic resonance imaging to describe the brain connectivity of each subject. This formulates a multi-view multi-task sparse learning problem and it is solved by a novel Sparse-MVTC method. Specifically, we treat each task as a central task and other tasks as the auxiliary ones. We then consider the task-task and view-view relations between the central task and each auxiliary task. We can use this task-centralized strategy for a highly efficient solution. The comprehensive experiments on the ABIDE database demonstrate that our proposed Sparse-MVTC method can significantly outperform the existing classification methods in ASD diagnosis.

1 Introduction

Autism spectrum disorder (ASD) is a major mental disorder for childhood. The computer-assisted diagnosis of ASD using neuroimaging data is highly desired, especially before abnormal behaviors of the patients turn observable. In recent years, resting-state functional magnetic resonance imaging (rs-fMRI) has become a pivotal tool in understanding the mechanism of ASD, as researchers can identify many disease-related biomarkers. However, it is non-trivial to extract features from the noisy rs-fMRI data, select the effective biomarkers, and learn the classification model for the diagnosis of the disease [1].

Functional connectivity (FC), which measures the correlation of the temporal BOLD signals in different brain regions and encodes the functional connection of the structurally segregated brain regions, is often adopted for feature extraction in rs-fMRI

© Springer International Publishing AG 2017
Q. Wang et al. (Eds.): MLMI 2017, LNCS 10541, pp. 159–167, 2017.
DOI: 10.1007/978-3-319-67389-9_19

analysis [2]. By computing FCs between many regions, one may derive a large matrix to represent the FC network. Since the pathology of ASD may disrupt the FC network, we are expected to utilize these correlation-based FC measures to diagnose the disease.

Note that the correlation-based FC is not the only metric to present the brain functional network. For example, Zhang *et al.* have proposed high-order functional connectivity (HOFC) [3], in which the connectivity of the brain regions is defined by the correlation of correlations. Specifically, given a region under consideration, its correlation feature vector is first calculated, i.e., following the conventional FC analysis method, to record its correlations with all other regions in the brain. After that, a high-level correlation is calculated between the correlation feature vectors of two regions, thus resulting in their in-between HOFC. This HOFC measure has shown its advantages, including the sensitivity to group difference, individual variability, and prominent modular structures [3]. To this end, for diagnosing ASD, we may extract both FC and HOFC measures from the rs-fMRI data of a certain subject, and treat them as two different views of connectivity features.

Recent studies show that ASD is an age- and sex-related neurodevelopmental disorder. For example, ASD patients differ from normal controls in the intrinsic FCs of the default mode networks, while the differences vary with ages [4, 5]. Besides, Alaerts *et al.* have found that males and females have different neural expressions of ASD, i.e., characterized by the predominant hypo-connectivity patterns in males while the hyper-connectivity patterns in females [6]. In order to account for these findings, one may partition the subjects into different age/sex groups naturally. Then, each group can be treated as a task, such that the ASD diagnosis upon all groups can be solved by the multi-task learning.

Since FC and HOFC act as two different views of connectivity features, they can be utilized simultaneously in the multi-view learning [7, 8]. In this way, the computer-assisted ASD diagnosis can be formulated as a *multi-view multi-task* (MVMT) learning problem. Higher classification accuracy is presumably achievable, once the learning upon all tasks with coupled views of connectivity features is jointly conducted in a proper way.

The solution to the MVMT learning, however, is non-trivial. For example, Zhang *et al.* has proposed regMVMT for multi-task learning on the multi-view data, in which co-regularization and task-task relationships are considered simultaneously [9]. Although the solution of regMVMT is a close-form analytically, it involves an inverse operation of a large matrix that strongly limits the actual usage of this method, especially when the number of the tasks is large.

In this work, we propose a novel sparse multi-view task-centralized classification method (Sparse-MVTC) [9, 10], in which the task-centralized learning mechanism helps handle a large number of tasks. Specifically, we decompose the multi-view classification problem into multiple age/sex-related tasks, each of which can be solved by regressing the ASD diagnosis from imaging features via sparse learning. Then, we introduce the task-centralized strategy by picking up a certain task as a central task and treating all others as the auxiliary tasks. By further considering the relationship between the central task and each auxiliary task, the joint sparse learning will lead to a set of classifiers that correspond to individual central/auxiliary tasks. Moreover, since the central task can be selected in turn, the above procedure of the joint sparse learning can be repeated for multiple times, thus resulting in multiple classifiers for each task. By integrating all the classifiers of each task, we are able to attain high-performance diagnosis accordingly. We do not find any similar work reported before.

We will detail the proposed Sparse-MVTC method and its solution in Sect. 2. In particular, the task-centralized strategy in our method considers the relationship between the central task and each auxiliary task only. The relationship across auxiliary tasks is neglected for easy computation. Regarding the task-task relationship, we devise novel terms in sparse learning to account for the joint feature selection and weighting between the central and the auxiliary tasks, as well as the consistency across the multi-view features. In Sect. 3, we apply our method to ASD diagnosis and present the experimental results on the multi-center ABIDE dataset. We conclude this work in Sect. 4.

2   Method

2.1   Sparse Multi-view Task-Centralized (Sparse-MVTC) Learning

For ASD diagnosis, we partition all subjects into T groups according to their age/sex information. Each group corresponds to a supervised learning task, as V views of features are assumed available per subject. In the t-th task ($t = 1, 2, \ldots, T$), we have N_t subjects $\{\mathbf{x}_i, y_i\}_{i=1}^{N_t}$ for training. Here, $\mathbf{x}_i = \left(\left(\mathbf{x}_i^1\right)', \cdots, \left(\mathbf{x}_i^V\right)' \right)' \in \mathbb{R}^D$ is a vector including all V-view features for the i-th subject. Each view has D_v features ($D = \sum\limits_{v=1}^{V} D_v$). $y_i \in \{-1, 1\}$ is the class label of $\mathbf{x}_i$ (e.g., "-1" for healthy controls, and "1" for ASD patients). Let $\mathbf{X}_t = [\mathbf{x}_1, \cdots, \mathbf{x}_{N_t}]' \in \mathbb{R}^{N_t \times D}$ and $\mathbf{y}_t = (y_1, \cdots, y_{N_t})$ be the data matrix and the training label vector for the t-th task, respectively. The vector $\mathbf{w}_t^v \in \mathbb{R}^{D_v}$ indicates the weights of all features in the v-th view with respect to the t-th task. We further define $\mathbf{w}_t = \left(\left(\mathbf{w}_t^1\right)', \cdots, \left(\mathbf{w}_t^V\right)' \right)' \in \mathbb{R}^D$ and $\mathbf{W} = [\mathbf{w}_1, \cdots, \mathbf{w}_T] \in \mathbb{R}^{D \times T}$.

We pick up one task as a central task and treat all others as the auxiliary tasks. Suppose that the t-th ($t = 1, 2, \cdots, T$) task is the central task. The sparse learning upon all tasks (i.e., Sparse-MVTC) is formulated as the following optimization problem

$$\min_{\mathbf{W}} \left(\sum_{u=1}^{T} \frac{1}{N_u} \left\| \mathbf{y}_u - \sum_{v=1}^{V} \mathbf{X}_u^v \mathbf{w}_u^v \right\|^2 + R\left(\mathbf{w}_t; \{\mathbf{w}_s\}_{s=1,s\neq t}^{T} \right) \right), \tag{1}$$

where N_u is the number of the training subjects in the u-th task, and $R\left(\mathbf{w}_t; \{\mathbf{w}_s\}_{s=1,s\neq t}^{T} \right)$ is a regularization to encode the relationship between the central task and each auxiliary task in the multi-view setting. In particular, we devise three terms for the regularization $R\left(\mathbf{w}_t; \{\mathbf{w}_s\}_{s=1,s\neq t}^{T} \right)$, i.e., $R = \gamma R_1 + \eta R_2 + \theta R_3$, where γ, η and θ are non-negative scalars to control the respective regularization terms, R_1, R_2, and R_3.

Joint task-task feature selection: To conduct feature selection jointly between the central task and each auxiliary task, we adopt

$$R_1\left(\mathbf{w}_t; \{\mathbf{w}_s\}_{s=1,s\neq t}^T\right) = \sum_{\substack{s=1 \\ s \neq t}}^{T} c_{s,t} \sum_{v=1}^{V} \left\|\mathbf{W}_{s,t}^v\right\|_{2,1}, \tag{2}$$

where $\mathbf{W}_{s,t}^v = [\mathbf{w}_s^v, \mathbf{w}_t^v] \in \mathbb{R}^{D_v \times 2}$ and $c_{s,t}$ measures the similarity between the two tasks s and t. If two tasks are similar, they should select similar features by sparse learning. To this end, we compute the coefficient as $c_{s,t} = \exp\left(-\|\bar{\mathbf{X}}_t - \bar{\mathbf{X}}\|_s^2/\sigma^2\right)$, where $\bar{\mathbf{X}}_t = \sum_{i=1}^{N_t} \mathbf{x}_i/N_t$, $\bar{\mathbf{X}}_s = \sum_{i=1}^{N_s} \mathbf{x}_i/N_s$ and $\sigma^2 = \sum_{i=1}^{N_s}\sum_{j=1}^{N_t} \mathbf{x}_i - \mathbf{x}_j^2/N_s N_t$.

Joint task-task feature weighting: Besides joint feature selection, we assume that, if the central task is similar with a certain auxiliary task, their jointly selected features should share similar weights when regressing the disease labels. To this end, we propose the regularization term R_2 for the joint task-task feature weighting:

$$R_2\left(\mathbf{w}_t; \{\mathbf{w}_s\}_{s=1,s\neq t}^T\right) = \sum_{\substack{s=1, \\ s \neq t}}^{T} c_{s,t} \sum_{v=1}^{V} \left\|\mathbf{w}_s^v - \mathbf{w}_t^v\right\|^2. \tag{3}$$

Note that $c_{s,t}$ encodes the similarity between the central task and the auxiliary task, as defined above.

Consistency of view-view predictability: It is important to effectively integrate the two views of features for ASD diagnosis. In the multi-view learning, the discriminant functions for different views of a subject tend to yield the same classification result. Therefore, we devise the following regularization term to ensure the consistency:

$$R_3\left(\mathbf{w}_t; \{\mathbf{w}_s\}_{s=1,s\neq t}^T\right) = \sum_{u=1}^{T} \frac{1}{N_u} \sum_{i,j=1}^{V} \left\|\mathbf{X}_u^i \mathbf{w}_u^i - \mathbf{X}_u^j \mathbf{w}_u^j\right\|^2. \tag{4}$$

2.2   Iterative Optimization in Sparse-MVTC

With the above three regularization terms, we now aim to minimize the following objective function for the proposed Sparse-MVTC method:

$$J(\mathbf{w}_t, \{\mathbf{w}_s\}) = \sum_{u=1}^{T} \frac{1}{N_u} \left\|\mathbf{y}_u - \sum_{v=1}^{V} \mathbf{X}_u^v \mathbf{w}_u^v\right\|^2 + \gamma \sum_{\substack{s=1, \\ s \neq t}}^{T} c_{s,t} \sum_{v=1}^{V} tr(\mathbf{W}_{s,t}^{v'} \Lambda_{s,t}^v \mathbf{W}_{s,t}^v) +$$

$$\eta \sum_{\substack{s=1, \\ s \neq t}}^{T} c_{s,t} \sum_{v=1}^{V} \left\|\mathbf{w}_s^v - \mathbf{w}_t^v\right\|^2 + \theta \sum_{u=1}^{T} \frac{1}{N_k} \sum_{i,j=1}^{V} \left\|\mathbf{X}_u^i \mathbf{w}_u^i - \mathbf{X}_u^j \mathbf{w}_u^j\right\|^2$$

$$\tag{5}$$

Here, we replace $\left\|\mathbf{W}_{s,t}^v\right\|_{2,1}$ with $\text{tr}(\mathbf{W}_{s,t}^v{}'\mathbf{\Lambda}_{s,t}^v\mathbf{W}_{s,t}^v)$, since the minimization upon the two terms are shown to be equivalent [11]. Specifically, $\mathbf{\Lambda}_{s,t}^v(v = 1,\cdots,V; s = 1,\cdots,T; s \neq t)$ is a $D_v \times D_v$ diagonal matrix with its i-th diagonal element being computed as $1/2\left\|(\mathbf{e}_i)'\mathbf{W}_{s,t}^v\right\|$. Note that $\mathbf{e}_i$ is a column vector with its i-th element as 1 and all others as zero.

In Eq. (5), the feature weights $\mathbf{w}_t$ for the central task and $\{\mathbf{w}_s\}$ for the auxiliary tasks, as well as $\left\{\mathbf{\Lambda}_{s,t}^v\right\}$, can be optimized alternatively, i.e., fixing any two of them and then optimizing the third one. The details are provided in the below.

(1) Fixing $\mathbf{w}_t$ and $\{\mathbf{w}_s\}$, we compute $\mathbf{\Lambda}_{s,t}^v$ with its i-th diagonal element as $1/2\left\|(\mathbf{e}_i)'\mathbf{W}_{s,t}^v\right\|$.

(2) Fixing $\left\{\mathbf{\Lambda}_{s,t}^v\right\}$ and $\mathbf{w}_t$, we compute $\mathbf{P}_s^v$, $\mathbf{Q}_s^v$ and $\mathbf{r}_s^v$ for each auxiliary task following:

$$\mathbf{P}_s^v = \left(\gamma c_{s,t}\mathbf{\Lambda}_{s,t}^v + \eta c_{s,t}\mathbf{I} + 2\theta\frac{1}{N_s}V(\mathbf{X}_s^v)'\mathbf{X}_s^v\right),$$
$$\mathbf{Q}_s^v = \left(\frac{1-2\theta}{N_s}\right)(\mathbf{X}_s^v)', \mathbf{r}_s^v = \frac{1}{N_s}(\mathbf{X}_s^v)'\mathbf{y}_s + \eta c_{s,t}\mathbf{w}_t^v. \tag{6}$$

We are then able to update $\{\mathbf{w}_s\}$ by:

$$\tilde{\mathbf{P}}_s = \begin{pmatrix} \mathbf{P}_s^1 & \cdots & 0 \\ \vdots & \ddots & \vdots \\ 0 & \cdots & \mathbf{P}_s^V \end{pmatrix}, \tilde{\mathbf{Q}}_s = \begin{pmatrix} \mathbf{Q}_s^1\mathbf{X}_s^1 & \cdots & \mathbf{Q}_s^1\mathbf{X}_s^V \\ \vdots & \ddots & \vdots \\ \mathbf{Q}_s^V\mathbf{X}_s^1 & \cdots & \mathbf{Q}_s^V\mathbf{X}_s^V \end{pmatrix}, \tilde{\mathbf{r}}_s = \begin{pmatrix} \mathbf{r}_s^1 & \cdots & \mathbf{r}_s^V \end{pmatrix}'$$

$$\tag{7}$$

$$\mathbf{w}_s = (\tilde{\mathbf{P}}_s + \tilde{\mathbf{Q}}_s)^{-1}\tilde{\mathbf{r}}_s. \tag{8}$$

(3) Similarly, we can fix $\left\{\mathbf{\Lambda}_{s,t}^v\right\}$ and $\{\mathbf{w}_s\}$, and optimize $\mathbf{w}_t$ by:

$$\mathbf{P}_t^v = \left(\gamma\sum_{\substack{s=1 \\ s \neq t}}^{T} c_{s,t}\mathbf{\Lambda}_{s,t}^v + \eta\sum_{\substack{s=1 \\ s \neq t}}^{T} c_{s,t}\mathbf{I} + 2\theta\frac{1}{N_t}M(\mathbf{X}_t^v)'\mathbf{X}_t^v\right),$$
$$\mathbf{Q}_t^v = \frac{1-2\theta}{N_t}(\mathbf{X}_t^v)'\sum_{i=1}^{V}\mathbf{X}_t^i\mathbf{w}_t^i, \mathbf{r}_t^v = \frac{1}{N_t}(\mathbf{X}_t^v)'\mathbf{y}_t + \eta\sum_{\substack{s=1 \\ s \neq t}}^{T} c_{s,t}\mathbf{w}_s^v, \tag{9}$$

$$\tilde{\mathbf{P}}_t = \begin{pmatrix} \mathbf{P}_t^1 & \cdots & 0 \\ \vdots & \ddots & \vdots \\ 0 & \cdots & \mathbf{P}_t^V \end{pmatrix}, \tilde{\mathbf{Q}}_t = \begin{pmatrix} \mathbf{Q}_t^1 \mathbf{X}_t^1 & \cdots & \mathbf{Q}_s^1 \mathbf{X}_t^V \\ \vdots & \ddots & \vdots \\ \mathbf{Q}_t^V \mathbf{X}_t^1 & \cdots & \mathbf{Q}_t^V \mathbf{X}_t^V \end{pmatrix}, \tilde{\mathbf{r}}_t = \begin{pmatrix} \mathbf{r}_t^1 & \cdots & \mathbf{r}_t^V \end{pmatrix}',$$

(10)

$$\mathbf{w}_t = \left(\tilde{\mathbf{P}}_t + \tilde{\mathbf{Q}}_t \right)^{-1} \tilde{\mathbf{r}}_t.$$

(11)

The optimization of the objective function in Eq. (5) is conducted by iteratively calling the three steps above. We abort from the optimization, once $\mathbf{W}$ tends to be stable.

Note that both $\left(\tilde{\mathbf{P}}_t + \tilde{\mathbf{Q}}_t \right)$ and $\left(\tilde{\mathbf{P}}_s + \tilde{\mathbf{Q}}_s \right)$ are $D \times D$ matrices. The bottleneck of the Sparse-MVTC method is thus the inverse of matrices in $\mathbf{w}_s = \left(\tilde{\mathbf{P}}_s + \tilde{\mathbf{Q}}_s \right)^{-1} \tilde{\mathbf{r}}_s$ (Eq. 8) and $\mathbf{w}_t = \left(\tilde{\mathbf{P}}_t + \tilde{\mathbf{Q}}_t \right)^{-1} \tilde{\mathbf{r}}_t$ (Eq. 11), each of which has the time complexity of $O(D^3)$. Compared to regMVMT [9] that also involves an inverse of a $TD \times TD$ matrix, Sparse-MVTC costs less computation time and less memory space, thus making Sparse-MVTC more suitable for MVMT applications with many tasks.

2.3   Ensemble Implementation of Sparse-MVTC

The training process in Sparse-MVTC determines the discriminant weights $\mathbf{W}$ for multi-view features. Once the weights are estimated, a testing subject can acquire the diagnosis accordingly. Moreover, in order to tackle the bias caused by the arbitrary selection of the central task, we pick up the central task in turn and repeat Sparse-MVTC for multiple times. In this way, for each task, there are T classifiers. Given the testing subject with known age/sex information, we can easily identify the classifiers corresponding to the respective group/task. The final diagnosis is thus obtained by averaging all the outputs of the respective classifiers, to which the testing subject belongs.

3   Experimental Results

3.1   Experimental Settings

In this study, we consider rs-fMRI scans acquired from two different imaging centers (i.e., NYU and UM-1 of ABIDE, http://fcon_1000.projects.nitrc.org/indi/abide/index. html). Both male and female subjects are included in our study and their ages vary from 6 to 40. We partition these subjects into different groups according to their age and sex information. We further extract FCs from rs-fMRI using the standard pipeline provided by DPARSF (http://rfmri.org/DPARSF). To measure the FCs between ROIs, the pairwise Pearson correlation coefficients are computed, which results in a 116×116 correlation matrix for each subject. After that, HOFC is computed following [3].

In our study, ASD diagnosis is performed by combining the two views of FC and HOFC. For both views, the upper triangles of the matrices are utilized due to the symmetry of the matrices. These measures are reshaped into a vector with 6670 elements. Prior to training, simple feature selection is conducted. Specifically, we select 300 FC features and 300 HOFC features using t-tests. All these features are further normalized regarding the z-score and used for subsequent computation.

We consider ASD diagnosis as the binary classification problem, with label '+1' for ASD patients and label '−1' for the healthy controls. We adopt a 10-fold nested cross-validation strategy to evaluate the performance of our proposed method. The nested cross-validation consists of a 5-fold inner loop that is used to determine the optimal parameters including γ, η, and θ automatically. Finally, we repeat the 10-fold nested cross-validation for 10 times to avoid the arbitrary bias of fold partitioning. We report the average statistics of all 10 repetitions.

3.2 Comparisons with State-of-the-Art Methods

We compare Sparse-MVTC with several popular classifiers. We consider the following experimental settings for CSVC [12] and M2SVC [13] under comparison (see Table 1).

Table 1. Summary of the methods under comparison.

Method	Description on the method	Data preparation
CSVC-S	C-SVC in LibSVM. Linear kernel is adopted	FC and HOFC features of each subject are concatenated
CSVC-J		
M2SVC-S	Multi-modal classification proposed by [13]	FC and HOFC features are regarded as one modality in M2SVC
M2SVC-J		
regMVMT	The regularized MVMT method proposed by [9]	FC and HOFC features are regarded as one view, respectively, and each group is regarded as one task
Sparse-MVTC	Our proposed method	

(1) CSVC-S and M2SVC-S: All groups are trained and tested separately. That is, there are T generated classifiers, each of which corresponds to a task.
(2) CSVC-J and M2SVC-J: All groups are combined together for joint training and testing. There is only a single classifier that is applied to all T groups.

Besides, we also compare our method with regMVMT, which is a typical MVMT learning method proposed in [9].

We report the classification performances of all methods in Table 2. One may observe that the proposed Sparse-MVTC method could achieve the best classification accuracy. Concerning all 279 subjects from both clinical centers, the performances are mostly comparable across the centers for our method.

Table 2. Performances of the nested 10-fold classifications for different methods.

	ACC	SEN	SPE	AUC	p-value
CSVC-S	0.588	0.729	0.402	0.566	<1e–3
CSVC-J	0.676	**0.775**	0.544	0.66	0.045
M2SVC-S	0.599	0.716	0.443	0.58	<1e–3
M2SVC-J	0.656	0.719	0.571	0.645	0.030
regMVMT	0.594	0.644	0.527	0.585	0.003
Sparse-MVTC	**0.688**	0.736	**0.625**	**0.680**	

Note that, in CSVC, both FC and HOFC features are concatenated into a long feature vector, by simply ignoring the view-view relationship. On the contrary, M2SVC fuses the multi-view features for the classification. However, both CSVC and M2SVC fail to consider the multi-task learning setting. Different from CSVC and M2SVC, our Sparse-MVTC method *not only* treats FC/HOFC features jointly, *but also* fully considers the task-task relations through the task-centralized strategy. In this way, we are able to obtain much better results than CSVC and M2SVC.

Sparse-MVTC performs joint feature selection and weighting between the central task and each auxiliary task. The regMVMT method also considers the task-task and the view-view relations. However, regMVMT does not require the selected features to be sparsely distributed. The experimental results show that Sparse-MVTC outperforms regMVMT significantly in terms of classification accuracy. This implies that the sparse feature selection helps overcome the overfitting problem on small training datasets, and contributes to higher performances of the discriminant classifiers.

Regarding the memory requirement, it might be hard to deploy regMVMT on an ordinary PC, since it needs an inverse operation of a 10800×10800 matrix. However, Sparse-MVTC reduces the scale to 600×600 matrices. The run-time is about 2 s for Sparse-MVTC and about 10 s for regMVMT on a computer with X5670 processor and 48 GB memory. It is evident to see the advantages of the task-centralized strategy on multi-task learning, especially for the case with many tasks.

4   Conclusion

ASD is a complex neurodevelopmental disorder, as the disease-related alterations in brain's functional connectivity vary according to age and sex. In this work, we formulate the computer-assisted ASD diagnosis as an MVMT learning problem, and propose a novel Sparse-MVTC method to enforce the strong regularizations upon the task-task and view-view relations. An iterative optimization is further schemed for Sparse-MVTC. Using ABIDE database, we achieve a significant performance improvement for diagnosing ASD, compared with state-of-the-art classification methods.

References

1. Anagnostou, E., Taylor, M.J.: Review of neuroimaging in autism spectrum disorders: what have we learned and where we go from here. Mol. Autism **2**, 1–9 (2011)
2. Greicius, M.: Resting-state functional connectivity in neuropsychiatric disorders. Curr. Opin. Neurol. **21**, 424–430 (2008)
3. Zhang, H., Chen, X., Shi, F., et al.: Topographical information-based high-order functional connectivity and its application in abnormality detection for mild cognitive impairment. J. Alzheimer's Dis. **54**, 1–18 (2016)
4. Wiggins, J.L., Peltier, S.J., Ashinoff, S., et al.: Using a self-organizing map algorithm to detect age-related changes in functional connectivity during rest in autism spectrum disorders. Brain Res. **1380**, 187–197 (2011)
5. Wiggins, J.L., Bedoyan, J.K., Peltier, S.J., et al.: The impact of serotonin transporter (5-HTTLPR) genotype on the development of resting-state functional connectivity in children and adolescents: a preliminary report. Neuroimage **59**, 2760–2770 (2012)
6. Alaerts, K., Swinnen, S.P., Wenderoth, N.: Sex differences in autism: a resting-state fMRI investigation of functional brain connectivity in males and females. Soc. Cogn. Affect. Neurosci. **11**, 1002–1016 (2016)
7. Sun, S.: A survey of multi-view machine learning. Neural Comput. Appl. **23**, 2031–2038 (2013)
8. Jiang, Y., Chung, F.-L., Wang, S., et al.: Collaborative fuzzy clustering from multiple weighted views. IEEE Trans. Cybern. **45**, 688–701 (2015)
9. Zhang, J., Huan, J.: Inductive multi-task learning with multiple view data. In: Proceedings of the 18th ACM SIGKDD International Conference on Knowledge Discovery and Data Mining, pp. 543–551 (2012)
10. He, J., Lawrence, R.: A graph-based framework for multi-task multi-view learning. In: Proceedings of the 28th International Conference on Machine Learning (ICML 2011), pp. 25–32 (2011)
11. Nie, F., Huang, H., et al.: Efficient and robust feature selection via joint $\ell_{2,1}$-norms minimization. In: Advances in Neural Information Processing Systems, pp. 1813–1821 (2010)
12. Chang, C.-C., Lin, C.-J.: LIBSVM: a library for support vector machine, 2001 (2012). http://www.csie.ntu.edu.tw/~cjlin/libsvm
13. Zhang, D., Wang, Y., Zhou, L., et al.: Multimodal classification of Alzheimer's disease and mild cognitive impairment. Neuroimage **55**, 856–867 (2011)

Inter-subject Similarity Guided Brain Network Modeling for MCI Diagnosis

Yu Zhang, Han Zhang, Xiaobo Chen, Mingxia Liu, Xiaofeng Zhu,
and Dinggang Shen[✉]

Department of Radiology and BRIC,
University of North Carolina at Chapel Hill, Chapel Hill, USA
dgshen@med.unc.edu

Abstract. Sparse representation-based brain network modeling, although popular, often results in relatively large inter-subject variability in network structures. This inevitably makes it difficult for inter-subject comparison, thus eventually deteriorating the generalization capability of personalized disease diagnosis. Accordingly, group sparse representation has been proposed to alleviate such limitation by jointly estimating connectivity weights for all subjects. However, the constructed brain networks based on this method often fail in providing satisfactory separability between the subjects from *different groups* (e.g., patients *vs.* normal controls), which will also affect the performance of computer-aided disease diagnosis. Based on the hypothesis that subjects from the same group should have larger similarity in their functional connectivity (FC) patterns than subjects from other groups, we propose an "inter-subject FC similarity-guided" group sparse network modeling method. In this method, we explicitly include the inter-subject FC similarity as a constraint to conduct group-wise FC network modeling, while retaining sufficient between-group differences in the resultant FC networks. This improves the separability of brain functional networks between different groups, thus facilitating better personalized brain disease diagnosis. Specifically, the inter-subject FC similarity is roughly estimated by comparing the Pearson's correlation based FC patterns of each brain region to other regions for each pair of the subjects. Then, this is implemented as an additional weighting term to ensure the adequate inter-subject FC differences between the subjects from different groups. Of note, our method retains the group sparsity constraint to ensure the overall consistency of the resultant individual brain networks. Experimental results show that our method achieves a balanced trade-off by *not only* generating the individually consistent FC networks, *but also* effectively maintaining the necessary group difference, thereby significantly improving connectomics-based diagnosis for mild cognitive impairment (MCI).

1 Introduction

Characterized by progressive perceptive and cognitive deficits, Alzheimer's disease (AD) is an irreversible neurological disease with no cure [1]. Mild cognitive impairment (MCI) is known as a prodromal stage of AD, and individuals with MCI tend to progress to AD at a rate of about 10–15% per year [2]. Early detection of MCI is of

© Springer International Publishing AG 2017
Q. Wang et al. (Eds.): MLMI 2017, LNCS 10541, pp. 168–175, 2017.
DOI: 10.1007/978-3-319-67389-9_20

great clinical significance, thus imaging-based diagnosis has attracted much attention in the past few years [3]. However, accurate MCI diagnosis is considerably challenging due to subtle brain anatomical and functional changes during this early stage [4, 5].

As an *in vivo* brain functional imaging technique, the resting-state functional magnetic resonance imaging (rs-fMRI) measures blood oxygenation level-dependent (BOLD) signals related to spontaneous neural activity when subject is in the natural rest. In recent years, rs-fMRI has been successfully applied to abnormality detection of various neurological diseases and psychiatric disorders, including schizophrenia, autism spectrum disorder, and AD/MCI [6]. The most-widely used methods with rs-fMRI are based on functional connectivity (FC), which measures temporal correlation of BOLD signals between any pair of brain regions. Based on FC between each pair of brain regions, the brain FC network can be constructed for characterizing the intrinsic functional architecture of the human brain and its abnormality caused by the possible pathological attack [7, 8]. Accurate construction of the brain FC network based on rs-fMRI is one of the most essential problems for more reliable early detection of MCI and also better understanding of potential biomarkers at the whole-brain systematical level [9].

Of various brain FC network modeling methods, the most widely-used one is Pearson's correlation (PC). Despite of its simplicity and biological intuitiveness, this method also suffers drawbacks that only pair-wise linear interactions are revealed without accounting for more complex influences from other brain regions. To solve this problem, sparse representation (SR) has been adopted for constructing sparse brain FC networks based on the observations that the brain network is largely sparse and the wiring is efficient and cost-effective [10]. Based on SR, the BOLD signals of a brain region can be represented by a linear combination of the signals from a small number of other brain regions, under a sparsity constraint by forcing insignificant connections to be zero. However, because of the data-driven nature, a potential issue of the SR is that it often results in brain networks with a relatively large inter-subject variability due to unpredicted interferences of rs-fMRI noise and artifact. This often leads to a consequence of poor generalization ability of a trained classifier for brain disease diagnosis and, more problematically, for MCI diagnosis because the subtle pathological changes in MCI could be overwhelmed by the large inter-subject variability [11]. Targeting at increasing inter-subject comparability, group sparse representation (GSR) has been proposed by jointly estimating the FC weights for all subjects using a group lasso constraint with $l_{2,1}$-norm [12]. This will make certain connectivity links in *all* subjects being zero or non-zero jointly, which alleviates inter-subject variability, but potentially sacrificing inter-subject separability especially for the subjects from different (e.g., patient and control) groups. Therefore, it will yield suboptimal classification performance when applied to brain disease diagnosis [3].

More recently, connectivity strength-weighted SR method was proposed for individual brain network construction by exploiting FC connectivity prior [13]. With guidance from connectivity strength of PC, the network modeled at the individual level achieved better biological meaning and yielded improved classification accuracy of MCI. One previous study about unsupervised cluster analysis on major depression [14] suggested that subjects from the same group often have larger FC similarity than those from different groups. Accordingly, in this study, we introduce such a prior into GSR-based brain FC network modeling to preserve systematical group difference, without losing the merit of inter-subject consistency in sparse learning framework. Specifically, we propose an "inter-subject FC similarity-guided group sparse" brain network modeling method to increase the between-group separability of FC networks, thus facilitating personalized brain disease diagnosis. In particular, the inter-subject similarity of FC networks is estimated by comparing the PC-based FC pattern of each brain region (i.e., the one-to-all FC pattern) between each pair of subjects. This inter-subject PC-based FC-pattern resemblance is then used as a weighting to form an additional constraint that could penalize those excessive "inter-subject differences in SR-weights" for subjects from the same group, while retaining the sufficient SR-weight differences between subjects from different groups. Next, we will show how this idea can be seamlessly integrated into the GSR-based brain network modeling. To validate the effectiveness of our proposed method, we carry out experiments by applying the new network modeling method to MCI patient identification, a challenging problem due to subtle pathological changes in MCI compared with large inter-subject variability. Results show that our method can *not only* effectively detect group difference, *but also* significantly improve the brain functional connectomics-based MCI diagnosis.

2   Methods

2.1   GSR for Brain Network Modeling

Suppose that $\mathbf{X}_i = [\mathbf{x}_i^1, \mathbf{x}_i^2, \ldots, \mathbf{x}_i^K]$ contains the mean time series of a total of K regions-of-interest (ROIs) for the i-th subject. Without loss of generality, let us assume that $\mathbf{x}_i^k$ has been de-meaned and variance-standardized (i.e., divided by the standard deviation). With PC, the brain FC network of each subject i can be roughly estimated by calculating the full correlation $\mathbf{C}_i = \mathbf{X}_i^T \mathbf{X}_i$, such that the k-th column $\mathbf{c}_i^k$ in $\mathbf{C}_i$ characterizes the functional interactions between the k-th ROI and all other ROIs (i.e., one-to-all FC-pattern of the k-th ROI for the i-th subject). Different from PC, SR estimates such a one-to-all FC-pattern $\mathbf{w}_i^k$ through linearly regressing BOLD signals from the k-th ROI $\mathbf{x}_i^k$ by BOLD signals of all other regions $\mathbf{X}_i^k$ using a l_1-norm sparse regularization:

$$\mathbf{w}_i^k = \arg\min_{\mathbf{w}_i^k} \frac{1}{2} \left\| \mathbf{x}_i^k - \mathbf{X}_i^k \mathbf{w}_i^k \right\|_2^2 + \lambda \left\| \mathbf{w}_i^k \right\|_1, \tag{1}$$

where λ is a regularization parameter controlling the sparsity of $\mathbf{w}_i^k$. SR models a brain network for each subject separately; such an independent modeling strategy may easily lead to relatively large inter-subject variability in $\mathbf{w}_i^k$. GSR-based FC network modeling can alleviate such a problem by jointly estimating non-zero connections across subjects via $l_{2,1}$-norm regularization-based group lasso:

$$\mathbf{W}^k = \arg\min_{\mathbf{W}^k} \sum_{i=1}^N \frac{1}{2} \left\| \mathbf{x}_i^k - \mathbf{X}_i^k \mathbf{w}_i^k \right\|_2^2 + \lambda \left\| \mathbf{W}^k \right\|_{2,1}, \tag{2}$$

where $\mathbf{W}^k = [\mathbf{w}_1^k, \mathbf{w}_2^k, \ldots, \mathbf{w}_N^k]$ consists of the one-to-all FC-patterns of the k-th ROI for all N subjects, and λ controls the amount of group sparsity. The brain networks modeled by GSR will share similar topological structures (by enforcing similar nonzero or zero connectivities for all subjects) to reduce inter-subject variability. However, an inherent problem of the GSR-based network modeling roots in the group lasso constrain term, which also sacrifices the potentially important between-group differences that often benefit the disease diagnosis. Thus, the suboptimal classification performance is achieved when applied to computer-aided disease diagnosis.

2.2   Inter-subject Similarity-Guided GSR for Brain Network Modeling

We propose to estimate inter-subject FC similarity based on PC values of the same FC-patterns between different subjects, and then use this as *a prior* to control the inter-subject similarity/difference in the final estimated FC. In the following, we explain how the constraint can be integrated into the GSR-based method for guiding the construction of better brain networks. Let $\mathbf{c}_i^k$ and $\mathbf{c}_j^k$ denote the regional FC-patterns (estimated by PC) of the k-th ROI for the i-th and the j-th subjects, respectively. A graph Laplacian [15, 16] is constructed with a similarity matrix $\mathbf{S}^k = [s_{ij}^k] \in \mathbb{R}^{N \times N}$ with $s_{ij}^k = \exp(-\left\|\mathbf{c}_i^k - \mathbf{c}_j^k\right\|_2^2 / \sigma)$ defining the pairwise similarity of subjects in terms of their FC patterns for the k-th ROI. For simplicity, we set the kernel width $\sigma = 1$ in our experiments. Then, a similarity-preserving regularization term can be defined to control the inter-subject similarity/difference as follows:

$$\Theta = \sum\nolimits_{i,j=1}^{N} s_{ij}^k \left\|\mathbf{w}_i^k - \mathbf{w}_j^k\right\|_2^2 = tr(\mathbf{W}^k \mathbf{L}^k (\mathbf{W}^k)^T), \tag{3}$$

where $\mathbf{L}^k = \mathbf{D}^k - \mathbf{S}^k$, and $\mathbf{D}^k \in \mathbb{R}^{N \times N}$ is a diagonal matrix with its diagonal elements defined as $d_{ii}^k = \sum_j s_{ij}^k$. By integrating the regularization term Θ into GSR, a new model for constructing brain network is derived as:

$$\mathbf{W}^k = \arg\min\nolimits_{\mathbf{W}^k} \sum\nolimits_{i=1}^{N} \frac{1}{2}\left\|\mathbf{x}_i^k - \mathbf{X}_i^k \mathbf{w}_i^k\right\|_2^2 + \lambda\left\|\mathbf{W}^k\right\|_{2,1} + tr(\mathbf{W}^k \mathbf{L}^k (\mathbf{W}^k)^T), \tag{4}$$

where λ_1 and λ_2 denote the regularization parameters for group sparsity and inter-subject FC-pattern similarity, respectively. In Eq. (4), by further adding the second regularization term Θ, we encourage inter-subject FC-pattern resemblance if their PC-based FC patterns are similar, and penalize inter-subject FC-pattern resemblance if their PC-based FC patterns are quite distinct. This will suppress within-group FC difference while retaining sufficient group differences. That is, the proposed new model will allow us to both achieve the good separability without losing the merit of group sparsity and promote the brain connectomics-based diagnosis. The optimization problem in Eq. (4) can be solved by an iterative approach, based on the accelerated proximal gradient algorithm [17]. Figure 1 illustrates the framework of our proposed inter-subject FC similarity constraint based GSR modeling. Specifically, for the i-th subject, the constructed brain network is formed as $\mathbf{G}_i = [\mathbf{w}_i^1, \mathbf{w}_i^2, \ldots, \mathbf{w}_i^K]$. Note that, the network matrix $\mathbf{G}_i$ is typically asymmetric. Thus, a symmetry operation $\mathbf{G}_i = (\mathbf{G}_i + \mathbf{G}_i^T)/2$ is further carried out to achieve the symmetric network.

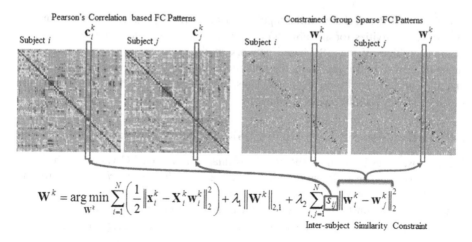

Fig. 1. Framework of our proposed brain network modeling method.

3 Experiments

3.1 Data Preprocessing

We use a publicly available Alzheimer's Disease Neuroimaging Initiative (ADNI) phase-2 dataset (http://adni.loni.usc.edu/) to evaluate our proposed brain FC network modeling method. Specifically, 52 normal control (NC) subjects and 52 MCI subjects with rs-fMRI data are selected. These selected subjects are age- and gender-matched, and were all scanned using 3.0T Philips scanners with the same imaging parameters. The rs-fMRI data of these subjects are preprocessed using SPM8 toolbox (http://www.fil.ion.ucl.ac.uk/spm/software/spm8/). In particular, the first three volumes of each rs-fMRI data are discarded for magnetization equilibrium. After head motion correction, the remaining rs-fMRI data are nonlinearly registered into Montreal Neurological Institute (MNI) space and further spatially smoothed by an isotropic Gaussian kernel with full-width-at-half-maximum (FWHM) of 6 mm. Of note, we do not perform data scrubbing (i.e., removing the rs-fMRI frames with larger than 0.5-mm frame-wise displacement), since this would introduce additional artifacts. However, the subjects with large frame-wise displacement for 2.5-min data are excluded in data screening. The rs-fMRI data are then parcellated into 116 ROIs based on the Automatic Anatomical Labeling (AAL) template. In each ROI, the mean time series is extracted and band-pass filtered (0.015–0.15 Hz); also, head motion parameters and the mean BOLD time series of both white matter and cerebrospinal fluid are regressed out for reducing the potential interference to the subsequent FC estimation.

3.2 Performance Evaluation

The upper triangle elements of the constructed brain network of each subject are concatenated to form a feature vector. The dimensionality of this feature vector is $116 \times (116 - 1)/2 = 6670$. Then, we carry out two-sample t-tests with a significance level of $p < 0.05$ to reduce the redundant features. Lasso [18] is further employed to select a small number of features with better discriminative ability. Finally, a support vector machine (SVM) with a linear kernel is trained on the selected features for MCI classification. The leave-one-out cross-validation (LOOCV) scheme is adopted for evaluation of diagnosis performance. In each fold of LOOCV procedure, an additional inner LOOCV is also carried out on the training data to determine the optimal hyper-parameters for the sparse regression (λ_1 and λ_2) as well as for the SVM. Classification performance is evaluated based on classification accuracy (ACC), area under ROC curve (AUC), sensitivity (SEN), and specificity (SPE). To further evaluate the effectiveness of our proposed framework, we have made extensive comparisons with the brain networks constructed by Pearson's correlation (PC), sparse representation (SR), group sparse representation (GSR), and our method, using the same dataset.

3.3   Experimental Results

Table 1 summarizes the classification results by different brain network modeling methods. Compared with PC, all of other sparse representation-based methods improved the classification accuracy. Among them, GSR performed better than SR, and our proposed method performed better than GSR. In particular, our proposed method produced the highest accuracy of 85.6%, with improvements of 21.2%, 15.4% and 7.7% compared with PC, SR, and GSR, respectively.

Table 1. Performance comparison of different network construction methods in MCI classification.

Method	ACC (%)	AUC	SEN (%)	SPE (%)
PC	64.4	0.709	61.5	67.3
SR	70.2	0.750	69.2	71.2
GSR	77.9	0.835	76.9	78.9
Proposed	**85.6**	**0.927**	**82.7**	**88.5**

To intuitively illustrate the superiority of our proposed network modeling method, we also present the separability values (r^2 value, with larger value indicating higher separability [19, 20]) between two groups, for each connection of the brain FC networks modeled using GSR (Fig. 2a) and our proposed method (Fig. 2b). Our method reveals larger and more group differences compared to the GSR-based method. Moreover, the potential biomarkers detected by our method are largely non-overlapped with those detected by GSR, indicating that including an additional constraint term has resulted in systematical changes of the constructed brain network. Our newly identified connectivities with large MCI/NC separability ($r^2 > 0.07$) mainly include three sets of connections: (1) within-hemisphere connections that specifically located in the left hemisphere (Fig. 2c), (2) inter-hemisphere connections (Fig. 2c), and (3) cerebro-cerebellar connections (Fig. 2d). Most of these connections involve brain regions at the frontal lobe, which indicates that the pathological changes of AD start from the frontal area.

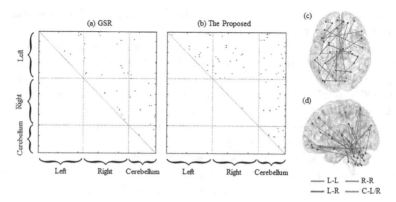

Fig. 2. Illustration of the separability matrices measured by r^2 values between the MCI and NC groups for the brain FC networks modeled by (a) GSR and (b) our proposed method, respectively. Here, only the r^2 values at the upper triangle are shown, since the matrices are symmetric. The blue points denote different biomarkers suggested by the two methods, while the red points denote the shared biomarkers by the two methods. Subfigures (c) and (d) depict the FC connectivities detected by our proposed method, where the connections of left-hemisphere (L-L), right hemisphere (R-R), and inter-hemisphere (L-R) are shown in (c) and the cerebro-cerebellar (C-L/R) connections are shown in (d).

4 Conclusion

In this paper, we propose a group-level brain network modeling method (i.e., with inter-subject similarity-guided group sparse representation) for better brain functional network construction. Experimental results show that our method is capable of improving network separability between different groups, which facilitates brain disease diagnosis. The effectiveness of our method has also been proven by significantly improving MCI classification, compared with the traditional Pearson's correlation or sparse representation based brain network modeling methods. All these suggest the promise of our method for future clinical brain imaging studies, especially for biomarker detection and personalized brain connectomics-based disease diagnosis.

Acknowledgements. This work is partially supported by NIH grants (EB006733, EB008374, EB009634, MH107815, AG041721, and AG042599).

References

1. Association, A.: Alzheimer's disease facts and figures. Alzheimers Dement. **9**(2), 208–245 (2013)
2. Gauthier, S., Reisberg, B., Zaudig, M., Petersen, R.C., Ritchie, K., Broich, K., Belleville, S., Brodaty, H., Bennett, D., Chertkow, H., Cummings, J.L.: Mild cognitive impairment. Lancet **367**(9518), 1262–1270 (2006)
3. Suk, H.I., Wee, C.Y., Lee, S.W., Shen, D.: Supervised discriminative group sparse representation for mild cognitive impairment diagnosis. Neuroinformatics **13**(3), 277–295 (2015)

4. Zhu, X., Suk, H.I., Wang, L., Lee, S.W., Shen, D.: A novel relational regularization feature selection method for joint regression and classification in AD diagnosis. Med. Image Anal. **38**, 205–214 (2017)
5. Zhu, X., Suk, H.I., Shen, D.: A novel matrix-similarity based loss function for joint regression and classification in AD diagnosis. NeuroImage **100**, 91–105 (2014)
6. Lee, M.H., Smyser, C.D., Shimony, J.S.: Resting-state fMRI: a review of methods and clinical applications. Am. J. Neuroradiol. **34**(10), 1866–1872 (2013)
7. Zhang, Y., Zhang, H., Chen, X., Lee, S.-W., Shen, D.: Hybrid high-order functional connectivity networks using resting-state functional MRI for mild cognitive impairment diagnosis. Scientific reports (2017)
8. Chen, X., Zhang, H., Lee, S.-W., Shen, D.: Hierarchical High-order functional connectivity networks and selective feature fusion for MCI classification. Neuroinformatics **15**, 271–284 (2017)
9. Chen, X., Zhang, H., Gao, Y., Wee, C.Y., Li, G., Shen, D.: High-order resting-state functional connectivity network for MCI classification. Hum. Brain Mapp. **37**(9), 3282–3296 (2016)
10. Lee, H., Lee, D.S., Kang, H., Kim, B.N., Chung, M.K.: Sparse brain network recovery under compressed sensing. IEEE Trans. Med. Imaging **30**(5), 1154–1165 (2011)
11. Yuan, M., Lin, Y.: Model selection and estimation in regression with grouped variables. J. R. Stat. Soc. Series B **68**(1), 49–67 (2006)
12. Wee, C.Y., Yap, P.T., Zhang, D., Wang, L., Shen, D.: Group-constrained sparse fMRI connectivity modeling for mild cognitive impairment identification. Brain Struct. Funct. **219**(2), 641–656 (2014)
13. Yu, R., Zhang, H., An, L., Chen, X., Wei, Z., Shen, D.: Connectivity strength-weighted sparse group representation-based brain network construction for MCI classification. Hum. Brain Mapp. **38**(5), 2370–2383 (2017)
14. Zeng, L.L., Shen, H., Liu, L., Hu, D.: Unsupervised classification of major depression using functional connectivity MRI. Hum. Brain Mapp. **35**(4), 1630–1641 (2014)
15. Zhou, T., Bhaskar, H., Liu, F., Yang, J.: Graph regularized and locality-constrained coding for robust visual tracking. IEEE Trans. Circuits Syst. Video Technol. (2016)
16. Zhu, X., Li, X., Zhang, S., Ju, C., Wu, X.: Robust joint graph sparse coding for unsupervised spectral feature selection. IEEE Trans. Neural Netw. Learn. Syst. **28**(6), 1263–1275 (2017)
17. Liu, M., Zhang, D., Shen, D.: View-centralized multi-atlas classification for Alzheimer's disease diagnosis. Hum. Brain Mapp. **36**(5), 1847–1865 (2015)
18. Zhang, Y., Zhou, G., Jin, J., Zhao, Q., Wang, X., Cichocki, A.: Aggregation of sparse linear discriminant analysis for event-related potential classification in brain-computer interface. Int. J. Neural Syst. **24**(1), 1450003 (2014)
19. Zhang, Y., Zhou, G., Zhao, Q., Jin, J., Wang, X., Cichocki, A.: Spatial-temporal discriminant analysis for ERP-based brain-computer interface. IEEE Trans. Neural Syst. Rehabil. Eng. **21**(2), 233–243 (2013)
20. Zhang, Y., Zhou, G., Jin, J., Zhao, Q., Wang, X., Cichocki, A.: Sparse Bayesian classification of EEG for brain-computer interface. IEEE Trans. Neural Netw. Learn. Syst. **27**(11), 2256–2267 (2016)

Scalable and Fault Tolerant Platform for Distributed Learning on Private Medical Data

Alborz Amir-Khalili[1]($\boxtimes$), Soheil Kianzad[2], Rafeef Abugharbieh[1], and Ivan Beschastnikh[2]

[1] Biomedical Signal and Image Computing Lab,
University of British Columbia, Vancouver, Canada
`alborza@ece.ubc.ca`

[2] Computer Science, University of British Columbia, Vancouver, Canada

Abstract. Medical image data is naturally distributed among clinical institutions. This partitioning, combined with security and privacy restrictions on medical data, imposes limitations on machine learning algorithms in clinical applications, especially for small and newly established institutions. We present InsuLearn: an intuitive and robust open-source (open-source code available at: https://github.com/ DistributedML/InsuLearn) platform designed to facilitate distributed learning (classification and regression) on medical image data, while preserving data security and privacy. InsuLearn is built on ensemble learning, in which statistical models are developed at each institution independently and combined at secure coordinator nodes. InsuLearn protocols are designed such that the liveness of the system is guaranteed as institutions join and leave the network. Coordination is implemented as a cluster of replicated state machines, making it tolerant to individual node failures. We demonstrate that InsuLearn successfully integrates accurate models for horizontally partitioned data while preserving privacy.

1 Introduction

State-of-the-art machine learning (ML) techniques have shown promise in medical image analysis. Performance of successful ML techniques, e.g., deep learning, is directly tied to the amount of data available during the training phase as more data allows the trained statistical model to account for rarely occurring patterns and increases specificity to outliers. Compared to natural image datasets, medical image datasets typically contain fewer instances as they are subject to certain restrictions, namely: (i) **privacy:** medical data are privacy-sensitive as access

This work is supported in part by the Institute for Computing, Information and Cognitive Systems (ICICS) at UBC.

Electronic supplementary material The online version of this chapter (doi:10. 1007/978-3-319-67389-9_21) contains supplementary material, which is available to authorized users.

© Springer International Publishing AG 2017
Q. Wang et al. (Eds.): MLMI 2017, LNCS 10541, pp. 176–184, 2017.
DOI: 10.1007/978-3-319-67389-9_21

to and transfer of patient data is restricted by privacy legislation; (ii) **distribution:** medical data are naturally distributed among different institutions; and (iii) **size:** medical image data requires considerable per-instance storage space and bandwidth for transfers between institutions. These restrictions limit medical data accessibility and constrain ML to data available at a single institution. This hurts collaboration and newly established, small, and rural institutions that do not have access to substantial datasets [1]. Unfortunately, most ML systems used by the medical image analysis community are not designed to overcome unique system requirements imposed by the restrictions above, which adds to the reluctance of clinical institutions to contribute data to these systems. All of the above points to a need for distributed ML systems that allow for multiple clinical data sources to contribute data without compromising data privacy.

Supporting data collaboration in a privacy-preserving way is challenging [2]. One solution is to generate a centralized *warehouse* that aggregates anonymized (sanitized) features extracted from different data sources. However, warehousing complicates data management and is ineffective at preventing adversaries from extracting sensitive information [3]. Furthermore, ethics review boards require a thorough audit of the proposed research before the sanitized data can be shared.

Private multi-party ML (PMPML) is an emerging alternative to warehousing, e.g., Google Inc. has recently revealed work in this space [4]. Among proposed PMPML methods, popular trends include: (T1) aggregation of privately learned models [1,5–7] or (T2) using distributed privacy-preserving solvers to iteratively train a global model [4,8]. Many T1 methods [5–7] require auxiliary publicly-available and annotated datasets, which limits their applicability. T2 methods, on the other hand, impose a predetermined global model that is sensitive to initialization and is thus difficult to design and refine. In contrast with T1 methods, T2 methods are designed for domains with more participants, i.e., smartphone users around the world [4] versus a few participating clinical institutions, and are thus ill-suited for the research and development of novel medical ML solutions.

To address the needs outlined above, we contribute **InsuLearn**: a scalable open-source solution that supports distributed T1 approaches in which every data source (node) privately trains local models that are then aggregated into a shared global model using an ensemble technique. InsuLearn does not require a publicly-available dataset and relies on other nodes to cross-validate locally trained models. As long as local models can be cross-validated at other nodes, InsuLearn does not impose any other requirements on the parameterization of the locally trained models. To our knowledge InsuLearn is the first open-source platform for the development of PMPML algorithms.

InsuLearn most closely resembles Li et al. [1] but, compared to InsuLearn, the peer-to-peer system of Li et al. is idealistic as: (i) It lacks a secure coordination node, implying that the local models trained at peers are known by all peers. This violates privacy since a malicious peer A can forward a crafted model to peer B and use B's response to infer data at B. (ii) The system was not implemented nor deployed on a real distributed system. (iii) The approach does not handle node/network failures, and does not discuss guarantees such as liveness, which is an ability of the system to make progress in spite of failures.

InsuLearn ensures data-security with built-in incentives to improve performance, deter abuse, and guarantee liveness as institutions join and leave the system. The key contributions of our work are: (i) We designed and implemented an open-source privacy-preserving distributed ML system that can interface with popular ML tools. (ii) We simultaneously improve privacy, fault tolerance, and liveness guarantees of the system by using replicated coordinator nodes. (iii) We propose a secure model aggregation scheme that is robust to noise and can be applied to popular classification and regression methods. (iv) We deployed our system prototype on Microsoft Azure cloud computing service to substantiate our claims regarding scalability and fault tolerance.

2   Methodology

InsuLearn uses ensemble learning techniques and supports different regression and classification tasks. Medical data is never transferred from one institution to another; instead, locally trained models are collected, sanitized, cross-validated, and aggregated into a global model with the help of coordinator nodes. InsuLearn is developed in Go, uses TCP for all network communication, and interfaces with the powerful ML toolboxes in MATLAB via MATLAB Engine C API[1]. This integration enables InsuLearn to deploy a wide selection of advanced ML algorithms and different ensemble strategies (e.g., boosting and bagging).

The basic representation of InsuLearn consists of a trusted secure coordinator node s_0 connected to $H = \{h_i : i = 1, 2, ..., N\}$ nodes representing N different institutions. We start with the following assumptions: (1) s_0 is secure, fault tolerant, and non-malicious; (2) h_i may be malicious, i.e., may try to infer information about data at other nodes and may upload false results (noise) into the system; and (3) malicious nodes do not collude and do not control the majority of the data across all the nodes. We first make the above assumptions and present our aggregation technique for generating a global model G from a set of locally trained models. We then present a more robust version of the system in which we relax the fault tolerance assumption of s_0 by replacing s_0 with a set $S = \{s_r : r = 1, 2, ..., R\}$ of R replicated coordinator nodes.

Model Aggregation: The goal is to generate a global predictor model $G(\mathbf{x}; \Theta) = \hat{\mathbf{y}}$ by aggregating a set of trained local predictor models $M = \{m(\mathbf{x}; \theta_i) = \hat{\mathbf{y}} : i = 1, 2, ..., N\}$ parametrized by $\Theta = \{\theta_i : i = 1, 2, ..., N\}$, where each θ_i is independently trained on a corresponding fraction of the data $X = \{\mathbf{x}_i : i = 1, 2, ..., N\}$ and labels $Y = \{\mathbf{y}_i : i = 1, 2, ..., N\}$ in the system. In this context, training entails finding parameters θ_i that minimize the error $\epsilon(\hat{\mathbf{y}}_i, \mathbf{y}_i)$ between label $\mathbf{y}_i$ and prediction $\hat{\mathbf{y}}_i$; this process may be expressed as

$$\underset{\theta_i}{\operatorname{argmin}} \ \epsilon(m(\mathbf{x}_i; \theta_i), \mathbf{y}_i). \tag{1}$$

The global model $G(\mathbf{x}; \Theta, W, D) = \sum_{\forall i} w_i m(\mathbf{x}; \theta_i) / \sum_{\forall i} w_i$, is defined as a weighted average of independently trained local models, where the weights $w_i \in W$

---

[1] Open-source code available at: https://github.com/DistributedML/InsuLearn.

$$w_i = d_i \sum_{\forall j} e^{-R_i(\epsilon(m(\mathbf{x}_j; \theta_i), \mathbf{y}_j))} \qquad (2)$$

are obtained from a combination representing the sample size $d_i \in D$ of local data $\mathbf{x}_i$ on which θ_i was trained and an exponential loss computed by a ranking function $R_i : \epsilon(m(\mathbf{x}_j; \theta_i), \mathbf{y}_j) \subset \mathbb{R} \to \mathbb{N}$, which captures the predictive performance of parameters θ_i on data $\mathbf{x}_j$ of node h_j using an error metric ϵ. To eliminate the contribution of poor performing or potentially malicious models, every weight w_i that is below the median value of all weights W is set to zero.

General System Protocol: The proposed aggregation approach requires all θ_i models to be cross-validated using the data $\mathbf{x}_i$ from all N nodes, which can be stored in a mapping of $E(i, j) : \mathbb{R}^{N \times N} \to \epsilon(m(\mathbf{x}_j; \theta_i), \mathbf{y}_j)$. E should not be made available to h_i as it may be malicious and use $E(i, j)$ to make inferences about the data $\mathbf{x}_j$ at h_j. We use the coordinator node s_0 as an intermediary for all interactions between H. This simplifies the burden and dependency between H as they become stateless (i.e., are not required to record preceding events in their interaction with the coordinator) by shifting all state information, aside from the state of sensitive data stored at each node, to s_0. Therefore, a node h_i in the system can only perform the following interactions with the coordinator:

(1) generate a new model and send $\{d_i, \theta_i\}$ to s_0;
(2) request and receive global model G from s_0; and
(3) receive and test incoming model parameters θ_* from s_0 by computing the error $\epsilon(m(\mathbf{x}_i; \theta_*), \mathbf{y}_i)$ and communicate the computed error back to s_0.

Since, h_i cannot associate θ_* with any other node in H^2, it cannot compromise the privacy of the other nodes. On the other hand, the stateful coordinator s_0 must maintain all state information. Specifically, s_0 must do the following:

(1) maintain a database of participating nodes H and associated $\{\Theta, D, E, W\}$;
(2) receive θ_i from h_i, anonymize $\theta_{i \to *}$ and forward θ_* to $h_j, \forall h_j \in H, j \neq i$;
(3) receive $\epsilon(m(\mathbf{x}_j; \theta_*), \mathbf{y}_j)$ from h_j and update $E(* \to i, j)$;
(4) commit changes to $\{\Theta, D, W\}$ after E is completed; and
(5) receive global model G requests from h_i, generate G, and send G to h_i.

The singular s_0 coordinator is impractical for real applications. If s_0 fails, all state information and progress by the system will be lost. Next, we detail improvements to achieve stronger liveness guarantees in InsuLearn.

Fault Tolerance: We make the coordinator fault tolerant by replacing s_0 with S, a cluster of R coordinators [9] that replicate copies of state $\{\Theta, D, E, W\}$. This replicated version of InsuLearn can survive up to $\lceil R/2 \rceil - 1$ coordinator failures (a necessary failures upper-bound for all majority-based consensus protocols). InsuLearn coordinators use the Raft consensus algorithm [10] to guarantee liveness and maintain strong consistency of replicated state. We use Raft because it has several well-tested, industry-standard, and open-source implementations.

---

² In fact h_i does not know the size of H nor the nodes in H.

Raft is a leader-based consensus algorithm. A leader is elected from S whose commands are confirmed and replicated by other replicas in S. In case a leader fails, Raft will elect a new leader without compromising liveness and the consistency of $\{\Theta, D, E, W\}$, which are replicated by all of the nodes in S.

Nodes contact any of the replicated coordinators to join the system. In case of a coordinator failure a node transparently switches to another coordinator. New nodes can join the system at any time.

Partial Model Update: The coordinators can process incoming local models $\{d_i, \theta_i\}$ and requests for G asynchronously as changes to $\{\Theta, D, W\}$ and aggregation into G is performed only by the leader. The leader coordinator does not commit changes to $\{\Theta, D, W\}$ until E is completed; meaning that θ_i in Θ and associated $\{W, D\}$ are not replaced or set to zero when a new θ_i is submitted by h_i until $\{d_i, \theta_i\}$ is tested by all other nodes in H.

InsuLearn incentivizes nodes to test the models of other nodes. It maintains a *testQueue* in S that prevents h_i from submitting new models until h_i has performed all of the pending tests. During operation, some of the test nodes may go offline or be slow to test θ_* (e.g., as a denial of service attack by a malicious h_i). In this situation, delaying the commit to $\{\Theta, D, W\}$ until all test node results are available may indefinitely block the system. InsuLearn coordinators overcome this problem by actively computing a running sum of test data size d_i over all nodes responding to tests on $\theta_{i \to *}$. A *partial commit* of a model update may then be performed if the associated sum exceeds a predetermined fraction, e.g., half of the total available distributed data $\sum_{\forall i} d_i$, followed by additional partial commits with subsequent updates to $E(i, .)$.

3   Results and Discussions

To assess the validity of the learned global model G, we test InsuLearn on a classification task using a skin segmentation dataset and a regression task using real Parkinson's telemonitoring data; both of which are publicly available from the UCI ML repository [11]. The skin segmentation dataset consists of a large binary classification problem containing 245,057 instances (50,000 of which were randomly selected for our experiments) with 3 attributes, and the telemonitoring data consists of 5,875 instances with 26 attributes. For both tasks 25% of the instances are randomly selected for testing and the remainder is used for training. Training set instances are randomly split across $N = 20$ nodes and then the training data is augmented with an additional 25% of random noise instances, which are distributed across the nodes.

We assess trade-offs associated with secured distributed learning by comparing regression and classification errors of our proposed approach to a naïve secure aggregation approach (where the weights are equal $w_i = 1/N$) and an unsecure warehouse approach (where we simply pool all data prior to training). Ten different built-in MATLAB classification and regression methods are used in our evaluation and the test errors are computed on 100 randomly distributed datasets, averaged, and presented Fig. 1. To test the effects of a deliberate attack

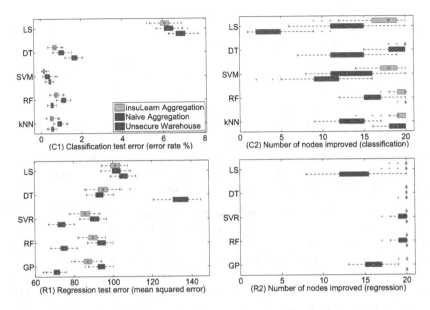

Fig. 1. Performance of three global model aggregation methods. Each method is tested using **(C1)** five different MATLAB classification and **(R1)** five regression functions on real data (randomly redistributed over 20 nodes and averaged over 100 trials). At each trial, the total number of nodes whose local model was improved upon by the global **(C2)** classification and **(R2)** regression model is also computed and presented. Results indicate that our proposed aggregation outperforms the naïve method.

on the system, we perform our experiments on (i) a case where noise is randomly distributed across all nodes (results shown in Fig. 1), and on (ii) a case where noise is injected into a single malicious node (results in supplementary material).

Model Aggregation Performance: The test results clearly demonstrate a reduction in test error with InsuLearn's aggregation scheme over the naïve approach for all learning models except for decision tree (DT) regression (C1 in Fig. 1). In each experiment we also computed the total number of nodes whose local model was improved upon by the global model (C2 and R2 in Fig. 1) and observed that, compared to the naïve global model, more nodes benefited from the global model learned by InsuLearn. InsuLearn outperforms the warehouse approach on simpler models, i.e., least squares (LS) and DT, but this is due to the fact that LS and DT are weak learners that are improved by ensembling. Compared to more advanced methods that already incorporate ensembling like random forests (RF), kernel transformations like support vector regression (SVR), and Gaussian process (GP) optimization, the performance with InsuLearn is no better than warehousing. This is expected because of an unavoidable trade-off between data privacy and accuracy of the estimated model. In case of bagging, for example, the trade-off manifests in a loss of the ability to train on bootstrap samples from data that spans across multiple nodes. It is important to note that an improvement over locally trained models are not guaranteed, even with advanced methods implemented on the unsecure warehousing approach (e.g., RF classification on unsecure warehouse, Fig. 1 C2).

It is also important to note that our proposed approach is generic and can be applied to *all* classification and regression methods. Tailoring the aggregation scheme to each method may improve performance but our generic approach is sufficient to aggregate the different local models into one.

As expected, the distribution of noise did not effect the warehouse approach. On the other hand, while our proposed method performs marginally better in LS tests when noise is injected at a single node, performance drops for more complicated models when noise is not randomly distributed. However, the performance of our proposed method is still better than the naïve approach.

Scalability: We simulated a real deployment of InsuLearn by deploying it on the Microsoft Azure cloud to measure scalability and fault tolerance. Coordinators and nodes were deployed, each in an independent, identical DS1_V2 virtual machine with 1 core and 3.5 GB of memory and connected over a virtual network. To test the scalability of the system, we set the number of coordinators $R = 7$ and scaled the total number of emulated institutions $N = \{10, 30, 50, 70, 100\}$. The behavior at each node was automated with a state machine that restricts the node to only submit its local model once to the system. Nodes were added to the system with a randomized $\delta \in (0, 2)$ minute delay from the start of the coordinators. We measured the time it took to generate a complete global model, encapsulating models from all N nodes, over 5 independent runs and observed linear performance scaling with N (Fig. 2a). Model testing at nodes is independent and nodes can perform training in parallel. Idempotent communication and commutative update operations protect the system from a large number of highly concurrent nodes and improves InsuLearn's scalability.

Fault Tolerance: To assess fault tolerance, we fixed $R = 7$ and $N = 30$, updated the state machines to emulate random intermittent fail-and-restart with frequency γ_H for nodes that have pushed their models to the coordinators, and

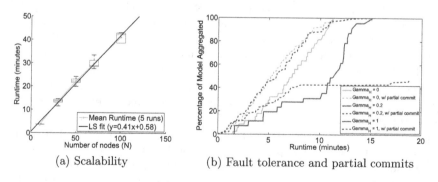

(a) Scalability   (b) Fault tolerance and partial commits

Fig. 2. (a) Scalability of InsuLearn with number of nodes, and (b) the advantage of partial commits during node failures.

measured progress in terms of percentage of global model G committed over the run of the system (Fig. 2b). We tested the system for cases where $\gamma_H = \{0, 0.2, 1\}$ failures per minutes and with/without the partial commit feature to see how partial commits affect the global model update rate. We observed that once the fail-and-start frequency surpasses a certain rate, progress in the system halts as nodes leave as soon as they submit their local models while there is not sufficient time to train on new models before the next failure. However, with the partial commit feature, a significant portion of the change to G is preserved.

Security: InsuLearn assumes that coordinators in S are secure. Although coordinators only know the results of the tests and sources of committed model, they can obtain more knowledge by manipulating test requests. For example, a rogue coordinator can ask a node h_i to test a number of malicious models and thereby infer information about data at h_i. Solving this problem requires nodes to detect and reject suspicious requests. One solution is to use a Byzantine fault tolerance algorithm such as PBFT [12]. In this approach a node checks that a consensus among coordinators has been reached prior to testing the model. A PBFT-based system with $3t$ coordinators can withstand t malicious coordinators. However, the extra rounds of communication would impose a substantial performance penalty.

4   Conclusions

We presented a fault tolerant distributed PMPML system called InsuLearn in which, with the exception of the anonymized local model, no information from one node is shared with other nodes. We compared InsuLearn against an unsecure warehousing and naïve model averaging approaches and showed that InsuLearn is fault tolerant and has reliable performance, surpassing a naïve aggregation approach. Our work shows the feasibility of ML on highly sensitive distributed medical image data. We hope that our open-source GitHub project will be adopted by others and encourage the development of an accessible and secure distributed ML toolkit that can facilitate medical research that is otherwise impractical.

References

1. Li, Y., Bai, C., Reddy, C.K.: A distributed ensemble approach for mining healthcare data under privacy constraints. Inf. Sci. **330**, 245–259 (2016)
2. Ohno-Machado, L.: To share or not to share: that is not the question. Sci. Trans. Med. **4**(165), 165cm15 (2012)
3. Fabian, B., Göthling, T.: Privacy-preserving data warehousing. Int. J. Bus. Intell. Data Min. **10**(4), 297–336 (2015)
4. McMahan, H.B., Moore, E., Ramage, D., Hampson, S., Arcas, B.A.: Communication-efficient learning of deep networks from decentralized data. In: Artificial Intelligence and Statistics (2016)
5. Hamm, J., Cao, P., Belkin, M.: Learning privately from multiparty data. In: International Conference on Machine Learning, pp. 555–563 (2016)

6. Xie, L., Plis, S., Sarwate, A.D.: Data-weighted ensemble learning for privacy-preserving distributed learning. In: ICASSP, pp. 2309–2313. IEEE (2016)
7. Wu, Y., Jiang, X., Kim, J., Ohno-Machado, L.: Grid Binary LOgistic REgression (GLORE): building shared models without sharing data. J. Am. Med. Inform. Assoc. **19**(5), 758–764 (2012)
8. Shokri, R., Shmatikov, V.: Privacy-preserving deep learning. In: Computer and Communications Security, pp. 1310–1321. ACM (2015)
9. Schneider, F.B.: Implementing fault-tolerant services using the state machine approach: a tutorial. ACM Comput. Surv. **22**(4), 299–319 (1990)
10. Ongaro, D., Ousterhout, J.K.: In search of an understandable consensus algorithm. In: USENIX Annual Technical Conference, pp. 305–319 (2014)
11. Lichman, M.: UCI machine learning repository (2013)
12. Castro, M., Liskov, B.: Practical byzantine fault tolerance and proactive recovery. ACM Trans. Comput. Syst. **20**(4), 398–461 (2002)

Triple-Crossing 2.5D Convolutional Neural Network for Detecting Neuronal Arbours in 3D Microscopic Images

Siqi Liu[1]([✉]), Donghao Zhang[1], Yang Song[1], Hanchuan Peng[2], and Weidong Cai[1]

[1] School of Information Technologies, University of Sydney, Sydney, NSW, Australia
siqi.liu@sydney.edu.au
[2] Allen Institute for Brain Science, Seattle, WA, USA

Abstract. The automatic analysis of the 3D optical microscopic images containing neuron cells remains one of the central challenges in the modern computational neuroscience. The varying image qualities make the accurate detection of the curvilinear neuronal arbours elusive. The high computational cost raised by large 3D image volumes also makes the conventional filter-bank learning methods impractical. We present a novel Triple-Crossing (TC) 2.5D convolutional neural network to detect the neuronal arbours in large 3D microscopic volumes with a reasonable computational cost. The network is trained to output a regression map that indicates the presence of the neuronal arbours. The proposed methods can be used as a pre-processing step in an automated neuronal circuit reconstruction pipeline, which enables the collection of large-scale neuron morphological datasets. In our experiments, we show that the proposed methods could effectively eliminate dense background noises and fix the gaps along neuronal arbours. The proposed methods could also outperform the original 2.5D neural network regarding the training efficiency as well as the generalisation performance.

1 Introduction

Characterising the 3D morphology of a neuron, including its dendritic and axonal arbours, is central to determining its phenotype identity, connectivity, synaptic integration, firing properties, and ultimately its role in the neuronal circuit. To acquire the neuronal morphological data, 3D optical microscopic images were acquired to capture the curvilinear arbours and the blob-shaped soma of neuron cells. Detecting both structure types from the noisy image background is essential to accurately reconstruct the 3D neuron morphological models for neuron morphology studies. However, though the location of soma is normally easy to determine, the imaging artefacts make the accurate detection of the curvilinear arbours difficult. Such artefacts are dense noises and unevenly distributed intensities along the neuronal arbours which are normally caused by the fundamental limits of light microscopic imaging [8].

© Springer International Publishing AG 2017
Q. Wang et al. (Eds.): MLMI 2017, LNCS 10541, pp. 185–193, 2017.
DOI: 10.1007/978-3-319-67389-9_22

Hand-crafted filters were used to detect curvilinear structures with multi-scale anisotropic filters using the image gradient and Hessian information [4,5,7]. However, the performance of such hand-crafted filters could be limited in challenging cases as well as sensitive to the hyper-parameters. Recently, patch-based learning methods have been shown to outperform the hand-crafted filters by training either a binary voxel classifier [2] or a continuous centreline distance transform [12]. However, these learning based methods could be elusive to scale to 3D for practical use due to the enormous computational cost of performing 3D convolution and storing volumetric image descriptors.

The 2.5D Convolutional Neural Network (2.5D CNN) provides an alternative end-to-end learning approach to reduce the computational cost in the patch-based 3D image learning tasks [12]. The 2.5D CNN uses three orthogonal 2D slices of each 3D patch as the inputs for a 2D CNN. The convolutional kernel weights are shared among three input slices at the first convolutional layer. 2.5D CNN could make the 3D dense prediction feasible by using fewer parameters and allowing more augmented data samples for better model generalisation. However, the missing voxel information from the diagonal directions might constrain the performance of the 2.5D CNN.

In this paper, we present the Triple-Crossing (TC) 2.5D CNN for detecting neuronal arbours in 3D optical microscopic images. The proposed methods are effective in eliminating most of the background noises as well as fixing the arbours with broken shapes. To include more 3D contextual information than the previous 2.5D CNN, the sampling scheme of TC 2.5D patch consists of 9 slices centred at the voxel of interest. Also, the residual blocks [6] are used in the proposed network architecture to prevent network training from prematurity. In addition, to directly train deep networks with microscopic images which vastly vary in object intensities, we use the gradient-based intensity normalisation for volume histogram matching [11]. The proposed method was evaluated with a large number of patches extracted from 3D volumes containing neurons from different species. The results showed the networks trained by the proposed method can converge to lower costs than the previous 2.5D CNN and generalise

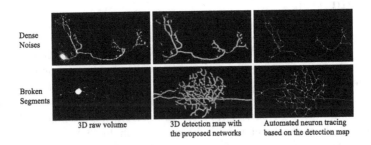

Fig. 1. The visual inspections of the neuronal arbours detected by the Triple-Crossing 2.5D Network (middle) and the automated neuron tracing based on the detection map (right). The proposed method is effective for eliminating the majority of dense noises and fixing the broken arbours.

better in predicting the unseen volumes. Some example effects and the application on neuron tracing of the proposed method are shown in Fig. 1.

2   Methods

2.1   Scale-Space Distance Transform of Neuronal Centreline

To automatically detect the neuronal arbours, a machine learning model can be designed to highlight the neuronal arbours of interests and suppress the background. Though intuitively the problem can be formed as a binary classification task, annotating a precise binary label map on large 3D image volumes is labour intensive. Since the neuronal arbours are generally curvilinear, it is relatively easier to obtain the validated neuronal tree models, in which the edges represent the approximated centrelines of neuronal arbours.

   To generate the ground truth for this learning task, we use a manually traced neuron model to generate a synthetic centreline transform $d(p, r)$ with the Scale-Space Distance Transform [12]

$$d(p, r) = \begin{cases} e^{\alpha \cdot (1 - \frac{D_C(p,r)}{d_M})} - 1 & \text{for } D(p, r) \leq d_M \\ 0 & \text{otherwise} \end{cases} \tag{1}$$

where $D(p, r)$ is a scaled distance transform at the 3D coordinate p with r as the arbour radius estimated in the input image. $D_C(p, r)$ is the scale space distance transform defined as:

$$D_C(p, r) = \|p - p'\|_2^2 + k(r - r') \tag{2}$$

where p' and r' are respectively the coordinate and the radius of the closest point on the neuronal centreline. Here, k, α and d_M are the free parameters chosen according to different datasets. We use $d(p, r)$ as the ground truth regression map for training the deep networks. $d(p, r)$ is only an approximate estimate of the presence of neuronal arbours since the manually annotated neuronal models do not guarantee to define precise neuronal centrelines. Thus, the predicted volume is used for segmenting the neuron from the noisy background by applying a fixed threshold (40%) in our study. The exact neuronal centrelines can be obtained with neuron tracing pipelines based on the segmentation volume.

2.2   Triple-Crossing Patches for 2.5D CNN

In the patch-based 3D learning tasks, 3D patches x_i with size K^3 are sampled from a 3D volume V to represent the contextual information surrounding the i-th voxel. To reduce the computational cost and the required amount of data for 3D learning, 2.5D CNN [10] uses three orthogonal 3D slices $\{x_{i1}, x_{i2}, x_{i3}\}$ centred at the i-th voxel to represent the 3D blocks as shown in Fig. 2(a), reducing the patch size from K^3 to $3K$. 2.5D CNN shares the same architecture as 2D CNN by using $\{x_{i1}, x_{i2}, x_{i3}\}$ as different input channels for 2D CNN. Thus, the hidden

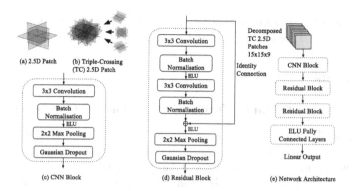

Fig. 2. The illustration of (a) the 2.5D patch and (b) the proposed Triple-Crossing (TC) 2.5D patch containing 9 slices. The diagonal slices in TC patches provide more contextual information than the 2.5D patches. The neural network architecture used is shown in (e) with the CNN block and the residual block depicted in (c) and (d) respectively.

receptive fields of the 2.5D CNN are jointly learnt based on all the three input slices. However, the performance of 2.5D patches might be constrained by the missing contextual information from the diagonal directions.

We propose to train the 2.5D CNN with the Triple-Crossing (TC) 2.5D patch which contains 9 slices instead of 3. The initial 3 sampling grids G_{XY}^1, G_{YZ}^1, G_{XZ}^1 with size $K \times K$ are formed on the planes perpendicular to the Z, X and Y axises. Then each grid is rotated by $-\pi/4$ and $\pi/4$ to form G_{XY}^2, G_{YZ}^2, G_{XZ}^2 and G_{XY}^3, G_{YZ}^3, G_{XZ}^3 respectively. The TC 2.5D patch x_{ij} is obtained as $x_{ij} = V(G_i)$, where $V(.)$ represents the 3D grid interpolation and G_i is the TC grids corresponding to the i-th patch. To speed up the formation of G_i, we initialise G' centred at the origin with size $15 \times 15 \times 9$ firstly and then apply 3D transformations to G' for rotation, translation and scaling before interpolating the TC 2.5D patches with data augmentation. We found it practical to fix the scale of the sampling scheme within the same volume since CNN is capable of learning receptive fields for different scales. However, the data augmentation with 3D rotations is important for the curvilinear structure detection. CNN would otherwise be overfitted since most of the receptive fields are trained to be sensitive to few directions.

2.3   Triple-Crossing 2.5D CNNs with Residual-Blocks

The TC 2.5D patch x_{ij} sampled at the i-th 3D coordinate with the j-th augmented observation can be used as the input channels for a 2D CNN. The proposed network consists of 1 initial CNN block, 2 residual blocks and a single linear output to predict the value map described in Sect. 2.1. The number of blocks was chosen by considering the balance between the learning capability and the computational cost. The output values from different observations at the same voxel are averaged. We use receptive fields of size 3×3 for all the convolutional layers. Inside the initial CNN block shown in Fig. 2(c), we use a convolutional layer with 64 receptive fields followed by a batch normalisation. The number of receptive fields is doubled in each higher convolutional layer. The normalised hidden feature maps are nonlinearly transformed with the Exponential Linear Units (ELU) [3] instead of ReLU for faster speed and better generalisation. 2×2 Max-pooling is applied after ELU. To avoid the training from over-fitting, a 25% Gaussian Dropout rate is applied.

With the depth of CNN increasing, the training and validation accuracy tend to saturate or become worse due to the degradation problem [6]. To address the degradation problem, we add the residual blocks, depicted in Fig. 2(d), [6] on top of the first convolutional layer. A residual block fits a mapping of $F(x) := H(x) - x$ by recasting it to $H(x) = F(x) + x$ using a shortcut identity connection, where $H(x)$ is the residual representation. x represents the inputs from a previous layer and $F(x)$ represents a weighted convolutional layer. The identity connections are helpful to increase the information flow across layers at different depths for refining the 2.5D representations. The entire network architecture is depicted in Fig. 2(e). The networks are optimised with the RMSProp algorithm.

2.4   Gradient-Based Intensity Normalisation

The normalisation of image intensities is essential to successfully train neural networks directly from voxels. However, the standard intensity normalisation methods perform poorly for confocal microscopic images, since the object density can vary remarkably between different images, even within the same dataset. Before training and predicting using the proposed neural network, we apply the gradient based intensity normalisation (GIN) [11] to normalise the intensity values of all images. In GIN, we firstly choose a reference volume from the training set, and then extract its gradient based intensity profile p_i as:

$$p_i = \sum_{g=0}^{R-1} g b_{ig} / \sum_{g=0}^{R-1} b_{ig} \tag{3}$$

where g is the gradient magnitude index of the image; R is the total level of grey scale intensity values; b_{ig} is computed as the number of occurrences of image pixels with intensity i and gradient magnitude g. This profile is invariant to change in the total number of voxels for the given intensity value i, depending only on the distribution of gradient values of those voxels. The intensities of all the other training images and future unseen images are mapped to the profile p_i with the fundamental histogram matching before sampling the TC 2.5D patches.

3   Experiments and Results

The neural network architectures were implemented with TensorFlow [1]. The code used in our experiments including the TC 2.5D patch extraction and deep network training will be released publicly. To evaluate the proposed methods,

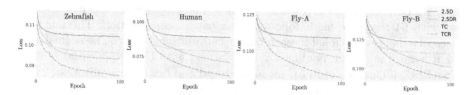

Fig. 3. The training convergence plots of the compared methods in 4 datasets. The training losses present were obtained with 100 epochs in the first leave-one-volume-out trial.

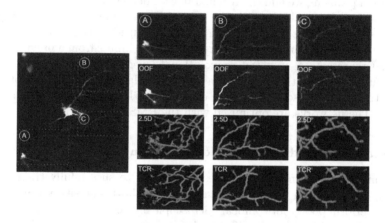

Fig. 4. Left: a low quality volume of a zebrafish adult neuron; Right: three sub-regions in each column for comparing the effects of different approaches including the optimal oriented flux (OOF), 2.5D CNN (2.5D) and the Triple-Crossing 2.5D CNN with residual blocks (TCR). The proposed TCR is capable of detecting the curvilinear structures as well as eliminating the background noises.

we extract a large number of patches from four challenging datasets from the BigNeuron repository which are publicly available [9]. obtained from a brain research institute. Each dataset contains five 3D volumes of single neurons from different animals, including the zebrafish, human and two datasets of fly (Fly-A and Fly-B) captured using different imaging pipelines. The volumes come with various sizes. Each 3D volume is accompanied with a 3D neuron model manually annotated and validated by at least three neuroscientists. The 3D models were used for synthesising the ground truth value map described in Sect. 2.1. The parameters k, α and d_M were fixed as 1, 6 and 5.

We evaluated the proposed method with respectively 2.5D patches and TC 2.5D patches. We also compared the deep CNNs with and without residual blocks described in Sect. 2.3. The sequential networks (2.5D and TC) and the residual networks (2.5DR and TCR) had approximately the same amount of parameters with 5 CNN blocks. The network architectures and the training settings were held consistent across different datasets.

All the compared CNN models were directly trained and tested on the raw voxels with the gradient based intensity normalisation described in Sect. 2.4. 60000 locations were sampled with 3 random rotations in each volume for training, resulting in 9×10^6 2.5D or Triple-Crossing 2.5D training patches for every dataset. We ensured that half of the training set have non-zero ground truth values. For testing volumes, the patches were obtained on the voxels with intensities above 0 with 3 random rotations. To evaluate the generalisation performance of the proposed methods, the leave-one-volume-out evaluation was used on each dataset, ensuring the patches in each volume were only predicted with a network trained using the patches from different volumes. The patches were cached and queried using HDF5 files. All the experiments were performed with the computing nodes containing one Nvidia Tesla K40 GPU and 128 GB RAM.

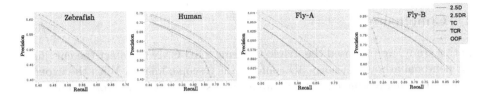

Fig. 5. The precision recall curves of different methods in 4 datasets. The curves were obtained by adjusting a tolerance threshold on the predicted regression maps. The regions with $d(p, r) < d_M/2$ in the ground truth volumes were considered as the ground truth segmentation.

The training losses of the networks are shown in Fig. 3. In all four datasets, TC 2.5D CNNs could fit faster eventually to a lower cost than the 2.5D CNNs. Though the residual networks (2.5DR and TCR) fit slightly slowly in the early epochs, the losses of both 2.5DR and TCR were able to keep descending after the sequential CNNs (2.5D and TC) converged to a plateau.

We show the visual inspection of a testing volume in Fig. 4. The proposed method (TCR) was capable of fixing the curvilinear structures with broken segments as well as eliminating more false positive points than the 2.5D network. To evaluate the generalisation performance of the proposed method on segmenting 3D volumes, the regions with $d(p, r) < d_M/2$ in the 3D ground truth maps were considered as the ground truth segmentation for each testing volume. We generated the precision-recall (PR) curves as shown in Fig. 5 by varying a tolerance threshold on the predicted volumes, ranging from 0% to 100% of the predicted domain. The PR curves were averaged across the five leave-one-volume-out trials. The results with either precision or recall lower than 0.4 were excluded from Fig. 5 to discard the predicted segmentation maps that were practically unusable. The proposed TC 2.5D patches generalised better than the 2.5D patches in the unseen volumes from all the four datasets with higher precision and recall values. In the datasets with zebrafish and human neurons, the TCR approach achieved the best testing performance. In the other two datasets with fly neurons, the sequential CNN with TC 2.5D patches performed slightly better than the residual networks, since the large inter-volume variance in two fly datasets might make the residual blocks easier to be overfitted. The performance of the residual networks might be further improved when more annotated neuron images become available. The CNN based methods greatly outperformed the conventional OOF filter in all datasets.

We evaluated the prediction time (ms/patch) by averaging approximately 1.32×10^8 total predictions from 4 datasets. The average patch prediction time of 2.5D CNN and TC 2.5D CNN were respectively 0.782 ms and 0.835 ms. A slightly longer prediction time was observed since only the size of the input layer weight was different. With the residual blocks, the patch prediction time of 2.5DR and TCR methods were 0.968 ms and 0.982 ms respectively. The additional time cost was introduced by the shortcut connections.

4 Conclusion

In this study, we proposed the Triple-Crossing 2.5D CNN to detect the curvilinear neuronal arbours in noisy 3D confocal microscopic images. With the experiments involving a large number of patches, we showed that the proposed Triple-Crossing 2.5D CNN could outperform the previous 2.5D CNN.

References

1. Abadi, M., Agarwal, A., Barham, P., et al.: TensorFlow: large-scale machine learning on heterogeneous distributed systems. arxiv:1603.04467 (2015)
2. Becker, C., Rigamonti, R., Lepetit, V., Fua, P.: Supervised feature learning for curvilinear structure segmentation. In: Mori, K., Sakuma, I., Sato, Y., Barillot, C., Navab, N. (eds.) MICCAI 2013. LNCS, vol. 8149, pp. 526–533. Springer, Heidelberg (2013). doi:10.1007/978-3-642-40811-3_66
3. Clevert, D.A., Unterthiner, T., Hochreiter, S.: Fast and accurate deep network learning by exponential linear units (ELUs). arxiv:1511.07289 (2015)
4. Frangi, A.F., Niessen, W.J., Vincken, K.L., Viergever, M.A.: Multiscale vessel enhancement filtering. In: Wells, W.M., Colchester, A., Delp, S. (eds.) MICCAI 1998. LNCS, vol. 1496, pp. 130–137. Springer, Heidelberg (1998). doi:10.1007/BFb0056195
5. Hannink, J., Duits, R., Bekkers, E.: Crossing-preserving multi-scale vesselness. In: Golland, P., Hata, N., Barillot, C., Hornegger, J., Howe, R. (eds.) MICCAI 2014. LNCS, vol. 8674, pp. 603–610. Springer, Cham (2014). doi:10.1007/978-3-319-10470-6_75
6. He, K., Zhang, X., Ren, S., Sun, J.: Deep residual learning for image recognition. In: CVPR, pp. 770–778 (2016)
7. Law, M.W.K., Chung, A.C.S.: Three dimensional curvilinear structure detection using optimally oriented flux. In: Forsyth, D., Torr, P., Zisserman, A. (eds.) ECCV 2008. LNCS, vol. 5305, pp. 368–382. Springer, Heidelberg (2008). doi:10.1007/978-3-540-88693-8_27
8. Pawley, J.B.: Fundamental limits in confocal microscopy. In: Pawley, J.B. (ed.) Handbook of Biological Confocal Microscopy, pp. 20–42. Springer, Boston (2006)

9. Peng, H., Hawrylycz, M., Roskams, J., Hill, S., Spruston, N., Meijering, E., Ascoli, G.A.: BigNeuron: large-scale 3D neuron reconstruction from optical microscopy images. Neuron **87**(2), 252–256 (2015)

10. Roth, H.R., Lu, L., Liu, J., Yao, J., Seff, A., Cherry, K., Kim, L., Summers, R.M.: Improving computer-aided detection using convolutional neural networks and random view aggregation. IEEE Trans. Med. Imaging **35**(5), 1170–1181 (2016)

11. Sintorn, I.M., Bischof, L., Jackway, P., Haggarty, S., Buckley, M.: Gradient based intensity normalization. J. Microsc. **240**(3), 249–258 (2010)

12. Sironi, A., Turetken, E., Lepetit, V., Fua, P.: Multiscale centerline detection. IEEE Trans. Pattern Anal. Mach. Intell. **38**(7), 1327–1341 (2016)

Longitudinally-Consistent Parcellation of Infant Population Cortical Surfaces Based on Functional Connectivity

Junyi Yan[1,3], Yu Meng[2,3], Gang Li[3], Weili Lin[3], Dazhe Zhao[1], and Dinggang Shen[3(✉)]

[1] Key Laboratory of Medical Image Computing of Ministry of Education, Northeastern University, Shenyang, China
[2] Department of Computer Science, University of North Carolina at Chapel Hill, Chapel Hill, NC, USA
[3] Department of Radiology and BRIC, University of North Carolina at Chapel Hill, Chapel Hill, NC, USA
dgshen@med.unc.edu

Abstract. Parcellation of the human cerebral cortex into functionally distinct and meaningful regions is important for understanding the human brain. Although there are plenty of studies focusing on functional parcellation for adults, longitudinally-consistent functional parcellation of the rapidly developing infant cerebral cortex at multiple ages is still critically missing for understanding early brain development. Due to the dramatic changes of the cortical structure and function in infants, it is challenging to both capture the meaningful changes of the boundaries of functional regions and keep the parcellation as longitudinally-consistent as possible. To address this problem, we propose a longitudinally-consistent framework to jointly parcellate a population of infant cortical surfaces at multiple ages. Specifically, first, a population-average representation of the functional connectivity profile is constructed at each vertex at each age. Second, the correlation of functional connectivity profiles between any two vertices on the average cortical surfaces is computed. Notably, this correlation computation is performed *not only* within the same age *but also* across different ages, weighted based on the age difference, thus forming a large comprehensive similarity matrix. Such similarity measurements encourage to assign similar vertices to the same parcels, even for the vertices on the average cortical surfaces from different ages, and thus hold the longitudinal consistency. Finally, we apply the spectral clustering method on the large similarity matrix to generate an initial joint parcellation for all average surfaces, and further employ a graph cuts method to produce the spatially-smooth longitudinally-consistent parcellations. The proposed method was applied to a longitudinal infant brain MRI dataset to jointly parcellate infant cortical surfaces at 7 different time points in the first 2 years of age. The results show that our parcellations *not only* capture the evolution of functional boundaries *but also* preserve the longitudinal consistency.

Keywords: Longitudinal parcellation · Infant brain · Functional connectivity

© Springer International Publishing AG 2017
Q. Wang et al. (Eds.): MLMI 2017, LNCS 10541, pp. 194–202, 2017.
DOI: 10.1007/978-3-319-67389-9_23

1 Introduction

Parcellation of the human cerebral cortex into functionally distinct and meaningful regions is a fundamental step in understanding the brain development, aging, and disorders. For example, accurate parcellation could help better compare the results across different studies, illustrate functional organization of the brain, and benefit many neuroimaging studies [1]. Resting-state functional magnetic resonance imaging (R-fMRI) allows researchers to parcellate the cerebral cortex based on the functional connectivity, and many methods have been proposed to generate the parcellation maps for both individual level and population level in adults [1–4]. Longitudinal parcellation of the rapidly developing infant cerebral cortex at multiple ages is very important for understanding the early functional development of the human brain. Several methods have been developed for longitudinal parcellation of cortical surfaces based on the anatomical sulcal-gyral patterns [5, 6], however, to the best of our knowledge, no previous studies dealt with the problem of longitudinal cortical parcellation based on functional connectives. Another limitation of the previous studies [5, 6] is that they all assumed that the number of parcels is the same across ages. However, due to the rapid development of infant brains, functional regions may change dramatically in the early age, and thus different number of regions in cortical surface parcellations is expected across ages to capture the development of functional regions. In fact, the inherently complex changes during early brain development and high noise in the infant fMRI could result in very inconsistent parcellations at different ages, making it difficult to accurately locate the functional regions and their correspondences across ages.

In this paper, we propose a longitudinally-consistent parcellation method to *jointly* parcellate a population of infant cortical surfaces with multiple time points (ages) during the first 24 months of age, based on R-fMRI. Given a population of infant cortical surfaces that have been aligned and resampled in the space of age-matched population-average surfaces [7], *first*, for each vertex on each cortical surface, a functional connectivity profile is built by calculating the correlations between functional signals of this vertex and the functional signals of each of 642 uniformly-distributed seeds on the cortical surface. Since our goal is to construct a population-level parcellation for each age, all subjects' functional connectivity profiles at the same age are further averaged, thus producing an age-specific population-average representation of the functional connectivity profile for each vertex on the average surface. *Second*, the correlation of population-average functional connectivity profiles between any two vertices on the average cortical surfaces is computed. Notably, we compute the correlation of functional connectivity profiles of vertices *not only* within the same age *but also* across different ages. This enables our method to assign similar vertices into the same parcels, even for the vertices on the average surfaces of different ages, and thus make the parcellations longitudinally-consistent. All correlation values are further adjusted by a weight according to the age difference to form a large comprehensive similarity matrix. Herein, we assign a smaller weight to the correlation value when the age difference is large, as intuitively the functional connectivity profiles of two faraway time points should not strongly affect each other's parcellation. *Finally*, we leverage a spectral clustering method on the large comprehensive similarity matrix to generate an initial parcellation for all longitudinal average surfaces, and further employ a graph cuts method to refine the results to produce spatially-smooth and longitudinally-consistent cortical parcellations.

2   Methods

Subjects and Image Acquisition. Multimodal MR images for 40 healthy infants were acquired by a Siemens 3T head-only scanner. For each infant, the scans were scheduled at 0, 3, 6, 9, 12, 18, and 24 months of age. All infants were scanned during natural sleep without sedation. Specifically, T1-weighted (T1w) MR images with 144 sagittal slices were acquired with the parameters: TR = 1900 ms, TE = 4.38 ms, and resolution = $1 \times 1 \times 1$ mm^3. T2-weighted (T2w) MR images with 64 axial slices were acquired with the parameters: TR = 7380 ms, TE = 119 ms, and resolution = $1.25 \times 1.25 \times 1.95$ mm^3. Resting-state fMRI with 150 volumes, each with 33 slices, were acquired with the parameters: TR = 2000 ms, TE = 32 ms, and resolution = $4 \times 4 \times 4$ mm^3.

Cortical Surface Mapping. All T1w and T2w MRIs were processed using an infant-specific pipeline [7]. Specifically, T1w and T2w images were rigidly aligned, skull-stripped, intensity inhomogeneity corrected, tissue segmented, and topology corrected. Cortical surfaces were reconstructed and mapped onto a spherical space, and vertex-wise cortical correspondences along ages and across subjects were established by intra-subject and inter-subject spherical registration and cortical surface resampling [5]. For each time point, an age-matched population-average cortical surface was built for displaying the parcellation results. Resting-state fMRI were processed using the procedures in [8]. Resampled cortical surfaces were then transformed onto the R-fMRI space based on the rigid alignment between T2w image and R-fMRI. For each R-fMRI, the functional signals were sampled at the positions of 2562 vertices on the middle cortical surface of each hemisphere, and then spatially smoothed. Note that the cortical surface was initially in high resolution with 163,842 vertices for each hemisphere. Due to the low resolution of R-fMRI (1/64 of T1w image), 2562 ($\approx$ 163842/64) vertices on the cortical surface were sufficiently accurate to capture all R-fMRI time series.

Representation of Population-level Functional Connectivity Profiles. To effectively capture the functional connectivity patterns, 642 vertices were selected uniformly on the cortical surface as seeds. Then, the Pearson's correlation of the R-fMRI time series between each vertex on each cortical surface and each seed is calculated. In this way, a 2562 × 642 functional connectivity profiling matrix was constructed for each cortical surface. Here, each row in this matrix was a feature vector, representing the correlation values between a specific vertex and each of 642 seeds. For each age, the profiling matrices of all individuals in the same age were averaged together for creating an age-specific representation of population-level functional connectivity profiles.

Construction of Comprehensive Similarity Matrix. To jointly parcellate all age-specific average cortical surface at 7 different time points (ages), we *not only* measured the similarity of vertices within the same age in terms of functional connectivity

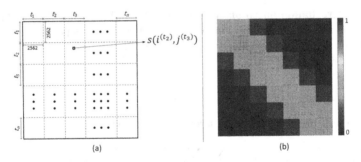

Fig. 1. An illustration of the large comprehensive similarity matrix of n ($n = 7$ in this study) time points (a) and the heat map of the correlation matrix for the real data (b).

profiles, *but also* measured the similarity of vertices across different ages. This helped group both vertices in the same age and vertices across different ages, thus leading to longitudinally-consistent results. Such similarity values formed a large comprehensive similarity matrix, as shown in Fig. 1. Specifically, the similarity between the vertex i at the age t_x and the vertex j at the age t_y ($t_x \neq t_y$) is defined as:

$$s\left(i^{(t_x)}, j^{(t_y)}\right) = corr\left(i^{(t_x)}, j^{(t_y)}\right) \cdot \exp\left(-\left|t_x - t_y\right|\right) \cdot \frac{2}{\left|t_x - t_y\right|} \tag{1}$$

Herein, the term $corr\left(i^{(t_x)}, j^{(t_y)}\right)$ is the correlation of the population-level functional connectivity profiles between the vertex i at the age t_x and the vertex j at the age t_y, measuring their similarity in functional connectivity patterns. The correlation is shifted to the range (0,1). The term $\exp\left(-\left|t_x - t_y\right|\right) \cdot \frac{2}{\left|t_x - t_y\right|}$ adjusts the similarity based on the age difference. When $t_x = t_y$, we set $s\left(i^{(t_x)}, j^{(t_y)}\right) = corr\left(i^{(t_x)}, j^{(t_y)}\right)$. Intuitively, vertices that are close in age are expected to be more related in longitudinal parcellation than those faraway in age.

Deriving Initial Parcellation based on Spectral Clustering. The comprehensive similarity matrix, which encodes the similarity between any two vertices at any two ages on the longitudinal average cortical surfaces, was fed into the Spectral Clustering algorithm [9], to generate an initial *joint* parcellation of all ages. Notably, functionally-corresponding regions across different ages will be largely in the same cluster, thus leading to relatively longitudinally consistent parcellations. However, the initial parcellations may not be spatially smooth due to the noise and the lack of spatial constraint in the similarity estimation. Of note, we did not impose any spatial constraint in the matrix, because functionally similar vertices may distribute in multiple spatially discontinuous cortical regions. Note that the proposed method requires to pre-define the number of expected regions, in order to use Spectral Clustering algorithm. Since we had no prior knowledge, we tried different number of clusters, and evaluated the quality of parcellation results both by visual checking and a quantitative measure, namely silhouette coefficient. More details will be discussed in the Results section.

Improving Parcellation based on Graph Cuts. To further refine the parcellation, we formulated this task as an optimization problem that minimizes an energy of a Markov random field, which can be solved by the Graph Cuts algorithm [10]. The energy function is defined as:

$$E = E_d + E_s + E_t \tag{2}$$

The first term E_d is a data fitting term and computed as:

$$E_d = \sum_x \sum_i -\log(p_{i^{(t_x)},c}) \tag{3}$$

where $p_{i^{(t_x)},c}$ is the probability of assigning a vertex i at time point t_x to the region c. We assume that the probability of assigning a vertex to a cluster is proportional to the similarity of functional connectivity profiles between the vertex and the cluster centroid by Spectral Clustering, formulated as:

$$p_{i^{(t_x)},c} = \frac{s(i^{t_x}, h_c)}{\sum_z s(i^{(t_x)}, h_z)} \tag{4}$$

where h_c is the average functional connectivity profile of the centroid of cluster c and h_z is the average functional connectivity profile of the centroid of cluster z (z represent all cluster regions). The second term E_s measures the spatial smoothness of the parcellation, which is computed as:

$$E_s = \lambda_s \sum_x \sum_{(i,j)\in N_s} s\left(i^{(t_x)}, j^{(t_x)}\right) \cdot \delta(c_{i^{(t_x)}}, c_{j^{(t_x)}}) \tag{5}$$

where N_s is a set of all one-ring neighboring vertex pairs on an age-specific average cortical surface; $\delta(c_{i^{(t_x)}}, c_{j^{(t_x)}})$ is an indicator of the cost of assigning vertex $i^{(t_x)}$ to parcel $c_{i^{(t_x)}}$ and assigning vertex $j^{(t_x)}$ to parcel $c_{j^{(t_x)}}$. $\delta(c_{i^{(t_x)}}, c_{j^{(t_x)}})$ is 1, when $c_{i^{(t_x)}} \neq c_{j^{(t_x)}}$, and is 0, when $c_{i^{(t_x)}} = c_{j^{(t_x)}}$. The parameter λ_s controls the degree of spatial smoothness. Ideally, for two neighboring vertices with different labels, this cost will be large, if their functional connectivity profiles are similar; while the cost is small, if their functional connectivity profiles are very different. The third term E_t measures the longitudinal consistency of cortical vertices at neighboring time points. It is computed as:

$$E_t = \lambda_t \sum_{(x,y)\in N_t} \sum_i s\left(i^{(t_x)}, i^{(t_y)}\right) \cdot \delta(c_{i^{(t_x)}}, c_{i^{(t_y)}}) \tag{6}$$

where N_t is a set of all neighboring pairs of time points, and λ_t controls the degree of longitudinal consistency. Similarly, for the two temporally-corresponding vertices with different labels, this cost will be large, if their functional connectivity profiles are similar; while this cost is small, if their functional connectivity profiles are very different.

3   Results

We applied the proposed method to a longitudinal infant brain MRI dataset to jointly parcellate population-average cortical surfaces at 7 different ages. Since our method needs to specify the expected number of parcels, we repeated our experiment multiple times with different parcel numbers from 10 to 50. The result with parcel number of 18 is demonstrated in the first two rows of Fig. 2. When the parcel number is 18, the sum of silhouette coefficient of 7 time points is largest. For example, there are 3 parcels from birth to 6 months, 4 parcels from 9 to 12 months, and 5 parcels from 18 to 24 months. As shown in Fig. 2, the proposed method generates relatively consistent parcellations across ages, and also captures the evolution of the functional regions. For example, it can be seen that the region "a" in Fig. 2 extends from the temporal pole along the temporal area to the supra-marginal area during the first 12 months, and further splits into two regions from 12 to 18 months. We can also see that the region "b" appears from 9 months of age, and keeps expending to 24 months of age.

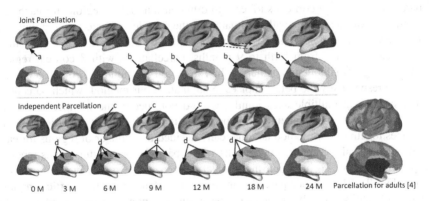

Fig. 2. Parcellation of population-average cortical surfaces at the 7 time points during the 24 months of age, shown on the inflated surfaces. The first two rows show the results of the proposed method that parcellates cortical surfaces at multiple time points jointly. The 3rd and 4th rows show the results produced by parcellation of each age independently. The right column shows a population-based parcellation of adults [4]. (Color figure online)

To illustrate the advantage of the proposed method, we also parcellated the population-average cortical surface atlas for each age *independently*, while keeping the same number of regions at each age as the joint parcellation in Fig. 2. As shown in the 3rd and 4th rows of Fig. 2, the results of independent parcellation at each age are very noisy and longitudinally inconsistent. For example, the region "c" in Fig. 2 varies dramatically from 6 to 12 months. From 3 to 18 months, the region "d" in Fig. 2 changes from 3 parcels into 4 parcels, and then reverses to 3 parcels (red, pink, and green), of which the pink parcel is missing 3 months later and comes back again after 6 months. One possible reason of such irregular changes of parcellation is the noisy signals existing in the R-fMRIs of each age. This example also indicates that our proposed joint parcellation method is robust to this kind of noise.

As a spectral clustering algorithm was used for parcellation, we need to define the number of regions. However, as mentioned, we had no prior knowledge about how many functional regions were expected for parcellation of the infant cerebral cortex from birth to 24 months of age. To decide the number of regions, we first parcellated average cortical surfaces into a different number of regions at each age independently, and then employed the silhouette coefficient as a quantitative index to help find the right number of regions. The silhouette coefficient is defined as:

$$sil(i) = \frac{d'(i) - d(i)}{\max\{d(i), d'(i)\}} \qquad (7)$$

where $d(i)$ is the average dissimilarity of vertex i with all other data within the same cortical region; $d'(i)$ is the shortest average dissimilarity of vertex i to any other cortical regions except the region include vertex i, to which vertex i does not belong. The dissimilarity between two vertices i and j is equal to $1 - s(i, j)$.

Table 1 reports the mean silhouette coefficients and its standard errors of the means for parcellating average cortical surface into different number of regions for each age. Standard error of means is usually estimated by the sample estimate of the population standard deviation (sample standard deviation) divided by the square root of the sample size. We can see that, from birth to 9 months, parcellations with 3 cortical regions achieve the highest silhouette coefficient. In 12, 18 and 24 months, 7, 6 and 5 cortical regions are respectively the better choices. Note that, in our method, which parcellates cortical surfaces at multiple ages jointly, we did not specify the number of cortical regions for each age independently. By specifying the total number of cortical regions for all ages together, our method automatically decided the number of regions for each age. We also visually compared our results with a parcellation of adult brains reported in a previous study [4], in which the cortical surface was parceled into 7 functional regions (Fig. 2). Though our parcellation results of infants have less cortical regions than that of adults, their boundaries of the cortical regions are consistent in many locations.

Table 1. Mean silhouette coefficients and standard errors of means for the parcellations using different number of parcels.

No. of regions	Age (month)						
	0	3	6	9	12	18	24
2	0.304 ± 0.003	0.400 ± 0.003	0.394 ± 0.003	0.329 ± 0.003	0.289 ± 0.003	0.334 ± 0.003	0.303 ± 0.003
3	**0.418** ± 0.004	**0.441** ± 0.003	**0.402** ± 0.004	**0.367** ± 0.003	0.328 ± 0.003	0.326 ± 0.003	0.367 ± 0.003
4	0.383 ± 0.004	0.385 ± 0.005	0.354 ± 0.004	0.309 ± 0.003	**0.345** ± 0.003	**0.352** ± 0.003	**0.373** ± 0.004
5	0.365 ± 0.005	0.324 ± 0.005	0.340 ± 0.005	0.310 ± 0.004	0.313 ± 0.004	0.331 ± 0.004	0.348 ± 0.004
6	0.326 ± 0.005	0.311 ± 0.006	0.334 ± 0.006	0.330 ± 0.004	0.330 ± 0.004	0.311 ± 0.004	0.341 ± 0.004
7	0.301 ± 0.005	0.261 ± 0.007	0.314 ± 0.006	0.315 ± 0.004	0.332 ± 0.004	0.295 ± 0.004	0.333 ± 0.005
8	0.271 ± 0.005	0.226 ± 0.007	0.348 ± 0.005	0.344 ± 0.005	0.337 ± 0.005	0.303 ± 0.005	0.319 ± 0.004
9	0.255 ± 0.006	0.213 ± 0.007	0.352 ± 0.006	0.331 ± 0.005	0.325 ± 0.004	0.323 ± 0.005	0.322 ± 0.005
10	0.271 ± 0.006	0.160 ± 0.006	0.303 ± 0.005	0.334 ± 0.005	0.334 ± 0.006	0.326 ± 0.005	0.282 ± 0.006

Joint Parcellation

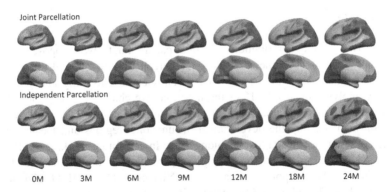

Independent Parcellation

OM   3M   6M   9M   12M   18M   24M

Fig. 3. Partition the cortical surfaces into more regions. The first two rows show the results of the proposed method that parcellates cortical surfaces at multiple time points jointly. The 3rd and 4th rows show the results produced by parcellation of each age independently. The region number of 7 time points during the 24 months of age is 7, 8, 9, 9, 6, 8, and 6, respectively.

Table 2. Quantitative measurement of parcellation consistency between neighboring time points, in terms of Rand Index.

Method	0-3 mon.	3-6 mon.	6-9 mon.	9-12 mon.	12-18 mon.	18-24 mon.
Individual	0.87	0.88	0.88	0.87	0.86	0.86
Ours	**0.89**	**0.89**	**0.91**	**0.89**	**0.91**	**0.87**

We also partitioned the cortical surfaces into more cortical regions. As shown in the first two rows of Fig. 3, 7, 8, 9, 9, 6, 8, and 6 cortical regions are automatically recognized for the cortical surfaces at 0, 3, 6, 9, 12, 18, and 24 months of age, when setting the parcel number as 33 using the proposed longitudinally-consistent parcellation method. For comparison, age independent parcellation results are also provided in the third and fourth rows in Fig. 3, with the same number of cortical regions as our results. To quantitatively evaluate the degree of longitudinal consistency, we adopt Rand Index [11] to measure the parcellation consistency between each pair of neighboring time points. As reported in Table 2, our longitudinal parcellation results achieved higher Rand Index than the independent parcellation results, indicating that our method produces longitudinally more consistent parcellations.

Note that, as shown in Fig. 3, the cortical parcels develop regionally differently. Specifically, from birth to 9 months, there are 2-3 parcels in the frontal cortex and only 1 parcel in the region around the central sulcus. At 12 months, the parcels in the frontal cortex merge together, while the parcel around the central sulcus splits into more parcels. This observation is largely consistent with the previous study of infant brain networks [12], which reported more functional connections in the frontal area than in central area of the neonatal brain.

4 Conclusion

There are two major contributions in this paper. First, we proposed a novel longitudinally-consistent framework for joint parcellation of cortical surfaces of a population of infants at multiple ages, based on spectral clustering and graph cuts. Second, by applying our method, for the first time, we charted the longitudinal functional parcellation maps of infant cortical surfaces during the first 2 years of age. These parcellation maps capture the development of functional regions and meanwhile preserve the consistency of parcellations along ages. In our future work, we will further extensively validate our method and apply our parcellations to neuroscience studies.

This work is also supported in part by an NIH grant (1U01MH110274) and the efforts of the UNC/UMN Baby Connectome Project Consortium.

References

1. Glasser, M.F., Coalson, T.S., Robinson, E.C., et al.: A multi-modal parcellation of human cerebral cortex. Nature **536**, 171–178 (2016)
2. Fan, L., Li, H., Zhuo, J., et al.: The human brainnetome atlas: a new brain atlas based on connectional architecture. Cereb. Cortex **26**, 3508–3526 (2016)
3. Wang, D., Buckner, R.L., Fox, M.D., et al.: Parcellating cortical functional networks in individuals. Nat. Neurosci. **18**, 1853–1860 (2015)
4. Yeo, B.T., Krienen, F.M., Sepulcre, J., et al.: The organization of the human cerebral cortex estimated by intrinsic functional connectivity. J. Neurophysiol. **106**, 1125–1165 (2011)
5. Li, G., Wang, L., Shi, F., et al.: Simultaneous and consistent labeling of longitudinal dynamic developing cortical surfaces in infants. Med. Image Anal. **18**, 1274–1289 (2014)
6. Li, G., Shen, D.: Consistent sulcal parcellation of longitudinal cortical surfaces. NeuroImage **57**, 76–88 (2011)
7. Li, G., Wang, L., Shi, F., et al.: Construction of 4D high-definition cortical surface atlases of infants: Methods and applications. Med. Image Anal. **25**, 22–36 (2015)
8. Gao, W., Alcauter, S., Elton, A., et al.: Functional network development during the first year: relative sequence and socioeconomic correlations. Cereb. Cortex **25**, 2919–2928 (2015)
9. von Luxburg, U.: A tutorial on spectral clustering. Stat. Comput. **17**, 395–416 (2007)
10. Boykov, Y., Kolmogorov, V.: An experimental comparison of min-cut/max-flow algorithms for energy minimization in vision. IEEE Trans. Pattern Anal. Mach. Intell. **26**, 1124–1137 (2004)
11. Rand, W.M.: Objective criteria for the evaluation of clustering methods. J. Am. Stat. Assoc. **66**, 846–850 (1971)
12. Gao, W., Gilmore, J.H., Giovanello, K.S., et al.: Temporal and spatial evolution of brain network topology during the first two years of life. PLoS ONE **6**, e25278 (2011)

Gradient Boosted Trees for Corrective Learning

Baris U. Oguz, Russell T. Shinohara, Paul A. Yushkevich, and Ipek Oguz[✉]

University Pennsylvania, Philadelphia, PA 19104, USA
ipekoguz@mail.med.upenn.edu

Abstract. Random forests (RF) have long been a widely popular method in medical image analysis. Meanwhile, the closely related gradient boosted trees (GBT) have not become a mainstream tool in medical imaging despite their attractive performance, perhaps due to their computational cost. In this paper, we leverage the recent availability of an efficient open-source GBT implementation to illustrate the GBT method in a corrective learning framework, in application to the segmentation of the caudate nucleus, putamen and hippocampus. The size and shape of these structures are used to derive important biomarkers in many neurological and psychiatric conditions. However, the large variability in deep gray matter appearance makes their automated segmentation from MRI scans a challenging task. We propose using GBT to improve existing segmentation methods. We begin with an existing 'host' segmentation method to create an estimate surface. Based on this estimate, a surface-based sampling scheme is used to construct a set of candidate locations. GBT models are trained on features derived from the candidate locations, including spatial coordinates, image intensity, texture, and gradient magnitude. The classification probabilities from the GBT models are used to calculate a final surface estimate. The method is evaluated on a public dataset, with a 2-fold cross-validation. We use a multi-atlas approach and FreeSurfer as host segmentation methods. The mean reduction in surface distance error metric for FreeSurfer was $0.2 - 0.3$ mm, whereas for multi-atlas segmentation, it was 0.1mm for each of caudate, putamen and hippocampus. Importantly, our approach outperformed an RF model trained on the same features ($p < 0.05$ on all measures). Our method is readily generalizable and can be applied to a wide range of medical image segmentation problems and allows any segmentation method to be used as input.

Keywords: Gradient boosted trees · Segmentation · MRI · Subcortical

1 Introduction

Deep gray matter atrophy is an important feature of many neurodegenerative diseases. In particular, the volumes of the caudate nucleus and the putamen are among the strongest predictors of motor disease onset in Huntington's disease [11]. Hippocampus may also be implicated in Huntington's and is also highly relevant in other neurodegenerative diseases such as Alzheimer's [24]. However,

© Springer International Publishing AG 2017
Q. Wang et al. (Eds.): MLMI 2017, LNCS 10541, pp. 203–211, 2017.
DOI: 10.1007/978-3-319-67389-9_24

the automated segmentation of these structures from MRI scans is challenging due to the large variability in their appearance, especially in the presence of neurodegeneration. Many approaches have been proposed, including probability-atlas approaches [6], Bayesian models of shape and appearance [13], surface-based graph cuts [12], and multi-atlas label fusion [20]. However, none of these methods are perfect, and the errors they make can often be of a systematic nature reflecting the bias of each approach. Wang et al. [19] have proposed a learning-based wrapper method to learn and correct for this systematic segmentation error of 'host' segmentation methods, which was further developed by Tustison et al. [17] in the context of hippocampal subfields. We propose a similar approach based on gradient boosted trees in a surface-based sampling setup.

Gradient boosting was first proposed in [7]. GBT models build ensembles of decision trees, and apply the boosting principle to learn a tree structure where each new tree is built to approximate the negative gradient of the empirical loss function in order to correct the errors made by previous trees in the ensemble. These trees are typically weak learners, i.e., the size of the individual trees is typically kept small. Furthermore, in each iteration of the training phase, only a random subsample of the data instances (rows) and features (columns) are used, in order to prevent overfitting [8]. The final prediction is calculated by combining the individual predictions with coefficients learned during the training phase. This is in contrast to random forests (RF), another tree-based ensemble model, where full-grown trees are built and their predictions are combined uniformly.

Novelty. Although GBT models have been studied for over a decade, their use in practice has been limited until recently, mainly due to their computational cost. We use XGBoost[1], which is an efficient and open source implementation of GBT models, first released in 2014. Unlike the popular RF approach, there has only been a few previous studies using GBT in the general medical image analysis field [2,3,21], and even fewer in 3D medical image segmentation. A notable exception is the work of Bakas et al. [1] who use GBT to refine brain tumor segmentation. Here, we show that GBT models outperform RF models trained on identical feature sets. While the current study is focused on corrective learning for deep gray matter structures, our results highlight that GBT models have potential for improving many medical image analysis problems where RF's are commonly used.

2   Methods

We propose using gradient boosted trees (GBT) to learn the appearance model of the caudate nucleus, putamen and hippocampus from human brain MRI and to improve the accuracy of existing segmentation methods. The automated pipeline begins with T1-weighted MRI images and applies the 'host' initial segmentation method to create an initial surface estimate for these subcortical structures. Next, a surface-based sampling process is used to construct a set of candidate

---

[1] http://xgboost.readthedocs.io/en/latest/.

locations for the vertices using this estimate as the base mesh. Raw numerical features are extracted at each candidate location, including spatial coordinates, image intensities, gradient magnitudes and texture. GBT classifiers are trained on an augmented set of features, labeling the node closest to the true surface in each column as the positive class. Finally, the classification probabilities from the GBT models are used as weights to calculate a final surface estimate.

2.1 Host Segmentation Methods

We use two different host methods to illustrate our segmentation correction algorithm. (1) **Multi-atlas.** Each training image was deformably registered[2] to the target image [23]. The manual segmentations for the training images were warped to the target image using these transformations. A consensus segmentation was achieved using the Joint Label Fusion (JLF) algorithm [20]. (2) **FreeSurfer.** FreeSurfer formulates subcortical segmentation as a Bayesian parameter estimation problem and leverages a probabilistic atlas to classify each voxel [6]. FreeSurfer v5.3 was used with the default settings and no manual interventions.

2.2 Construction of Candidate Locations

Given the initial segmentation results, a surface model was created using the marching cubes algorithm and smoothed for 25 iterations with a sinc filter. The resulting model was used as the base mesh. Starting with the base mesh, a column was constructed at each surface vertex, with the column consisting of 30 candidate locations (15 inside, 15 outside) at 0.15 mm intervals. The idea is to use the machine learning algorithm to move each surface vertex along the corresponding column to deform the surface into a more accurate configuration, similar to surface-based graphs [12,22] and active shape models [5]. The paths of the columns were determined following the electric lines of field [12,22] and were smoothed using Kochanek splines [10] for better geometric behavior.

2.3 Raw Feature Set

We begin with a series of pre-processing steps to reduce the variability between the image intensities. First, N4 bias correction [18] was used to remove inhomogeneity across the spatial domain, after skull-stripping with BET [15] for increased effectiveness. The WhiteStripe intensity normalization algorithm [14] was applied to the N4 results to normalize intensities across subjects. Finally, a non-local means filter [16] was applied to reduce noise. The intensity normalization (BET+N4+WhiteStripe) and noise filtering (BET+N4+WhiteStripe+NLM) results contributed 2 normalization features at each location.

Classical texture features [4,9] were computed using normalized gray-level co-occurrence matrices (GLCM). Given $g(i,j)$ elements of the GLCM

---

[2] https://github.com/pyushkevich/greedy.

matrix, and their weighted pixel average $\mu = \sum i \cdot g(i,j)$ and variance $\sigma = \sum (i - \mu)^2 \cdot g(i,j)$, 8 texture features were computed: energy ($\sum (g(i,j)^2)$), entropy ($\sum g(i,j)\log(g(i,j))$), correlation ($\sum \frac{(i-\mu)(j-\mu)g(i,j)}{\sigma^2}$), difference moment ($\sum \frac{1}{1+(i-j)^2} g(i,j)$), inertia, also known as contrast ($\sum (i - j)^2 g(i,j)$), cluster shade ($\sum ((i - \mu) + (j - \mu))^3 g(i,j)$), cluster prominence ($\sum ((i - \mu) + (j - \mu))^4 g(i,j)$) and Haralick's correlation ($\frac{\sum (i,j)g(i,j)-\mu^2}{\sigma^2}$). The GLCM was computed in each of 13 possible directions in a 3×3 neighborhood, resulting in a total of $8 \times 13 = 104$ texture features at each graph node location.

The anatomy surrounding deep brain structures is very heterogeneous; thus, the image appearance near the surface can vary for different regions. To encourage the trained model to capture these regional properties, we parcellate each surface into regions of interest (ROIs) and use the ROIs as a feature. We compute the bounding box of each base mesh surface, and divide it into 3 equal sections along the P-A axis and 2 equal sections along the I-S axis. The subdivision along the L-R axis was done based on the orientation of the surface normal vector. Thus, each vertex was assigned to one of $3 \times 2 \times 2 = 24$ ROIs.

The mean μ and standard deviation σ of intensity for each structure were determined from the host segmentation. Then, we use $((I - \mu)/\sigma)$ at each node as a proxy surface confidence feature.

In addition to the normalization and texture features, 12 raw features were thus extracted for each candidate location. 8 of these are node based (spatial coordinates of the node (3), node height along graph column, image intensity, intensity diff, gradient magnitude, surface confidence), and 4 are shared by all nodes in a given column (surface normal direction (3), ROI).

The features for the training set were created using the same process on the training set. The only difference was that in the multi-atlas experiment, for each training subject, the remaining N-1 training subjects were used as atlases.

2.4 Feature Engineering

For each node, we create 4 vectors in Euclidean space from the node to its 2 neighboring nodes up and down the column. We calculate the length of each vector (4 features), and the angles between each pair of vectors (6 features). Note that the angles encode approximate local curvature. Combined with the original 8 node-based raw features, this produces 18 raw features.

These features, however, may still vary in magnitude despite the normalization steps with WhiteStripe and N4. In order to prevent overfitting to the wrong signal, these features are normalized by min-max scaling, both per subject and per column (36 features). For the 8 original raw features, we also include the difference of the normalized values of the current node with 2 neighboring nodes up and down the column (64 features). The 4 column-based features are included as is, resulting in 104 base features. Thus, we have 104 base features + 2 normalization features + 104 texture features, resulting in a total of 210 features per location. Two nodes at each end of the column do not have enough neighbors; the values for these features are duplicated from the end node.

2.5   Gradient Boosted Trees

For each of the left/right caudate/putamen/hippocampus structures, a GBT model is trained on features described above. For each column in the sample set, the node that is closest to the true surface is labeled as the positive class. All other nodes in the column are labeled as the negative class.

Model parameter tuning is performed separately for each of the 6 structures, optimizing the mean surface distance over inner cross-validation folds; logarithmic loss and area under the receiver operating characteristic curve were also monitored during this phase. In the XGBoost implementation, the following parameters were used for all testing subjects, for all structures: 'colsample by level' = 0.05, 'learning rate' = 0.6, 'max depth' = 4, 'min child weight' = 10, 'n estimators' = 100, 'subsample' = 0.8. All other parameters were left at default values. We note that the number of parameters that need to be tuned is dramatically smaller than more complicated models such as deep learning methods, where number and type of layers as well as nodes per layer, connections between layers, activation functions, etc. need to be fine-tuned.

The final surface is fitted via a surface-based graph cut [12] using the probability output from the GBT model as weights. While this does not strongly affect the quantitative performance, it results in smoother surfaces.

3   Experimental Methods

3.1   Data and Cross-Validation

The method is evaluated on the MICCAI 2012 Multi-Atlas Segmentation Challenge dataset, consisting of T1-w MR images from 35 subjects. For each subject, manual segmentations of various regions, including the left and right caudate nuclei, putamen and hippocampi, were provided as part of the Challenge.

Given the relatively low number of subjects, a simple train/test split could lead to overfitting to the samples in the test set. GBT and other tree-based ensembles (e.g., RFs) are more prone to overfitting than linear models without a proper validation scheme. It has been extensively argued in the machine learning literature that overfit models will produce superficially good results on the test set they were tuned on, but will fail to generalize to new unseen data.

To prevent this, we use a two-fold cross-validation setup. We split the 35 subjects as 15 train/20 test, identical to the original Challenge for comparability with previous methods, and a second fold with the reversed setup (20 train/15 test). The whole automated pipeline is applied to the raw data in each cross-validation fold, to prevent contamination between folds. We tuned our method using cross-validation within the inner folds; after this tuning step within the training set, a single set of parameters was used to generate results on all test subjects (in the outer folds), across all structures (left/right caudate/putamen/hippocampus). Random forests (RF) models have also been trained on the same 210 features for each structure, using similar parameter tuning methods.

3.2 Evaluation Metrics

Mean vertex-to-surface distance between estimated surface and reference manual segmentation (for symmetry, distance from estimated to truth and vice versa are averaged) were used to evaluate the models. In the context of this surface-based analysis framework, we consider this a more appropriate metric than volumetric overlap measures such as Dice.

4 Results

Table 1 presents the surface-to-surface distance for the raw FreeSurfer results, and for corrective learning using GBT and RF. For each structure, for both metrics, both the GBT and the RF corrective learning led to statistically significant improvements ($p < 1e^{-4}$) over the raw FS results. Furthermore, the GBT corrective learning results were significantly more accurate than RF corrective learning results in every t-test ($p < 1e^{-4}$).

Table 1. Surface-to-surface error, with FreeSurfer as host. Mean ± std. dev. are shown. Differences between all pairs of methods were statistically significant.

Distance	FreeSurfer (Host)			FreeSurfer + RF Bias Correction			FreeSurfer + GBT Bias Correction		
Structure	Fold1	Fold2	Fold1+Fold2	Fold1	Fold2	Fold1+Fold2	Fold1	Fold2	Fold1+Fold2
LCaudate	0.87 ± 0.28	0.70 ± 0.09	0.80 ± 0.24	0.76 ± 0.29	0.59 ± 0.09	0.69 ± 0.24	0.68 ± 0.30	0.50 ± 0.09	0.60 ± 0.25
RCaudate	0.95 ± 0.21	1.07 ± 0.91	1.00 ± 0.61	0.86 ± 0.22	0.96 ± 0.91	0.90 ± 0.61	0.75 ± 0.23	0.84 ± 0.89	0.79 ± 0.60
LPutamen	1.09 ± 0.14	1.11 ± 0.10	1.10 ± 0.12	0.92 ± 0.13	0.94 ± 0.09	0.93 ± 0.11	0.77 ± 0.12	0.76 ± 0.10	0.76 ± 0.11
RPutamen	0.95 ± 0.15	1.14 ± 0.51	1.03 ± 0.36	0.78 ± 0.12	0.98 ± 0.50	0.86 ± 0.35	0.65 ± 0.11	0.81 ± 0.51	0.72 ± 0.35
LHippocampus	0.85 ± 0.18	0.83 ± 0.12	0.84 ± 0.16	0.78 ± 0.17	0.76 ± 0.11	0.77 ± 0.14	0.69 ± 0.16	0.65 ± 0.09	0.67 ± 0.14
RHippocampus	0.80 ± 0.08	1.01 ± 0.77	0.89 ± 0.51	0.73 ± 0.07	0.94 ± 0.78	0.82 ± 0.52	0.65 ± 0.07	0.84 ± 0.78	0.73 ± 0.51

Table 2 presents similar results using joint label fusion (JLF) as host method. Both the GBT and the RF corrective learning led to statistically significant improvements ($p < 0.002$) over the raw JLF results across the board. Furthermore, the GBT corrective learning results were significantly more accurate than RF corrective learning results in every t-test ($p < 0.04$).

Figure 1 shows qualitative results comparing the raw input segmentations and the GBT corrective learning results for two subjects. For FreeSurfer input, the improvement is especially pronounced for the lateral surface of the putamen, where our approach successfully fixes leakage into the neighboring external

Table 2. Surface-to-surface error, with joint label fusion as host. Mean ± std. dev. are shown. Differences between all pairs of methods were statistically significant.

Distance	Joint Label Fusion (Host)			JLF + RF Bias Correction			JLF + GBT Bias Correction		
Structure	Fold1	Fold2	Fold1+Fold2	Fold1	Fold2	Fold1+Fold2	Fold1	Fold2	Fold1+Fold2
LCaudate	0.50 ± 0.16	0.42 ± 0.08	0.47 ± 0.13	0.43 ± 0.15	0.34 ± 0.05	0.39 ± 0.13	0.39 ± 0.16	0.30 ± 0.04	0.35 ± 0.13
RCaudate	0.57 ± 0.22	0.40 ± 0.06	0.50 ± 0.19	0.51 ± 0.22	0.33 ± 0.04	0.44 ± 0.19	0.45 ± 0.22	0.29 ± 0.03	0.38 ± 0.19
LPutamen	0.46 ± 0.11	0.42 ± 0.03	0.44 ± 0.09	0.40 ± 0.12	0.36 ± 0.03	0.38 ± 0.09	0.35 ± 0.13	0.29 ± 0.03	0.32 ± 0.10
RPutamen	0.41 ± 0.12	0.35 ± 0.02	0.38 ± 0.10	0.39 ± 0.13	0.33 ± 0.03	0.36 ± 0.10	0.35 ± 0.13	0.29 ± 0.03	0.32 ± 0.10
LHippocampus	0.54 ± 0.14	0.50 ± 0.06	0.52 ± 0.11	0.52 ± 0.13	0.48 ± 0.06	0.50 ± 0.11	0.48 ± 0.12	0.43 ± 0.06	0.46 ± 0.10
RHippocampus	0.52 ± 0.10	0.50 ± 0.06	0.51 ± 0.08	0.50 ± 0.09	0.47 ± 0.06	0.48 ± 0.08	0.47 ± 0.08	0.43 ± 0.06	0.45 ± 0.08

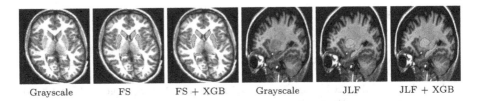

Grayscale   FS   FS + XGB   Grayscale   JLF   JLF + XGB

Fig. 1. Qualitative bias correction results for FreeSurfer (**left**) and joint label fusion (**right**). The reference manual segmentation is shown in solid yellow, whereas the automated segmentations are shown as pink outlines. (Color figure online)

capsule white matter. For the JLF input, our method successfully fixes an under-segmentation problem for the putamen.

Each GBT model for each left-right pair of structures takes around 15 min in total for both training and predicting the probabilities. The RF run time was about twice longer than the GBT run time.

Note that the JLF+GBT performance is superior to FS+GBT result in the reported metrics. This is presumably due to differences in host methodologies: while JLF uses the training data which has similar characteristics and segmentation protocol, FS uses its own external training data, which may be less compatible with the testing data.

5   Discussion

Our results show the proposed GBT-based corrective learning approach can be successfully applied to learn and correct systematic errors in input 'host' segmentation algorithms, leading to a substantial boost in accuracy. Importantly, the results of the GBT-based learning were significantly more accurate than a comparable RF-based learning approach trained on identical features. Given the popularity of the RF model in the medical image analysis community, this data suggests that GBT models may also offer improvements in other machine learning applications in medical image analysis.

We note that while the current experiments focused on the caudate, putamen and hippocampus which are of specific interest in Huntington's disease studies, the methods we propose are readily generalizable and can be used to learn and correct errors in other structures, given a suitable host segmentation algorithm.

The current ROI choice is based on a coarse heuristic, and a more sophisticated parcellation based on an atlas initialization or clustering of columns based on intensity similarity and spatial proximity may further enhance the performance. Exploring these issues as well as additional feature sets such as SIFT features remains as future work.

Acknowledgments. This work was supported, in part, by NIH grants NINDS R01NS094456, NIBIB R01EB017255, NINDS R01NS085211 and NINDS R21NS093349.

References

1. Bakas, S., et al.: GLISTRboost: combining multimodal MRI segmentation, registration, and biophysical tumor growth modeling with gradient boosting machines for glioma segmentation. In: Crimi, A., Menze, B., Maier, O., Reyes, M., Handels, H. (eds.) BrainLes 2015. LNCS, vol. 9556, pp. 144–155. Springer, Cham (2016). doi:10.1007/978-3-319-30858-6_13
2. Becker, C., Rigamonti, R., Lepetit, V., Fua, P.: Supervised feature learning for curvilinear structure segmentation. In: Mori, K., Sakuma, I., Sato, Y., Barillot, C., Navab, N. (eds.) MICCAI 2013. LNCS, vol. 8149, pp. 526–533. Springer, Heidelberg (2013). doi:10.1007/978-3-642-40811-3_66
3. Cao, G., Ding, J., Duan, Y., Tu, L., Xu, J., Xu, D.: Classification of tongue images based on doublet and color space dictionary. In: IEEE BIBM, pp. 1170–1175 (2016)
4. Conners, R.W., Harlow, C.A.: A theoretical comparison of texture algorithms. IEEE PAMI 2(3), 204–222 (1980)
5. Cristinacce, D., Cootes, T.F.: Boosted regression active shape models. BMVC 2, 880–889 (2007)
6. Fischl, B., Salat, D.H., Busa, E., Albert, M., Dieterich, M., Haselgrove, C., van der Kouwe, A., Killiany, R., Kennedy, D., Klaveness, S., Montillo, A., Makris, N., Rosen, B., Dale, A.M.: Whole brain segmentation: automated labeling of neuroanatomical structures in the human brain. Neuron 33(3), 341–355 (2002)
7. Friedman, J.H.: Greedy function approximation: a gradient boosting machine. Ann. Stat. 29(5), 1189–1232 (2001)
8. Friedman, J.H.: Stochastic gradient boosting. Comput. Stat. Data Anal. 38(4), 367–378 (2002)
9. Haralick, R.M., Shanmugam, K., Dinstein, I.: Textural Features for Image Classification. IEEE Trans. Syst. Man Cybern. B Cybern. 6, 610–621 (1973)
10. Kochanek, D.H.U., Bartels, R.H., Kochanek, D.H.U., Bartels, R.H.: Interpolating splines with local tension, continuity, and bias control, vol. 18. ACM (1984)
11. Long, J.D., Paulsen, J.S., Marder, K., Zhang, Y., Kim, J.I., Mills, J.A.: Researchers of the PREDICT-HD Huntington's study group: tracking motor impairments in the progression of Huntington's disease. Mov. Disord. 29(3), 311–319 (2014)
12. Oguz, I., Kashyap, S., Wang, H., Yushkevich, P., Sonka, M.: Globally optimal label fusion with shape priors. In: Ourselin, S., Joskowicz, L., Sabuncu, M.R., Unal, G., Wells, W. (eds.) MICCAI 2016. LNCS, vol. 9901, pp. 538–546. Springer, Cham (2016). doi:10.1007/978-3-319-46723-8_62
13. Patenaude, B., Smith, S.M., Kennedy, D.N., Jenkinson, M.: A Bayesian model of shape and appearance for subcortical brain segmentation. NeuroImage 56(3), 907–922 (2011)
14. Shinohara, R.T., Sweeney, E.M., Goldsmith, J., Shiee, N., Mateen, F.J., Calabresi, P.A., Jarso, S., Pham, D.L., Reich, D.S., Crainiceanu, C.M.: Statistical normalization techniques for MRI. NeuroImage Clin. 6, 9–19 (2014)
15. Smith, S.M.: Fast robust automated brain extraction. HBM 17(3), 143–155 (2002)
16. Tristán-Vega, A., García-Pérez, V., Aja-Fernández, S., Westin, C.F.: Efficient and robust nonlocal means denoising of MR data based on salient features matching. Comput. Methods Programs Biomed. 105(2), 131–144 (2012)
17. Tustison, N., Avants, B., Wang, H., Yassa, M.: Multi-atlas intensity and label fusion with supervised segmentation refinement for the parcellation of hippocampal subfields. In: The 13th International Conference on Alzheimer's and Parkinson's Diseases Abstract 029 (2017)

18. Tustison, N., Avants, B., Cook, P., Zheng, Y., Egan, A., Yushkevich, P., Gee, J.: N4ITK: improved N3 bias correction. IEEE TMI **29**(6), 1310–1320 (2010)
19. Wang, H., Das, S.R., Suh, J.W., Altinay, M., Pluta, J., Craige, C., Avants, B., Yushkevich, P.A.: ADNI: A learning-based wrapper method to correct systematic errors in automatic image segmentation: consistently improved performance in hippocampus, cortex and brain segmentation. NeuroImage **55**(3), 968–985 (2011)
20. Wang, H., Suh, J.W., Das, S.R., Pluta, J., Craige, C., Yushkevich, P.A.: Multi-Atlas Segmentation with Joint Label Fusion. IEEE PAMI **35**(3), 611–623 (2012)
21. Yang, T., Chen, W., Cao, G.: Automated classification of neonatal amplitude-integrated EEG based on gradient boosting method. Biomed. Signal Process. Control **28**, 50–57 (2016)
22. Yin, Y., Zhang, X., Williams, R., Wu, X., Anderson, D.D., Sonka, M.: LOGISMOS-layered optimal graph image segmentation of multiple objects and surfaces: cartilage segmentation in the knee joint. IEEE TMI **29**(12), 2023–2037 (2010)
23. Yushkevich, P.A., Pluta, J., Wang, H., Wisse, L.E., Das, S., Wolk, D.: Fast automatic segmentation of hippocampal subfields and medial temporal lobe subregions in 3 Tesla and 7 Tesla T2-weighted MRI. Alzheimer's & Dementia. J. Alzheimer's Assoc. **12**(7), 126–127 (2016)
24. Yushkevich, P.A., Pluta, J.B., Wang, H., Xie, L., Ding, S.L., Gertje, E.C., Mancuso, L., Kliot, D., Das, S.R., Wolk, D.A.: Automated volumetry and regional thickness analysis of hippocampal subfields and medial temporal cortical structures in mild cognitive impairment. Hum. Brain Mapp. **36**(1), 258–287 (2015)

Self-paced Convolutional Neural Network for Computer Aided Detection in Medical Imaging Analysis

Xiang Li[1]($\boxtimes$), Aoxiao Zhong[2], Ming Lin[3], Ning Guo[1], Mu Sun[4],
Arkadiusz Sitek[4], Jieping Ye[3], James Thrall[1], and Quanzheng Li[1]

[1] Massachusetts General Hospital, Boston, USA
xli60@mgh.harvard.edu
[2] Zhejiang University, Hangzhou, China
[3] University of Michigan, Ann Arbor, USA
[4] Beijing Institute of Technology, Beijing, China

Abstract. Tissue characterization has long been an important component of Computer Aided Diagnosis (CAD) systems for automatic lesion detection and further clinical planning. Motivated by the superior performance of deep learning methods on various computer vision problems, there has been increasing work applying deep learning to medical image analysis. However, the development of a robust and reliable deep learning model for computer-aided diagnosis is still highly challenging due to the combination of the high heterogeneity in the medical images and the relative lack of training samples. Specifically, annotation and labeling of the medical images is much more expensive and time-consuming than other applications and often involves manual labor from multiple domain experts. In this work, we propose a multi-stage, self-paced learning framework utilizing a convolutional neural network (CNN) to classify Computed Tomography (CT) image patches. The key contribution of this approach is that we augment the size of training samples by refining the unlabeled instances with a self-paced learning CNN. By implementing the framework on high performance computing servers including the NVIDIA DGX1 machine, we obtained the experimental result, showing that the self-pace boosted network consisntly outperformed the original network even with very scarce manual labels. The performance gain indicates that applications with limited training samples such as medical image analysis can benefit from using the proposed framework.

Keywords: Deep learning · Self-paced learning · Medical image analysis

1 Introduction

In medical image analysis, tissue characterization and classification are among the most important components in a Computer Aided Diagnosis (CAD) system. An accurate and robust tissue classifier is one of the ultimate goals for many radiology applications. In recent years, impressive improvements on various computer vision problems have been reported using deep learning-based models over traditional machine learning and

© Springer International Publishing AG 2017
Q. Wang et al. (Eds.): MLMI 2017, LNCS 10541, pp. 212–219, 2017.
DOI: 10.1007/978-3-319-67389-9_25

statistical methods. Specifically, Convolutional Neural Networks (CNN) have shown superior capabilities in extracting the low to high-level image features needed to perform the classification with the deep neural networks. These successes have motivated the increasing application of deep learning for medical image analysis [1–4]. However, it has also been recognized that deep learning models (and actually most of the learning-based methods) are far more difficult to be successfully applied on medical image analysis comparing with the natural image analysis. One of the main challenges arises from the limited number of labeled samples for training the model [5], as annotation and labeling of medical images is a highly time consuming and labor-intensive work. Also, medical images are highly heterogeneous both on an individual-level and population-level. The combination effect of these two limitations severely degrades the robustness of the models and the reproducibility of the learning results.

On the other hand, the availability and size of medical images on public domains have been increasing very fast over the past few years. However most of them are not annotated as these databases are usually provided for general purpose of use, and annotation is extremely costly. Consequently, there exist huge discrepancies between the large number of datasets to be analyzed and the very limited number of available annotations to be used as training data. In response to the challenge of the lack of training samples, and the success of self-paced learning in optimizing the learning procedure [6–8] and curriculum development [9], we propose the self-paced Convolutional Neural Network (spCNN) framework which is able to identify unlabeled image patches as "virtual" training samples. These virtual samples are then mixed with the original manually-labeled samples to retrain a new network. By introducing the virtual samples, we can practically obtain any number of training samples by increasing the computational load of the machines in exchange for the (much more expensive) human labor work. We tested the performance of both the raw CNN trained only from manually-labeled samples and the CNN retrained on the mixed training samples, by applying them both to another benchmark testing dataset labeled by a different group of experts. The classification results show that the accuracy of the spCNN framework is consistently improved by 10% with the help of the virtual samples.

2   Materials and Methods

2.1   Method Overview

In this work, we propose the self-paced Convolution Neural Network (spCNN) framework in order to improve the accuracy and robustness of the learned model beyond the information provided from the initially limited training data. The major contribution and novelty of the proposed framework is that it leverages the large amount of new, unlabeled data as potential new training samples for the retraining. The new training samples are called "virtual samples" in contrast to the original manually-labeled samples. Specifically, class labels and the distribution of prediction accuracies of the samples in the new dataset are estimated by bootstrapping CNNs. Image patches with significant different prediction probabilities across labels are then pooled together with the original training data for retraining a new CNN. A conceptual diagram of the framework design is illustrated in Fig. 1.

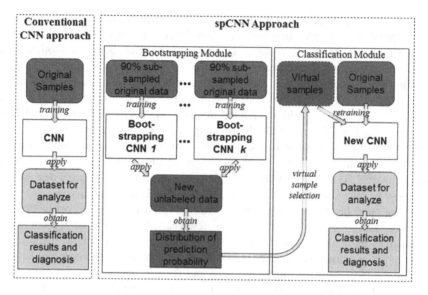

Fig. 1. Left: Illustration of the conventional CNN approach of performing image classification. Right: Illustration of the spCNN framework consists of the main "Classification Module" similar to the conventional approach, and the "Bootstrapping Module" which provides the extra training data through virtual sample selection based on the bootstrapping CNNs performed on the new unlabeled data.

2.2   Architecture of the CNN Applied in the Framework

The CNN model used in the proposed framework is implemented in Caffe [10], and its architecture is shown in Fig. 2. Image patches of size 36×36 are convolved by 4 convolutional layers. The kernel size of all convolutional layers is set to 3. Based on the principles introduced in [1] that the number of kernels in each layer shall be proportional to the area of its receptive field (in this work, from 3×3 in the first layer to 6×6 in the fourth layer), we set the number of kernels in the four layers as 45, 80, 125 and 180 respectively. Each convolutional layer is followed by a maximum pooling layer. The extracted features are then fed into three fully connected layers, with the number of neurons being 1080, 360 and 3. These numbers are proportional (6 and 2 times) to the number of features (180), based on the empirical rules reported in [1]. The first two fully connected layers are equipped with dropout layers [11] with probability of 50%. Both the convolutional layers and the fully connected layers use the activation function of LeakyReLU [12].

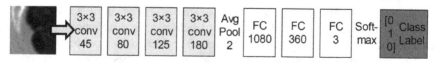

Fig. 2. Architecture of the CNN used in the proposed framework. Each convolutional layer and fully-connected layer is followed by a LeakyReLU activation function.

2.3   Bootstrapping Module for Virtual Sample Selection

The key challenge of the spCNN framework is how to correctly select the image patches from the new dataset into the virtual samples: labels of the patches could be wrongfully assigned by the initially trained CNN which is clearly not desired. Specifically, it has been observed in both our experiments and in previous work [8] that the errors of the model could be quickly accumulated during the retraining and eventually lead to a performance decrease. On the other hand, we will also want to push the boundary of the retraining dataset beyond the original manual annotations, which often involves image patches with higher uncertainty of the accuracy from the network. In other words, the framework needs to balance between the original manually-labeled samples and the latterly identified virtual samples.

Thus, in this work we apply a 10-folds bootstrapping scheme to estimate the empirical distribution of the predication probabilities of the new samples, and select the most suitable samples automatically according to the statistical testing. Specifically, we perform random subsampling for 10 times to obtain 10 sets of 90% of the original training data, which are 360 patches for each class for a total of 1080 patches. These 10 sets of data are then used to train the bootstrapping networks. Patches in the new dataset are then classified by each of the 10 networks, resulting in 10 sets of class labels and prediction probabilities for each patch, illustrated in Fig. 3. It could be found that while certain patches (e.g. the first two patches in Fig. 3) in the new dataset can be easily classified with high prediction probabilities and low variability from all the bootstrapping networks, there are cases where the classification uncertainty is much

	Sample 1			Sample 2			Sample 3		
	I	II	III	I	II	III	I	II	III
Run1	0.0%	0.5%	99.4%	0.0%	0.1%	99.9%	0.1%	10.2%	89.7%
Run2	0.0%	0.1%	99.9%	0.0%	0.1%	99.9%	0.0%	1.7%	98.3%
Run3	0.1%	0.8%	99.1%	0.0%	0.3%	99.6%	0.0%	21.0%	79.0%
Run4	0.2%	7.0%	92.8%	0.0%	0.2%	99.7%	0.1%	5.6%	94.3%
Run5	0.0%	0.3%	99.7%	0.0%	0.2%	99.8%	0.1%	28.4%	71.5%
Run6	0.1%	3.6%	96.2%	0.0%	0.1%	99.9%	0.1%	0.6%	99.4%
Run7	0.1%	1.4%	98.4%	0.0%	0.0%	99.9%	0.1%	4.0%	96.0%
Run8	0.0%	0.3%	99.6%	0.0%	0.1%	99.9%	0.1%	3.2%	96.7%
Run9	0.1%	1.1%	98.8%	0.0%	0.1%	99.8%	0.3%	16.3%	83.4%
Run10	0.1%	0.6%	99.4%	0.0%	0.1%	99.9%	0.0%	3.3%	96.6%

Fig. 3. Illustration of the 10-folds bootstrapping results of the new data on 3 example image patches. Captions of the table columns (I, II and III) indicate the prediction probability of the given patch belonging to the corresponding class.

higher (e.g. the third patch). Visual inspection indicates that the third image patch lies on the boundary between the normal lung tissue and regions outside of lung, which is definitely a good candidate to be included in the retraining process. As reported in [13], the sheer number of training samples does not help too much for training the network especially if they come from a homogeneous population. It is the samples that are not encountered before will actually lead to better performance. Based to such observations, in this work, for each of the 10×3 prediction probability matrix of the given image patch estimated by the bootstrapping CNNs, we will perform two two-sample t-tests (as there are totally 3 labels), aiming to find whether the label with highest average prediction probability is significantly higher than the other two labels. The two p-values produced by the t-tests from each patch will be then aggregated and further analyzed by the false discovery rate (FDR) control. Here we employed the FDR to minimize the possibility that the huge number of testing performed could lead to increased false positives (i.e. unfitting patches). Patches with significantly different prediction probabilities across the 3 labels will be selected as virtual samples for retraining the new CNN.

3 Experimental Results

3.1 Data Acquisition and Preprocessing

In this work, we use the data from the COPDGene database [14] sponsored by NIH, which aims to investigate the CT phenotypes in Chronic Obstructive Pulmonary Disease (COPD) and other lung diseases. For the purpose of testing and validating the proposed model, we mainly focus on pulmonary emphysema, defined as the permanent enlargement of airspaces distal to the terminal bronchioles and the destruction of the alveolar walls. In the COPDGene database, 3-D volumetric images are acquired using 64-slice CT scanners during full inspiration, and then reconstructed using sub-millimeter slice thickness with smoothing and edge-enhancing filters. From the total of 10,000 subjects in the database from both normal and COPD population, 500 image slices from 150 subjects were manually annotated by a group of experts on our team for the three classes: airway (Class I), emphysema (Class II), and other lung tissue (Class III). For each of the 3 classes, 600 non-overlapping image patches of size 36×36 were extracted from the annotation results, constituting the samples for training (400 patches) and verification (200 patches). At the same time, from the new unlabeled dataset, 9600 patches were extracted and analyzed by the bootstrapping CNNs, constituting the candidates for virtual sample selection. Finally, 161 image slices from another 59 subjects were manually annotated by another group of experts. Totally 887 (Class I: 203, Class II: 192, Class III: 255) image patches were extracted from the annotated regions, which were used as the benchmark testing inputs for evaluating the model performance.

3.2   Performance Comparisons

By applying the bootstrapping module of the proposed spCNN framework on the 9600 image patches in the new dataset, we select the virtual samples according to the different significant level. We then retrain the new CNN models from the mixture of the virtual samples and the original manually-labeled samples. The new CNNs are then applied to classify the benchmark testing dataset. The model performance and the details of the virtual samples are summarized in Table 1. The results show that using the significant level $p = 0.05/0.1$ for the FDR-controlled statistical testing, spCNN can obtain as high as 10% of accuracy increase over the raw CNN model trained solely from the original manually-labeled samples. The classification accuracy which is near 90% is on the same level with the results from a similar lung CT image study using CNN as reported in [4]. Using a more conservative significant level ($p = 0.025$), fewer data will be selected, obtain similar levels of accuracy compared to the raw CNN without causing performance decrease.

Table 1. Comparison of the number of virtual samples selected (out of 9600 patches) as well as the classification accuracies among the raw CNN (first row) and spCNN under different significant levels for FDR-controlled statistical testing.

Model	Number of virtual samples	Accuracy
Original samples only	N/A	79.0%
$p = 0.025$	665	84.1%
$p = 0.05$	891	87.3%
$p = 0.1$	943	88.9%

As the current virtual sample selection in spCNN are empirically determined using bootstrapping scheme, one important question is whether the framework are robust enough to guide the virtual sample selection process under different models and/or different datasets. Limited by the size and scope of this manuscript, we only focused on the COPDGene dataset, yet test the spCNN performance using the same virtual sample selection method but different CNN architectures. Specifically, we have tried replacing the CNN architecture as introduced in 2.1 by the following designs: (1) Reducing the number of kernels in the convolutional layers as well as the number of neurons in the fully connected layers by half. (2) Increasing the number of kernels in the convolutional layers as well as the number of neurons in the fully connected layers by 50%. (3) Adding an extra fully connected layer with number of neurons of 180 before the last layer. (4) Removing the first 3×3 convolutional layer. The results show that, while the classification performance of the spCNN framework based on these 4 network architectures varies, in all of the cases using significant level of $p = 0.1$ will outperform other configurations, as well as the original CNN method.

3.3   Time Cost for the Virtual Sample Selection

As we previously discussed, the self-paced learning framework essentially exchanges human labor work with computational costs through the bootstrapping process. So, the time cost for training the bootstrapping CNNs could be an important factor for the proposed spCNN framework, especially for larger datasets and/or more complicated network architectures. Currently we deploy the framework on two platforms: one is an in-house server installed with two NVIDIA Tesla P-100 GPUs. The other is the NVIDIA DGX-1 deep learning system with eight P-100 GPUs interconnected with the NVIDIA NVLink. Time costs for training one bootstrapping CNN in the bootstrapping module, as well as for performing one forward-backward propagation using different hardware configurations are listed in Table 2.

Table 2. Time cost for training one CNN during bootstrapping ("per session", measured in seconds) and time cost for performing one forward-backward propagation ("per iteration", measured in milliseconds). All values are estimated by averaging from the time costs of running the CNN training for 100 times.

Configuration	per Session (s)	per Iteration (ms)
In-house, single GPU	50.63	5.01
In-house, 2 GPUs	50.92	5.00
DGX1, single GPU	44.46	4.41
DGX1, 2 GPUs	33.80	3.32
DGX1, 4 GPUs	27.84	2.66
DGX1, 8 GPUs	27.98	2.54

It can be seen that using the most advanced accelerator of NVIDIA DGX1, we can achieve a nearly 2-fold speed increase. It should be noted that the in-house sever shows a lowered running speed using two GPUs comparing with a single GPU, due to the fact that P2P DMA access between devices is needed for running Caffe in multiple-GPU mode. When the P2P access is not supported (as in our in-house server), data will need to be copied through hosts thus severely affect the performance. On the contrary, the DGX1 system is much better optimized for parallelizing the computational loads across multiple GPUs, showing the importance of the P2P DMA access and the NVIDIA NVLink technology. Also, we observe that using 8 GPUs in DGX1 does not result in better performance comparing with 4 GPUs even though the iteration time has been reduced, which is most likely due to the fact that the overhead for parallelization became dominant in the time cost for 8 GPUs. Considering the fact that the current CNN architecture is relatively simple, we envision that 8 GPUs will outperform other configurations in more complicated cases.

4   Conclusion and Discussion

In this work, we develop the self-paced scheme for identifying virtual samples from the unlabeled data and use them to retrain a new CNN, in order to overcome the problems of the lack of training samples. The FDR-controlled statistical testing for the virtual sample selection based on bootstrapping scheme shows that the current optimized threshold is around $p = 0.1$. Similar threshold could be used for analyzing the rest of the data within the COPDGene dataset as such inference is not affected by the number of classes nor the number of samples tested. We propose that the parameter tuning on the threshold is essentially the empirical characterization for the relationship between the distribution of the network outputs and the quality/confidence of the corresponding samples which is highly related with the nature of the dataset, and our self-paced learning scheme can leverage such relationship to help the training by expanding the solution space it can explore.

References

1. Anthimopoulos, M., Christodoulidis, S., Ebner, L., Christe, A., Mougiakakou, S.: Lung pattern classification for interstitial lung diseases using a deep convolutional neural network. IEEE Trans. Med. Imaging 35(5), 1207–1216 (2016)
2. Cireşan, D.C., Giusti, A., Gambardella, L.M., Schmidhuber, J.: Mitosis detection in breast cancer histology images with deep neural networks. In: Mori, K., Sakuma, I., Sato, Y., Barillot, C., Navab, N. (eds.) MICCAI 2013. LNCS, vol. 8150, pp. 411–418. Springer, Heidelberg (2013). doi:10.1007/978-3-642-40763-5_51
3. Shen, D., Wu, G., Suk, H.-I.: Deep learning in medical image analysis. Ann. Rev. Biomed. Eng. (2016)
4. Shin, H.C., Roth, H.R., Gao, M., Lu, L., Xu, Z., Nogues, I., Yao, J., Mollura, D., Summers, R.M.: Deep convolutional neural networks for computer-aided detection: CNN architectures, dataset characteristics and transfer learning. IEEE Trans. Med. Imaging 35(5), 1285–1298 (2016)
5. Greenspan, H., van Ginneken, B., Summers, R.M.: Guest editorial deep learning in medical imaging: overview and future promise of an exciting new technique. IEEE Trans. Med. Imaging 35(5), 1153–1159 (2016)
6. Jiang, L., Meng, D., Yu, S.-I., Lan, Z., Shan, S., Hauptmann, A.G.: Self-paced learning with diversity. In: Advances in Neural Information Processing Systems (NIPS) (2014)
7. Kumar, M.P., Packer, B., Koller, D.: Self-paced learning for latent variable models. In: Advances in Neural Information Processing Systems (NIPS) (2010)
8. Jiang, L., Meng, D., Zhao, Q., Shan, S., Hauptmann, A.G.: Self-paced curriculum learning. In: AAAI Conference on Artificial Intelligence (2015)
9. Bengio, Y., Louradour, J., Collobert, R., Weston, J.: Curriculum learning. In: International Conference on Machine Learning (ICML) (2009)
10. Jia, Y., Shelhamer, E., Donahue, J., Karayev, S., Long, J., Girshick, R., Guadarrama, S., Darrell, T.: Caffe: convolutional architecture for fast feature embedding. In: International Conference on Multimedia (ACM MM) (2014)
11. Srivastava, N., Hinton, G., Krizhevsky, A., Sutskever, I., Salakhutdinov, R.: Dropout: a simple way to prevent neural networks from overfitting. J. Mach. Learn. Res. 15, 1929–1958 (2014)
12. Maas, A.L., Hannun, A.Y., Ng, A.Y.: Rectifier nonlinearities improve neural network acoustic models. In: ICML Workshop on Deep Learning for Audio, Speech, and Language Processing (WDLASL) (2013)
13. Zhu, X., Vondrick, C., Fowlkes, C., Ramanan, D.: Do we need more training data? In: British Machine Vision Conference (2012)
14. Washko, G.R., Hunninghake, G.M., Fernandez, I.E., Nishino, M., Okajima, Y., Yamashiro, T., Ross, J.C., Estépar, R.S.J., Lynch, D.A., Brehm, J.M., Andriole, K.P., Diaz, A.A., Khorasani, R., D'Aco, K., Sciurba, F.C., Silverman, E.K., Hatabu, H., Rosas, I.O.: Lung volumes and emphysema in smokers with interstitial lung abnormalities. N. Engl. J. Med. 364(10), 897–906 (2011)

A Point Says a Lot: An Interactive Segmentation Method for MR Prostate via One-Point Labeling

Jinquan Sun[1], Yinghuan Shi[1], Yang Gao[1]([⊠]), and Dinggang Shen[2]

[1] State Key Laboratory for Novel Software Technology,
Nanjing University, Nanjing, China
gaoy@nju.edu.cn
[2] Department of Radiology and BRIC, UNC Chapel Hill, Chapel Hill, USA

Abstract. In this paper, we investigate if the MR prostate segmentation performance could be improved, by only providing one-point labeling information in the prostate region. To achieve this goal, by asking the physician to first click one point inside the prostate region, we present a novel segmentation method by simultaneously integrating the boundary detection results and the patch-based prediction. Particularly, since the clicked point belongs to the prostate, we first generate the location-prior maps, with two basic assumptions: (1) a point closer to the clicked point should be with higher probability to be the prostate voxel, (2) a point separated by more boundaries to the clicked point, will have lower chance to be the prostate voxel. We perform the Canny edge detector and obtain two location-prior maps from horizontal and vertical directions, respectively. Then, the obtained location-prior maps along with the original MR images are fed into a multi-channel fully convolutional network to conduct the patch-based prediction. With the obtained prostate-likelihood map, we employ a level-set method to achieve the final segmentation. We evaluate the performance of our method on 22 MR images collected from 22 different patients, with the manual delineation provided as the ground truth for evaluation. The experimental results not only show the promising performance of our method but also demonstrate the one-point labeling could largely enhance the results when a pure patch-based prediction fails.

1 Introduction

Prostate cancer is one of the most leading cause of male death [1]. Previous clinical studies demonstrate that the radiotherapy can provide effective treatment for prostate cancer. During the radiotherapy process, the prostate cancer tissues should be killed while the normal tissues could not be hurt at the same time. Therefore, an accurate prostate segmentation is significant from the clinical perspective, which indicates that the success of the radiotherapy highly depends on the accuracy of prostate segmentation. In fact, the segmentation of prostate is conventionally done by physician with slice-by-slice delineation, which is very time-consuming.

© Springer International Publishing AG 2017
Q. Wang et al. (Eds.): MLMI 2017, LNCS 10541, pp. 220–228, 2017.
DOI: 10.1007/978-3-319-67389-9_26

In recent years, many automatic prostate segmentation methods have been proposed with promising results for different modalities, *e.g.* CT and Ultrasound [2]. In this paper, we focus on segmentation of MR images. The prostate segmentation is a challenging task due to the low tissue contrast, irregular prostate motion, as well as large shape variation among different patients. Many previous attempts were developed to address the aforementioned challenges. Atlas-based prostate segmentation in MR images is popular in the last decade [3]. Also, prior information is employed to improve the segmentation performance. Gao *et al.* [4] incorporated both local image statistics and learnt shape prior to guide better segmentation. In [5] the spatial locations of the prostate identified via spectra are used as the initial ROI for a 2D Active Shape Model (ASM). These approaches largely depend on the discriminative ability of the hand-crafted features, with different types of features to choose and also lots of parameters to select. Fortuantely, in recent years, deep learning provides a more feasible way for learning good features. Liao *et al.* in [6] propose a deep learning framework using independent subspace analysis to extract useful features for segmentation.

However, the performance of these previous automatic segmentation methods largely depends on the consistency of sample distributions between training and testing images. A natural question is whether we could use a simple interaction from physicians to improve the performance. To overcome this issue, several interactive segmentation methods are presented by performing prostate segmentation with a few interactions from physician, although these methods are not specifically designed for segmentation in MR images. In [7], physician's interactive labeling information is first required to label a small set of prostate and non-prostate voxels, and then transductive Lasso is used to select the most discriminative features. Moreover, interactive methods based on prior knowledge of training data have been proposed: Park *et al.* [8] used the spatial relationship of adjacent patches to constrain the specific shapes of organs.

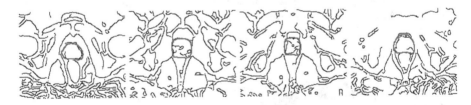

Fig. 1. Typical boundary image of our training data. The black curves denote the boundary detected by Canny edge detector. The red curves denote the ground-truth manual delineation. (Color figure online)

In this paper, a novel interactive method for MR prostate segmentation is proposed, by only requiring one-point interaction from physicians. This is motivated by the following two facts. First, for a new MR image, physician focuses on the region which has a high probability of being prostate, instead of wasting time on other regions. Second, the borders in image provide more information for segmentation than the inside regions. As what Fig. 1 conveys, although the exact boundary of prostate cannot be detected, the edges in image are useful to infer the location of prostate. Specifically, we first ask a physician to provide one point on the MR image, which is probably in the center of prostate. Then, we use Canny operator to obtain the detected edges. By simultaneously combining detected edges and one-point labeling information, we could obtain two prostate location-prior maps from the vertical and horizontal directions, respectively, with two basic assumptions: (1) a point closer to the clicked point should be with higher probability to be prostate voxel, (2) a point separated by more boundaries to the clicked point will have lower chance to be the prostate voxel. The location-prior maps are regarded as new channels and added to the original raw image. We finally train a multi-channel patch-based FCN [9] to perform the patch-based prediction, and employ the refinement for the final segmentation results.

2   Our Method

We now first present how to generate the location-prior maps and then illustrate details of network structure. Finally, we will introduce the result refinement for generating final segmentations. The pipeline of the whole framework is shown in Fig. 2.

Generating location-prior maps: For a new MR image, we ask the physician to roughly find the center of prostate for generating the location-prior maps. Please note that, we do not mean that the physician must find the true center of prostate, and the later evaluation also shows the robustness of our method to different initializations. Then more attention is paid to the regions extending from the center of prostate, especially those with border information. As what Fig. 1 conveys, partial edges of prostate can be detected by common edge detector (*i.e.*, Canny edge detector), which are close to the ground-truth manual delineation. Also, the borders of rectum and bladder can be detected at the same

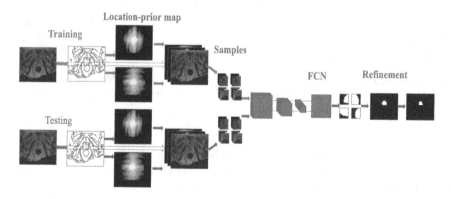

Fig. 2. Illustration of the pipeline of our method.

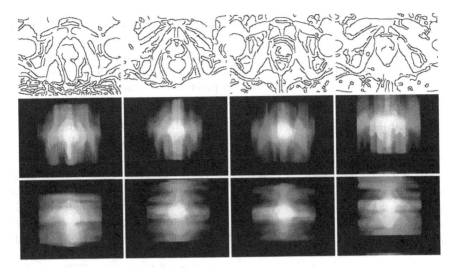

Fig. 3. Typical location-prior maps generated from our dataset. Images in first row are the border images obtained by Canny edge detector, while the second and the third are the location-prior maps obtained from vertical and horizontal directions, respectively.

time, which are in fact surrounding the prostate region. Although it is infeasible that all the images could provide relative clear and complete edge of prostate region, the border of other organs surrounding prostate is generally clear and can thus provide effective heuristic information for generating the location-prior maps. Figure 3 shows several typical examples.

For each testing image, we ask the physician to first provide one point to indicate the location of prostate, which is generally in the central area of prostate. For the sake of convenience, we take the point as a voxel in the image with exact coordinates. Please note that, the one point information for training images is given by calculating the mass center, since the manual delineation of training images are available during the training stage. Normally, to generate the prior-location maps, we follow the two basic assumptions: (1) a point closer to the clicked point should be with higher probability to be the prostate voxel, (2) a point separated by more boundaries to the clicked point will have lower chance to be the prostate voxel. After using Canny edge detector to detect all edges in the MR image, two horizontal and vertical rays are extended out from one-point voxel (we set the intensity value as 255) with the intensity reducing strategy as follows for each move: in the location-prior map, the intensity value is reduced by 1, and in particular, when the move crosses through a detected edge by Canny edge detector, the intensity value is reduced by 10. From each voxel in all lines, rays are extended with the same intensity reducing strategy as above. Then we use a median filter to smooth these two calculated images as the location-prior maps from two different directions, respectively. Finally, the original MR image along with the two location-prior maps are combined as a multi-channel image in the subsequent learning process.

Since different regions of prostate and non-prostate regions do not distribute uniformly, we sample patches from both prostate and non-prostate regions from training images as previous methods [10,11]. Typically, we sample patches in the following ways: (1) densely sampling the patches which locate inside the prostate region or are centered close to prostate boundary, and (2) sparsely sampling patches which are far from prostate boundary.

Table 1. Network structure.

Layer	Kernel	Pooling	Activation
Conv	$5 \times 5 \times 3 \times 32$	N.A.	Relu
Conv	$5 \times 5 \times 32 \times 32$	N.A.	Relu
Conv	$5 \times 5 \times 32 \times 64$	Max	Relu
Conv	$4 \times 4 \times 64 \times 64$	N.A.	Relu
Conv	$4 \times 4 \times 64 \times 2$	Upsample	Softmax

Neural network structure: To predict the prostate-likelihood for the patches from testing images, we design a multi-channel fully convolutional network inspired by FCN [9]. The traditional FCN [9] is modified to fit the small size input patches in our task. Specifically, the whole structure is similar to traditional FCN [9], but with fewer layers. Please refer to Table 1 for details. Training a deep neural network will be a challenging task when internal covariance shift problem happens [12]: the distribution of internal nodes changes when the parameter of previous layer is updated. Fortunately, batch normalization [12] provides an efficient way to tackle this issue. To avoid the above issue, we perform batch normalization towards reducing internal covariance shift. Typically, we add one batch normalization layer to each convolutional layer. We observe that, with batch normalization [12], the neural network will end up with a poor local optimum. The Adam [13] optimizer is employed for optimization, where initial learning rate is set 0.001 and other parameters keep default.

We implement our method with TensorFlow toolbox [14], on a PC with 3.7 GHz CPU, 128 GB RAM, and Nvidia Tesla K80 GPU. The number of epoch is set to 30. The running time for training requires 2 to 3 h. Currently, our method only takes 1–5 s to segment a new coming image.

Refinement: It is noteworthy that, in the training stage, for each image we randomly sample patches from the whole image to train our model, while, in the testing stage, we use a different sample pattern to choose patches fed into the neural network: a number of rays in equal degree intervals are extended from the one-point pixel labeled by physicians, we choose testing patches whose center point locates at these rays. Their responding segmentation will be integrated to forming the prostate likelihood map. Experiments show that, in this way, we can capture more precise boundaries of prostate. Since the patient-specific shape prior is not available, on the obtained prostate-likelihood maps, we perform the level-set method [15] to generate the final segmentations.

3   Experimental Results

Setting: Our dataset consists of 22 MR images, scanned from 22 different patients. The resolution of each MR image after image preprocessing is

$193 \times 152 \times 60$: the in-plane voxel size is $1 \times 1\,\mathrm{mm}^2$ and the inter-slice thickness is $1\,\mathrm{mm}$. The manual delineation results are available for each image that can be used as ground truth for evaluation. Meanwhile, for segmenting each testing image, we will first ask the physician to provide an additional one-point coordinate. We perform 2-fold cross validation on these 22 MR images. For evaluation metrics, we employ the Dice ratio and centroid distance (CD) along 3 directions (*i.e.*, lateral x-axis, anterior-posterior y-axis, and superior-inferior z-axis), which are widely used in previous studies [10, 11].

Table 2. Evaluation comparison with FCN.

	CD-x (mm)	CD-y (mm)	CD-z (mm)	Dice ratio
FCN	1.91 ± 2.63	1.31 ± 0.99	0.57 ± 0.37	0.71 ± 0.15
Our method	0.74 ± 0.48	0.49 ± 0.44	0.27 ± 0.19	0.84 ± 0.02

Qualitative results: Figure 4 shows the typical MR images in our dataset along with the detected prostate boundaries by our segmentation method (green) and manual rater (red). It is obvious that our method can achieve promising result.

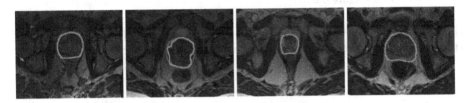

Fig. 4. Typical results. Red curves denote the manual delineation. Green curves denote the results obtained by our method. (Color figure online)

Figure 5 shows that, with the help of additional one-point information, compared to the traditional fully convolutional network, our method can locate prostate more precisely with a significant improvement.

Since the point provided from physician is important in our framework, it is necessary to evaluate how the point coordinates affect the segmentation result. As what Fig. 6 conveys, the coordinates of point truly have effect on the final segmentation result: the farther away from the center area of prostate, the worse

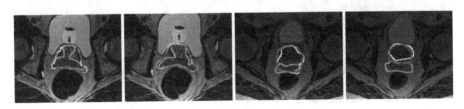

Fig. 5. Typical results of FCN and our method. Red, green, yellow curves denote the manual delineation, traditional FCN and our method, respectively. (Color figure online)

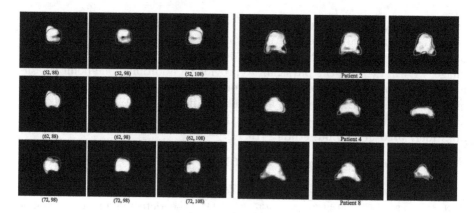

Fig. 6. Illustration of prostate likelihood maps. Left part demonstrates prostate likelihood maps when different point coordinates are given for the same image (i.e., initial coordinates of point are (62,98)). Right part illustrates the likelihood maps obtained by our method on prostates with irregular shapes. The red curves denote the manual delineation. (Color figure online)

the result will be. Besides, we plot a heatmap in Fig. 7 to illustrate the impact. It is noteworthy that, for this image, the Dice ratio by performing traditional FCN [9] is 0.85.

Table 3. Comparison with other state-of-the-art methods.

	Coup *et al.* [16]	Klein *et al.* [17]	Liao *et al.* [6]
Dice ratio	0.82 ± 0.03	0.83 ± 0.03	0.86 ± 0.02

Quantative results: Our method can obtain mean dice ratio of 0.84 ± 0.02 which is higher than 0.71 ± 0.15 achieved by traditional FCN [9]. Please refer to Fig. 7 for

the Dice ratio of each patient. Table 2 shows evaluation compared with traditional FCN [9].

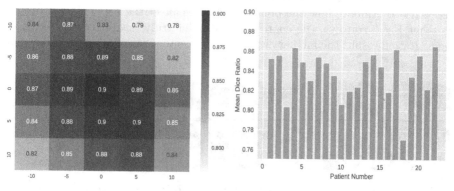

Fig. 7. (Left) Illustration of the Dice ratio values with changes of coordinates. (Right) The Dice ratio values for 22 individual patients in our dataset.

Due to the fact that neither executables nor the datasets of other works are publicly available, it is difficult for us to directly compare our method with other MR prostate segmentation method [6,16,17]. Thus, we only cite the results reported in their publications in Table 3 for reference. It is worth noting that our method can obtain competitive results compared with these state-of-art methods.

4   Conclusion

In this paper, we propose a novel interactive segmentation method for MR prostate, which can achieve the promising results with just one-point labeling from the physician. Specifically, we can make full use of provided interaction information by simultaneously incorporating the additional point labeling and detected edges, in order to generate two location-prior maps, from vertical and horizontal directions, respectively. Upon the obtained location-prior maps along with the original patches from MR images, a multi-channel patch-based fully convolutional network is then used for patch-based prediction. Finally, a level-set based refinement is performed for final segmentation results. The experimental results demonstrate the effectiveness of our method.

Acknowledgement. This work was supported by NSFC (61673203, 61432008), Nanjing Science and Technique Development Foundation (201503041), Young Elite Scientists Sponsorship Program by CAST (YESS 20160035) and NIH Grant (CA206100).

References

1. Cokkinides, V., Albano, J., Samuels, A., et al.: American Cancer Society: Cancer Facts and Figures. American Cancer Society, Atlanta (2005)
2. Ghose, S., Oliver, A., Mart, R., et al.: A survey of prostate segmentation methodologies in ultrasound, magnetic resonance and computed tomography images. Comput. Methods Programs Biomed. **108**(1), 262–287 (2012)
3. Klein, S., van der Heide, U.A., Lips, I.M., et al.: Automatic segmentation of the prostate in 3D MR images by atlas matching using localized mutual information. Med. Phys. **35**(4), 1407–1417 (2008)
4. Gao, Y., Sandhu, R., Fichtinger, G., et al.: A coupled global registration and segmentation framework with application to magnetic resonance prostate imagery. IEEE Trans. Med. Imaging **29**(10), 1781–1794 (2010)
5. Toth, R., Tiwari, P., Rosen, M., et al.: A magnetic resonance spectroscopy driven initialization scheme for active shape model based prostate segmentation. Med. Image Anal. **15**(2), 214–225 (2011)
6. Liao, S., Gao, Y., Oto, A., Shen, D.: Representation learning: a unified deep learning framework for automatic prostate MR segmentation. In: Mori, K., Sakuma, I., Sato, Y., Barillot, C., Navab, N. (eds.) MICCAI 2013. LNCS, vol. 8150, pp. 254–261. Springer, Heidelberg (2013). doi:10.1007/978-3-642-40763-5_32

7. Shi, Y., Liao, S., Gao, Y., Zhang, D., Gao, Y., Shen, D.: Transductive prostate segmentation for CT image guided radiotherapy. In: Wang, F., Shen, D., Yan, P., Suzuki, K. (eds.) MLMI 2012. LNCS, vol. 7588, pp. 1–9. Springer, Heidelberg (2012). doi:10.1007/978-3-642-35428-1_1

8. Park, S.H., Yun, I.D., Lee, S.U.: Data-driven interactive 3D medical image segmentation based on structured patch model. In: Gee, J.C., Joshi, S., Pohl, K.M., Wells, W.M., Zöllei, L. (eds.) IPMI 2013. LNCS, vol. 7917, pp. 196–207. Springer, Heidelberg (2013). doi:10.1007/978-3-642-38868-2_17

9. Long, J., Shelhamer, E., Darrell, T.: Fully convolutional networks for semantic segmentation. In: Proceedings of the IEEE Conference on Computer Vision and Pattern Recognition, pp. 3431–3440 (2015)

10. Shi, Y., Liao, S., Gao, Y., et al.: Prostate segmentation in CT images via spatial-constrained transductive lasso. In: Proceedings of the IEEE Conference on Computer Vision and Pattern Recognition, pp. 2227–2234 (2013)

11. Shi, Y., Gao, Y., Liao, S., et al.: Semi-automatic segmentation of prostate in CT images via coupled feature representation and spatial-constrained transductive lasso. IEEE Trans. Pattern Anal. Mach. Intell. 37(11), 2286–2303 (2015)

12. Ioffe, S., Szegedy, C.: Batch normalization: accelerating deep network training by reducing internal covariate shift. arXiv: 1502.03167 (2015)

13. Kingma, D., Ba, J.: Adam: A Method for Stochastic Optimization. arXiv: 1412.6980 (2014)

14. Abadi, M., Barham, P., Chen, J., et al.: TensorFlow: a system for large-scale machine learning. In: Proceedings of the 12th USENIX Symposium on Operating Systems Design and Implementation (OSDI), Savannah, Georgia, USA (2016)

15. Li, C., Xu, C., Gui, C., et al.: Distance regularized level set evolution and its application to image segmentation. IEEE Trans. Image Process. 19(12), 3243–3254 (2010)

16. Coupé, P., Manjnó, J.V., Fonov, V., et al.: Patch-based segmentation using expert priors: application to hippocampus and ventricle segmentation. NeuroImage 54(2), 940–954 (2011)

17. Klein, S., van der Heide, U.A., Lips, I.M., et al.: Automatic segmentation of the prostate in 3D MR images by atlas matching using localized mutual information. Med. Phys. 35(4), 1407–1417 (2008)

Collage CNN for Renal Cell Carcinoma Detection from CT

Mohammad Arafat Hussain[1]([✉]), Alborz Amir-Khalili[1], Ghassan Hamarneh[2], and Rafeef Abugharbieh[1]

[1] BiSICL, University of British Columbia, Vancouver, BC, Canada
{arafat,alborza,rafeef}@ece.ubc.ca
[2] Medical Image Analysis Lab, Simon Fraser University, Burnaby, BC, Canada
hamarneh@sfu.ca

Abstract. Renal cell carcinoma (RCC) is a common malignancy that accounts for a steadily increasing mortality rate worldwide. Widespread use of abdominal imaging in recent years, mainly CT and MRI, has significantly increased the detection rates of such cancers. However, detection still relies on a laborious manual process based on visual inspection of 2D image slices. In this paper, we propose an image collage based deep convolutional neural network (CNN) approach for automatic detection of pathological kidneys containing RCC. Our collage approach overcomes the absence of slice-wise training labels, enables slice-reshuffling based data augmentation, and offers favourable training time and performance compared to 3D CNNs. When validated on clinical CT datasets of 160 patients from the TCIA database, our method classified RCC cases vs. normal kidneys with 98% accuracy.

1 Introduction

Renal cell carcinomas (RCC) refer to a group of chemotherapy-resistant malignancies [1] that constitutes the most common type of kidney cancer in adults. Responsible for approximately 90% of cases of kidney cancers, RCCs accounted for an estimated 61,560 new patients and 14,080 deaths in the United States in 2015 alone [2]. In fact, North America and Europe have recently reported the highest numbers of new cases of renal tumor in the world [3]. This increased number of RCC over the past several years has been contributing to a steadily increasing mortality rate per unit population worldwide [4].

Although some patients with renal tumors present with clinical symptoms like flank pain, gross haematuria or palpable abdominal mass, the detection rate of renal tumours has significantly increased due to the widespread use of various types of abdominal imaging including ultrasonography, computed tomography (CT) and magnetic resonance imaging (MRI). Typically, tumour staging is accomplished with CT, which allows for assessment of local invasiveness, lymph node involvement, or other metastases. Nonetheless, more than 50% of RCCs are currently detected incidentally [4]. This RCC detection is typically carried out by radiologists through manual observation of abdominal image data. Although a

© Springer International Publishing AG 2017
Q. Wang et al. (Eds.): MLMI 2017, LNCS 10541, pp. 229–237, 2017.
DOI: 10.1007/978-3-319-67389-9_27

good number of studies have been carried out on kidney localization and anatomical analysis [5–9], to the best of our knowledge, there has been no study to date that focused on automatic discrimination between healthy vs. renal cell carcinoma kidneys. Such discrimination ability coupled with an automatic kidney localization procedure would be invaluable during targeted as well as incidental analysis of kidney health.

Medical image analysis has enjoyed significant performance improvements through the use of various machine learning (ML) algorithms over the past few years. Most of these algorithms are fully supervised, requiring a large number of annotated datasets for model learning and prediction accuracy analysis. Unlike two dimensional (2D) single- or three-channel data (e.g., gray-scale or color images), which are most commonly used in computer vision tasks, three dimensional (3D) medical data presents different sets of challenges for ML approaches. For example, tissue abnormalities such as tumors, cancers, nodules, stones etc. are most often localized within a small region of anatomy and do not span the whole image volume. Localization and analysis of abnormal tissue are thus typically carried out on the 2D image slices. For example, staging of kidney tumors is done through slice-based tumor analysis and manual boundary tracing. However, image tags or labels (e.g. healthy, cancerous etc.) are mostly assigned per image volume or per patient basis. Therefore, all slices of an image are by default labeled with a single tag, though not all slices may contain the abnormal tissue. This scenario makes 'single-instance' ML approaches, especially deep learning ones such as convolutional neural networks (CNNs), very difficult to train on the 2D slices, as the input slice often does not correspond to the assigned volume-based label. A typical solution for this problem is to use the full 3D image volume as a single-instance for learning. However, 3D CNNs are considerably more difficult to train as they contain significantly more parameters and consequently require many more training samples, necessitate the use of expensive GPUs with very large memory, and require a lot more time to converge.

An alternative approach to single-instance learning is multiple-instance learning (MIL) [10]. MIL is a variation on weakly supervised learning wherein the learner receives a set of labeled bags, or ensembles, each containing multiple instances. This scenario allows the learner to label a bag with a class even if some or most of the instances within it are not members of that class. Using this MIL approach, the objective of our RCC detection application can be formulated such that a labelled bag corresponds to a labeled CT volume, and the constituting instances within the bag correspond to the CT's 2D slices, some of which may contain RCC tumors while many may not. This reformulation allows us to correctly incorporate volume-based labels within an easy to train 2D slice-based CNN framework. In the context of deep learning on medical images, the joint benefits of MIL combined with the classification power of 2D CNNs have been recently demonstrated in a few applications including mammogram classification for breast cancer detection [11], identifying anatomical body parts [12], colon cancer classification based on histopathology images [13], and classification of large 2D microscopy images [14]. To the best of our knowledge, such an approach has not been implemented specifically on 3D kidney data and a novel representation of volumetric CT data is necessary in order to extend such techniques for detection of RCC in CT data.

In this paper, we propose a CNN based kidney classification method that makes use of a novel collage image representation. The image slices in a 3D volume are rearranged side-by-side into a virtual extended 2D image slice, which in turn correctly corresponds to the single available label for that dataset. Our approach is different from Zhu et al. [11] and Kraus et al. [14] as, instead of explicitly modelling MIL aggregation as a global pooling layer, we design the architecture of our CNN to implicitly learn a nonlinear relationship between the bag labels and feature representation of the encapsulated instances. Compared to the computationally expensive two stage (i.e. pre-train and boosting stages) CNN learning procedure adopted by Yan et al. [12], our single collage CNN is trained end-to-end and effectively performs efficient classification. Xu et al. [13] took the advantage of a fully supervised classifier (support vector machines) on the slice-wise labeled data along with an MIL procedure on the rest of the weekly labeled data. Our proposed collage also allows for data augmentation by random reshuffling of the locations of axial image slices within the collage; this augmentation also facilitates the training of the implicit relationship between bag labels and learn feature representation.

2   Materials and Methods

2.1   Data

Our clinical dataset consisted of 160 kidney scans of 160 patients accessed from The Cancer Imaging Archive (TCIA) database [15]. We used 80 healthy kidney samples from 80 patients who had one healthy kidney. The 80 pathological kidney samples used were from another 80 patient scans. Our dataset had variations in the scanner types, contrast administration, fields of view, spatial resolutions, and intensity (Hounsfield unit) ranges. The in-plane pixel size ranged from 0.58 to 1.50 mm and the slice thickness ranged from 1.5 to 5 mm. Of the 80 healthy and 80 carcinoma scans, we randomly chose 55 cases from each set to use for training and the remaining 25 for testing. Ground truth kidney RCC labels were also collected from the TCIA data records.

2.2   Collage Representation of 3D Image Data

Typically, renal tumors grow in different regions of the kidney and are clinically scored on the basis of their CT slice-based image features such as size, margin (well-define or ill-defined), composition (solid or cystic), necrosis, growth pattern (endophytic or exophytic), calcification etc. [16]. Of course not all kidney slices necessarily contain tumors, nonetheless clinical labels (healthy/pathological) are normally recorded on a kidney- or a patient-basis. Therefore, it is not possible to use slice-based inputs in the training of a CNN because the volume-based label is

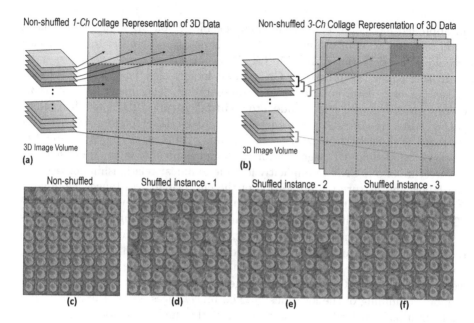

Non-shuffled *1-Ch* Collage Representation of 3D Data

Non-shuffled *3-Ch* Collage Representation of 3D Data

3D Image Volume
(a)

3D Image Volume
(b)

Non-shuffled   Shuffled instance - 1   Shuffled instance - 2   Shuffled instance - 3

(c)   (d)   (e)   (f)

Fig. 1. Schematic diagrams showing the non-shuffled (a) 1-channel and (b) 3-channels 2D collage representations of a 3D image volume. (c) An example 1-channel 2D collage image slice (512×512 pixel) containing 64 individual (non-shuffled) axial slices (64×64 pixel) of an actual kidney CT volume. The axially top and bottom slices (two corner slices in (c)) are colored to locate those in the randomly shuffled collages in (d)−(f).

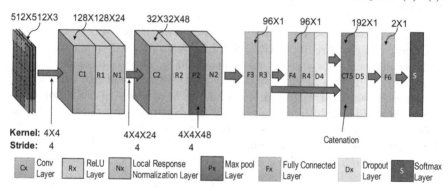

Fig. 2. The architecture of our collage deep convolutional neural network for pathological *vs.* healthy kidney classification. See Fig. 1 for the input image representation.

not applicable to all constituent axial slices. To address this challenge, we propose a novel approach where the slices within the 3D image are rearranged into an extended 2D image collage (Fig. 1). In a non-shuffled collage representation, each consecutive image slice (for 1-channel) or, a group of n consecutive image slices (for n-channels, where $n > 1$) along a particular direction are sequentially placed on a 2D plane, which is schematically shown for a 1-channel and a 3-channels ($n = 3$) image in Fig. 1(a) and (b), respectively. Note that we opt to keep the collage dimension square (i.e. 512×512 pixel) in this experiment, however it is not a necessity. This collage not only ensures meaningful correspondence to the volume's single label but also allows for invaluable data augmentation by simple random reshuffling of image slices as well as by rotation and flipping. A non-shuffled 2D image collage representing an actual kidney CT data and its shuffle-based three augmented collages are shown in Fig. 1(c) and (d)–(f), respectively. Note that we prepare our CNN input data in a process shown in Fig. 1(b), where we set $n = 3$. The resulting dimension of a single CNN input data is $512 \times 512 \times 3$ pixel and the output was either 0 (healthy) or 1 (pathological).

2.3   Pathological *vs* Healthy Kidney Classification

CNN Architecture. Our proposed CNN has seven layers excluding the input. All of these layers except the 5th layer (concatenation layer) contained trainable weights.

Layer C1 is a convolutional layer that filters the input image with 24 kernels of size $4\times4\times3$. Since we used collage-based image representation, we needed to carefully design our filter sizes and strides in a way that the convolutional (Cx) and max pooling (Px) filters do not overlap between two adjacent slices. To achieve this, we chose each edge size of the convolution filter to equal the stride in a particular layer. For example, the edge size of the convolution filter and the stride in the C1 layer were 4 and 4, respectively (Fig. 2). We chose a small convolutional filter size which tends to achieve better classification accuracy as demonstrated in [17].

Layer C2 is the second convolutional layer with forty eight $4\times4\times24$ kernels applied to the output of C1. Unlike C1, we used a max pooling (P2) of $4\times4\times48$ window in this layer to reduce the image size to 8×8 from 32×32.

The output of C2 is connected to a fully connected layer (F3), which contains 96 units. Similarly, a layer F4 contains 96 units and is fully connected to F3. We concatenated the units of F3 and F4 into CT5 in order to reduce possible information loss. This type of bypassing connections is typically suggested for better classification accuracy [18]. Note that the CT5 layer did not have any trainable weights.

The CT5 layer is connected to an F5 layer having 2 units. These units are connected to a softmax layer (S), which produces the relative probabilities for back-propagation and classification.

Solver. Our network was trained by minimizing the softmax loss between the desired and predicted labels. We used an optimization method called *Adam* [19]. All the parameters for this solver were set to the suggested default values, i.e. $\beta_1 = 0.9$, $\beta_2 = 0.999$, and $\epsilon = 10^{-8}$. We also employed a unit dropout (Dx) that drops 50% of units in both F4 and CT5 layers and used a weight decay of 0.005. The base learning rate was set to 0.01 and was decreased by a factor of

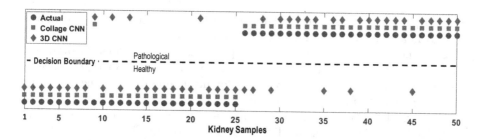

Fig. 3. Scatter plot showing the actual *vs.* predicted labels by the collage image-based and 3D CNNs.

0.1 to 0.0001 over 25000 iterations with a batch of 32 images processed at each iteration.

3   Results

We provide the classification accuracy results of our proposed collage image-based CNN as a bar plot in Fig. 3. We also compare our performance to that of a 3D CNN on the same plot. For the 3D CNN, we replaced the collage input (512×512×3 pixel) with the full 3D volume (64×64×64 pixel) of the kidney and performed 3D convolutions with a filter size of 4×4×64 with stride 4. For fair comparison, we chose the 3D volume dimension as 64×64×64 pixel, since each constituent axial slice in the collage was of 64×64 pixel. Other layer configurations remained the same as in Fig. 2. Both CNNs were implemented using *Caffe* [20]. The pre-processing of the data, visualizations, and comparisons were done in Matlab using the *MatCaffe* interface. Training was performed on a workstation with Intel 3.20 GHz Xeon processor, an Nvidia Quadro K600 GPU with 1 GB of VRAM, and 8 GB of host memory. Prior to generating the collage representation of the input data, we ensured a uniform voxel spacing in the image volume all axial, coronal and sagittal planes using interpolation. We manually defined the kidney ROI (sub)volume within the CT data in such a way that leaves an approximately 25% background area framing a kidney. Prior to training, both of the training and testing datasets were standardized.

In our experiments, we augmented the number of training samples by a factor of 40 by flipping and rotating the image slices as well as by random reshuffling the slice location within the collage. This augmentation process enabled by our novel image representation yielded a total of 4,400 2D image collages for training.

As demonstrated in Fig. 3, our proposed method succeeded in all but only one case out of 50 tested kidney samples, resulting in a classification accuracy of 98%. In comparison, the 3D convolution-based CNN failed in eight cases resulting in an accuracy of 80%.

Our preliminary results suggest that our proposed collage image representation may offer significant advantages for deep CNN-based classification tasks on 3D data. Our collage representation allows the convolution kernel to slide over all the axial 2D slices in a 3D volume, which is impossible in case of a 3D CNN. The training time of the collage CNN was approximately 5 h (on our basic machine) while the 3D CNN took approximately 7 h to converge. We also augmented the 3D data by using data rotation and flipping before feeding to the 3D CNN, and the performance of the 3D CNN is expected to be better than our collage CNN. But because of the better augmentation capability of the collage representation, it performed better compared to the 3D CNN in our experiment. Thus, the collage representation seems best suited in the insufficient annotated medical data scenario. It is worth noting that in order to improve the classification accuracy by the 3D CNN approach, one may possibly have to increase the convolution kernel size and/or decrease the stride size in order to capture more features from the image volume. However, this would drastically increase the number of trainable weights, which would necessitate the use of expensive GPUs with large memory, and would cost more time to converge.

4   Conclusions

In this paper, we proposed a novel collage image representation within a CNN based classification scheme to enable deep learning from sparsely labelled 3D datasets. We applied our proposed method on CT abdominal scans from the TCIA database to discriminate healthy from cancerous kidneys containing renal cell carcinoma. Our method enables efficient 2D slice-based learning in the absence of slice-based labels. In addition, the proposed collage inherently allows for easy data augmentation through random reshuffling of the locations of image slices within the collage, thus facilitating more efficient training of the implicit relationship between bag labels and feature representation in weekly supervised ML settings. Our approach was shown to be impressively effective (98% classification accuracy) on weakly labeled data on a small sized data base of 160 kidney CTs outperforming 3D CNNs, though the latter's performance could potentially be improved with significant increase in labeled data as well as computation cost. In future work, we plan to couple an automatic kidney localization setup prior to proceed our proposed classification to produce a fully automated end-to-end kidney discrimination clinical tool.

Acknowledgement. This work is supported in part by the Institute for Computing, Information and Cognitive Systems (ICICS) at UBC.

References

1. Cancer Genome Atlas Research Network: Comprehensive molecular characterization of clear cell renal cell carcinoma. Nature **499**(7456), 43–49 (2013)
2. Siegel, R.L., Miller, K.D., Jemal, A.: Cancer statistics. Cancer J. Clin. **65**(1), 5–29 (2015)
3. Ridge, C.A., Pua, B.B., Madoff, D.C.: Epidemiology and staging of renal cell carcinoma. Semin. Interv. Radiol. **31**(01), 003–008 (2014)

4. Escudier, B., Eisen, T., Porta, C., Patard, J.J., Khoo, V., Algaba, F., Mulders, P., Kataja, V., ESMO Guidelines Working Group: ESMO Clinical Practice Guidelines for diagnosis, treatment and follow-up. Ann. Oncol. 23(suppl 7), vii65-vii71 (2012)

5. Criminisi, A., Shotton, J., Robertson, D., Konukoglu, E.: Regression forests for efficient anatomy detection and localization in CT studies. In: Menze, B., Langs, G., Tu, Z., Criminisi, A. (eds.) MCV 2010. LNCS, vol. 6533, pp. 106–117. Springer, Heidelberg (2011). doi:10.1007/978-3-642-18421-5_11

6. Criminisi, A., Robertson, D., Konukoglu, E., Shotton, J., Pathak, S., White, S., Siddiqui, K.: Regression forests for efficient anatomy detection and localization in computed tomography scans. Med. Image Anal. 17(8), 1293–1303 (2013)

7. Cuingnet, R., Prevost, R., Lesage, D., Cohen, L.D., Mory, B., Ardon, R.: Automatic detection and segmentation of kidneys in 3D CT images using random forests. In: Ayache, N., Delingette, H., Golland, P., Mori, K. (eds.) MICCAI 2012. LNCS, vol. 7512, pp. 66–74. Springer, Heidelberg (2012). doi:10.1007/978-3-642-33454-2_9

8. Lu, X., Xu, D., Liu, D.: Robust 3D organ localization with dual learning architectures and fusion. In: Carneiro, G., Mateus, D., Peter, L., Bradley, A., Tavares, J.M.R.S., Belagiannis, V., Papa, J.P., Nascimento, J.C., Loog, M., Lu, Z., Cardoso, J.S., Cornebise, J. (eds.) LABELS/DLMIA -2016. LNCS, vol. 10008, pp. 12–20. Springer, Cham (2016). doi:10.1007/978-3-319-46976-8_2

9. Hussain, M.A., Hamarneh, G., O'Connell, T.W., Mohammed, M.F., Abugharbieh, R.: Segmentation-free estimation of kidney volumes in CT with dual regression forests. In: Wang, L., Adeli, E., Wang, Q., Shi, Y., Suk, H.-I. (eds.) MLMI 2016. LNCS, vol. 10019, pp. 156–163. Springer, Cham (2016). doi:10.1007/978-3-319-47157-0_19

10. Dietterich, T.G., Lathrop, R.H., Lozano-Pérez, T.: Solving the multiple instance problem with axis-parallel rectangles. Artif. Intell. 89(1), 31–71 (1997)

11. Zhu, W., Lou, Q., Vang, Y.S., Xie, X.: Deep Multi-instance Networks with Sparse Label Assignment for Whole Mammogram Classification. arXiv preprint arXiv:1612.05968 (2016)

12. Yan, Z., Zhan, Y., Peng, Z., Liao, S., Shinagawa, Y., Zhang, S., Metaxas, D.N., Zhou, X.S.: Multi-instance deep learning: discover discriminative local anatomies for bodypart recognition. IEEE Trans. Med. Imaging 35(5), 1332–1343 (2016)

13. Xu, Y., Mo, T., Feng, Q., Zhong, P., Lai, M., Eric, I., Chang, C.: Deep learning of feature representation with multiple instance learning for medical image analysis. In: IEEE International Conference on Acoustics, Speech and Signal Processing (ICASSP), pp. 1626–1630 (2014)

14. Kraus, O.Z., Ba, J.L., Frey, B.J.: Classifying and segmenting microscopy images with deep multiple instance learning. Bioinformatics 32(12), i52–i59 (2016)

15. Clark, K., Vendt, B., Smith, K., Freymann, J., Kirby, J., Koppel, P., Moore, S., Phillips, S., Maffitt, D., Pringle, M., Tarbox, L., Prior, F.: The cancer imaging archive (TCIA): maintaining and operating a public information repository. J. Digit. Imaging 26(6), 1045–1057 (2013)

16. Shinagare, A.B., Vikram, R., Jaffe, C., Akin, O., Kirby, J., Huang, E., Freymann, J., Sainani, N.I., Sadow, C.A., Bathala, T.K., Rubin, D.L.: Radiogenomics of clear cell renal cell carcinoma: preliminary findings of the cancer genome atlas–renal cell carcinoma (TCGA-RCC) imaging research group. Abdom. Imaging 40(6), 1684–1692 (2015)

17. Sermanet, P., Eigen, D., Zhang, X., Mathieu, M., Fergus, R., LeCun, Y.: OverFeat: integrated recognition, localization and detection using convolutional networks. In: Proceedings of ICLR (2014)

18. Sun, Y., Wang, X., Tang, X.: Deep learning face representation from predicting 10,000 classes. In: Proceedings of the IEEE Conference on Computer Vision and Pattern Recognition, pp. 1891–1898 (2014)
19. Kingma, D., Ba, J.: Adam: a method for stochastic optimization. In: 3rd International Conference for Learning Representations (2015)
20. Jia, Y., et al.: Caffe: convolutional architecture for fast feature embedding. In: ACM International Conference on Multimedia, pp. 675–678 (2014)

Aggregating Deep Convolutional Features for Melanoma Recognition in Dermoscopy Images

Zhen Yu[1], Xudong Jiang[2], Tianfu Wang[1], and Baiying Lei[1(✉)]

[1] National-Regional Key Technology Engineering Laboratory for Medical Ultrasound, School of Biomedical Engineering, Health Science Center, Shenzhen University, Shenzhen, China
leiby@szu.edu.cn
[2] School of Electric and Electronic Engineering, Nanyang Technological University, Singapore, Singapore

Abstract. **We present a novel framework for automated melanoma recognition in dermoscorpy images, which is a quite challenging task due to the high intra-class and low inter-class variations between melanoma and non-melanoma (benign).** The proposed framework shares merits of deep learning method and local descriptors encoding strategy. Specifically, the deep representations of a dermoscopy image are first extracted using a very deep residual neural network pre-trained on ImageNet. Then these local deep descriptors are aggregated by fisher vector (FV) encoding to build a holistic image representation. Finally, the encoded representations are classified using SVM. In contrast to previous studies with complex preprocessing and feature engineering or directly using existing deep learning architectures with fine-tuning on the skin datasets, our solution is simpler, more compact and capable of producing more discriminative features. Extensive experiments performed on ISBI 2016 Skin lesion challenge dataset corroborate the effectiveness of the proposed method, outperforming state-of-the-art approaches in all evaluation metrics.

Keywords: Dermoscopy image · Melanoma recognition · Residual network · Fisher vector

1 Introduction

Melanoma skin cancer is one of the most rapidly increasing and deadliest cancers in the world, which accounts for 79% of skin cancer deaths [1]. Early diagnosis is of great importance for treating this disease as it can be cured easily at early stages. To improve the diagnosis of this disease, dermoscopy has been introduced to assist dermatologists in clinical examination since it is a non-invasive skin imaging technique that provides clinicians high quality visual perception of skin lesion. Clinically, several heuristic approaches have been developed to enhance clinicians' ability to distinguish melanomas from benign nevi [3]. However, the correct diagnosis of a skin lesion is not trivial even for professionals. Furthermore, dermoscopic diagnosis made by human visual

© Springer International Publishing AG 2017
Q. Wang et al. (Eds.): MLMI 2017, LNCS 10541, pp. 238–246, 2017.
DOI: 10.1007/978-3-319-67389-9_28

inspection is often subjective. Hence, unsatisfactory accuracy and poor reproducibility are still intractable issues for diagnosing this disease.

To tackle these issues, numerous automatic algorithms were proposed for der-moscopic image analysis. Interested readers can refer to [9] for a comprehensive summary of related work over the past decades. Most of the existing studies have mainly focused on feature engineering and classification on images either implicitly or explicitly, assuming a lesion object in well condition. However, dermoscopy images may not always capture entire lesions, or lesion object occupies only a small part of an image, as shown in Fig. 1. Several studies proposed to adopt the bag-of-features (BoF) model (i.e. fisher vector, FV) with local features to handle complex situations [1, 9]. Although feature encoding in BoF model has been widely used in various classification tasks, hand-crafted features based diagnostic performance is still unsatisfactory due to the high intra-class and low inter-class variations between melanoma and non-melanoma.

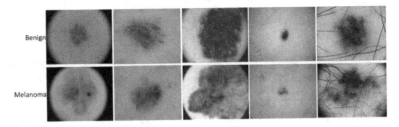

Fig. 1. Example dermoscopy image of skin lesions. There are low inter-class and high intra-class variations between the melanoma and non-melanoma (benign). The diagnosis of melanoma is non-trivial even for experienced clinicians.

Different from approaches that rely on the hand-crafted features, study in [12] demonstrated that transferred convolutional features can be utilized as generic visual representations, and convolutional neural network (CNN) architectures pre-trained on large ImageNet dataset also delivered promising results for other image recognition tasks even without retraining. To the end, transferred CNN features have also been applied in dermoscopy image classification in recent years [3, 4, 8]. By default, deep convolutional features are extracted from fully connected layers of a CNN model. Nevertheless, high-level CNN features are sensitive or vulnerable to geometric variations because they suffer from the paucity of descriptions of local patterns [2, 15]. For images with dramatic variations in viewpoint and scale, it would be a great challenge to perform classification directly using CNN features, not mention that in medical applications, these features are usually trained on limited training data. Several studies [5, 14, 15] were devoted to combining deep features with local descriptors encoding methods to beef up their discrimination capability and robustness. Although impressive improvement is achieved in some benchmarks, these approaches are highly computational intensive due to the adoption of sliding-windows to generate deep descriptors from local regions in original images or multi-scale pyramid pooling strategy to construct FV representations.

Motivated by [2, 17], in this work, we propose a novel, compact, and efficient framework based on very deep CNN and feature encoding strategy (FV encoding) for melanoma recognition in dermoscopy image (see Fig. 2). A very deep residual neural net-work (i.e. 50 layers) [7] pre-trained on ImageNet, is first applied to each input image, and then local deep descriptors are extracted from the dense activation maps of the last convolutional layer. These features are further encoded by FV into more invariant and discriminative representations. In addition, large scale of input images and special per image normalization are utilized to gain additional performance improvement. Experimental results demonstrate the effectiveness of our proposed approach.

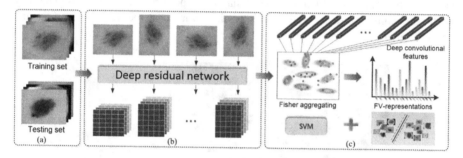

Fig. 2. Flowchart of proposed framework for melanoma recognition. (a) Dataset of dermoscopic lesion images. (b) Data augmentation and feature extraction. Local activations of intermediate layer are extracted as deep feature vectors. (c) FV encoding and classification.

2 Methodology

2.1 Image Preprocessing and Data Augmentation

Image preprocessing affects the performance of deep representations greatly as it takes the image characteristics into consideration. There is a huge variation in resolution of the skin lesion images dataset provided by ISBI 2016 challenge [6]. Resizing and cropping these images directly into required input size of CNN models may introduce object distortion and substantial information loss. Accordingly, in this study, we take relatively large images as inputs. For the skin lesion dataset, we resize each input image along the shortest side to a uniform scale (denoted as S for simplicity) while maintaining the aspect ratio. We also investigate the recognition performance with various values of S.

Typically, before processing by CNN, images are normalized by subtracting the mean pixel value calculated over the entire training dataset (denoted as all-img-mean). As a result, the RGB values are centered at zero. However, the lighting, skin tone and viewpoint of the skin lesion images vary greatly across the dataset, subtracting a uniform mean value does not well normalize individual image. Recent study [8] has illustrated this effect as well. To address this issue, we normalize each skin image by subtracting channel-wise average intensity values calculated over the individual image (denoted as per-img-mean). For the data augmentation, we rotate each resized image by four fixed angles ($0°$, $90°$, $180°$, and $270°$), and then pixel translation (with shift between -10 and 10 pixels) is randomly added over the rotated images. The deep features of these augmented images are aggregated into a single FV representation.

2.2 Extraction of Local Convolutional Features

Given a pre-trained network, an input skin lesion image $\mathcal{X}_i$ is first processed by the above-mentioned augmentation procedure, and thus we obtain four augmented images $\mathbb{X}_i = \{\mathcal{X}_{i1}, \mathcal{X}_{i2}, \mathcal{X}_{i3}, \mathcal{X}_{i4}\}$ for each skin image. These images are passed through the CNN model in a forward pass. In the l-th convolutional layer $\mathcal{L}_l$, we obtain $w_{ia}^l \times h_{ia}^l \times d^l$ spatial feature maps $\mathcal{M}_{ia}^l (a = 1, \ldots, 4)$, where w_{ia}^l and h_{ia}^l denote the width and height, respectively, d^l is the depth or channels of the current feature map. For brevity, we denote $\mathcal{N}_{ia}^l = w_{ia}^l \times h_{ia}^l$. It is worth noting that, for input images with different sizes, the size of the resulting feature maps can be different. Similar to [17], for activations at each location $c = (c_x, c_y)$, $1 \leq c_x \leq w_{ia}^l$ and $1 \leq c_y \leq h_{ia}^l$ in the feature map $\mathcal{M}_{ia}^l$, we obtain d^l-dimensional vector $f_{ia,c}^l \in \mathbb{R}^{d^l}$ which is considered as feature vector (local deep feature) in our study. Therefore, $\mathbb{N}_{ia}^l$ local deep feature vectors are obtained for each augmented image $\mathcal{X}_{ia}$. For i-th original skin lesion image $\mathcal{X}_i$, at convolutional layer $\mathcal{L}_l$ of the network, we obtain a set of deep features:

$$\mathbb{F}_i^l = \left\{ f_{i1,(1,1)}^l, \cdots f_{i4,(w_{i4}^l, h_{i4}^l)}^l \right\} \in \mathbb{R}^{\sum_{a=1}^4 \mathcal{N}_{ia}^l \times d^l}. \tag{1}$$

These features are encoded by FV into single representation for the final classification. In our study, considering the transferability and discrimination of the deep features, the output of last convolutional layer of the ResNet is adopted as local features.

2.3 Fisher Vector Encoding Strategy

Each local deep convolutional feature f_n^l extracted from layer $\mathcal{L}_l$, refers to a small region (receptive field) in the input image, and reflects the local distinction of that region. This is similar to traditional local descriptors. Since each image contains a set of deep features, and thus we propose to aggregate these local deep representations into a holistic representation using FV encoding. The FV encoding derived from fisher kernel is effective for encoding local features and has demonstrated excellent performance in image recognition [11].

To implement FV encoding, the popular Gaussian mixture model (GMM) is adopted to model the probability distribution of deep features. For the purpose of constructing a GMM with K components, a collection of skin images are sampled from the training set. The local deep descriptors of these images are then extracted and utilized to learn the parameters $\lambda = \{\pi_k, \mu_k, \sum_k, k = 1, 2, \ldots, K\}$, which includes the prior probability $\pi_k \in \mathbb{R}_+$ subjected to the constraint $\sum_1^K \pi_k = 1$, mean vector $\mu_k \in \mathbb{R}^{d^l}$, and covariance matrix $\sum_k \in \mathbb{R}^{d^l \times d^l}$ constrained to be diagonal. For a set of local deep features $\{\mathcal{F}_{i1}^l, \mathcal{F}_{i2}^l, \mathcal{F}_{i3}^l, \mathcal{F}_{i4}^l\}$ extracted from the augmented images regarding i-th skin lesion image, the first and second order differences of the GMM clusters are given by:

$$u_k = \frac{1}{N\sqrt{\pi_k}} \sum_{n=1}^{N} \mathcal{q}_{kn} \left(\frac{f_n^l - \mu_k}{\sum_k^{1/2}} \right), \tag{2}$$

$$v_k = \frac{1}{N\sqrt{2\pi_k}} \sum_{n=1}^{N} \mathcal{q}_{kn} \left[\frac{(f_n^l - \mu_k)^2}{\sum_k} - 1 \right], \, k = 1,2...K, \tag{3}$$

where $N = \sum_{a=1}^{4} \mathcal{N}_{ia}^l \times d^l$ represents the number of local deep descriptors of a skin image; $\mathcal{q}_{kn}$ denotes the soft-assignment of a certain feature vector f_n^l to cluster k. By concatenating u_k and v_k for all K components, we obtain the final FV representation Φ_i:

$$\Phi_i = \left[u_1^T, v_1^T, ... u_K^T, v_K^T \right]^T. \tag{4}$$

It is noteworthy that the dimensionality of deep feature vector is reduced by principle component analysis (PCA) before FV encoding because more Gaussian components are needed to capture the distribution of higher dimensional feature. For each FV representation, we further compute the improved FV by applying L2 and power normalization the same as that in [11].

2.4   Kernel-Based Classification

For the classification of the FV representations, we train a SVM classifier with Chi-squared (chi2) kernel. Although linear kernels are efficient for the classification, non-linear kernels tend to yield better performance and empirical studies have demonstrated the superiority of the chi2 kernel for image classification [11]. Prior to learning, the FV representations are further L2 normalized. During SVM training, the stochastic dual coordinate ascent algorithm is employed to minimize the regularized loss due to its efficiency and fast convergence rate.

3   Experimental Setting and Results

We validate our proposed method using ISBI 2016 challenge dataset of dermoscopic lesion images [6]. The dataset released in the challenge contains 1279 dermoscopic lesion images with corresponding class labels pre-partitioned into a training set of 900 images and a testing set of 379 images. There are two lesion categories in the dataset: melanoma and benign (non-melanoma). Approximately 20% of the dataset is melanoma (173 images in training set, 75 images in testing set). We obtain optimal hyper-parameters of SVM classifiers using cross-validation strategy on training data, then give final result on testing data. For performance metrics, we adopt the mean average precision (mAP), accuracy (Acc), area under receive operation curve (AUC), sensitivity (Sen) and specificity (Spec). All experiments are conducted on a 128G RAM computer with CPU Inter Xeon E5-2680 @ 2.70 GHz, GPU NVIDIA Quadro K4000.

We start by investigating the influence of image preprocessing. We carry out the experiment with different rescaled images and perform two normalizations (per-img-mean and all-img-mean). As seen from Fig. 3(a), in the case of adopting the normalization strategy of per-img-mean, the classification performance improves gradually as the scale increases, and remains stable after the scale reaches 448. When the scale is larger than 448, however, no significant improvement is observed, which indicates there is no gain of information with higher computational burden. For normalization with all-img-mean, the classification performance first increases as S increases. It reaches a peak at $S = 384$ followed by a steep fall. This demonstrates the superiority of per-img-mean over all-img-mean in normalizing lesion images with large S. By balancing the memory consumption and efficiency, we fix S as 448 in the following experiments.

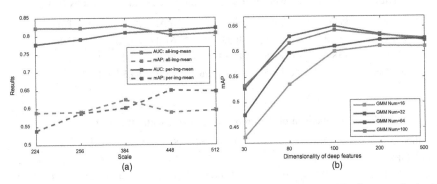

Fig. 3. Evaluation of proposed method on image preprocessing; (b) mAP of our method with varying number of Gaussians and dimensionality of deep features.

We conduct experiment to shed light on how parameters of FV encoding affect the classification performance. Apart from the size of GMM codebook, we also investigate the influence of PCA dimensionality of deep features. The result is illustrated in Fig. 3 (b). It can be observed that increasing the dimension of deep features yields significant improvements in performance of mAP initially. As the dimensionality becomes higher, mAP gradually drops in all GMM components setting, which indicates that the number of current Gaussians and the number of training samples are insufficient to model the distribution of higher dimensional features. In addition, we can see that the performance of larger GMM number setting (i.e. GMM Num = 100) outperforms the other fewer Gaussians in high dimensionality of 500, which suggests that increasing the number of GMM components can improve the performance. However, for larger number of GMM components, more training data is needed to estimate the GMM parameters. Furthermore, increasing Gaussian numbers under the case of high dimensional features leads to very high memory consumption and computational complexity. Hence, it is crucial to examine settings of GMM components and feature dimensionality, given the limited training data and computational platform.

Apart from the proposed ResNet-50, we explore two other CNN models including 8-layers AlexNet [10], and 16-layers VGGNet (VGG-16) [13] for performance comparison. All the models are pre-trained on ImageNet. We keep the same setting in the process of classification whenever possible for fair comparison. Table 1 shows the experimental results. Also, the average running time of each network for processing single lesion image is provided. Finally, in Table 2, we compare our result with the top ranked method in the challenge and method reported in the recent published literature [4, 16], our method is denoted as LDF-FV. For the fusion case, deep features are extracted from middle and last convolutional layers of ResNet-50, respectively. The final scores are given by averaging scores of two different level descriptors based FV representations.

Table 1. Impact of network architectures on the classification results (%).

Network	Parameter	Layer	Sen	Spec	mAP	Acc	AUC	Time
AlexNet	61 M	Conv5	40.00	95.72	61.37	84.70	82.08	0.94 s
VGG-16	138 M	Conv5_3	45.33	94.08	57.66	84.43	81.18	2.72 s
ResNet-50	25.6 M	Conv5_9	**45.33**	**96.71**	**65.08**	**86.54**	**81.49**	1.33 s

Table 2. Comparison of the proposed approach with other methods (%).

Method	Network	Dimension	Sen	Spec	mAP	Acc	AUC
DSIFT-FV	Na	12800	33.33	95.39	55.63	83.11	78.01
CNN-SVM [6]	ResNet-50	2048	40.00	95.39	58.42	84.43	81.82
CNNaug-SVM [12]	ResNet-50	2048	41.33	94.41	59.93	83.19	81.73
Fine-tuned CNN [12]	ResNet-50	Na	48.00	94.08	63.36	84.96	81.58
CUMED [7]	FCRN (DRN)-50	Na	50.70	94.10	63.70	85.50	80.40
Codella [6]	Ensemble models	Na	**69.30**	83.20	64.50	80.50	83.80
LDF-FV (ours)	ResNet-50	12800	45.33	96.71	65.08	86.54	81.49
LDF-FV (fusion)	ResNet-50	12800	42.67	**97.70**	**68.49**	**86.81**	**85.20**

4   Conclusion

In this paper, we propose a novel framework for dermoscopy image classification. It utilizes the state-of-the-art local descriptors encoding method (FV) to encode local convolutional features extracted from very deep residual network into holistic representations, which is more discriminative than hand-crafted descriptors and CNN features. Systematical and extensive experiments are performed to investigate a range of key elements that could affect the performance of our method. Experiments on the publicly available ISBI 2016 challenge skin lesion dataset show the promising results. Also, we compare the proposed framework with a number of existing well-established classification methods to further validate its superiority. Our future work will focus on studying the performance of our method on other applications and networks pre-trained on different datasets.

Acknowledgment. This work was supported partly by National Natural Science Foundation of China (Nos. 81571758, 61571304, 61402296, 61571304 and 61427806), National Key Research and Develop Program (No. 2016YFC0104703), Shenzhen Peacock Plan (NO. KQTD2016 053112051497), and the National Natural Science Foundation of Shenzhen University (No. 827000197).

References

1. Abder-Rahman, A.A., Deserno, T.M.: A systematic review of automated melanoma detection in dermatoscopic images and its ground truth data. In: Proceedings of SPIE Medical Imaging (2012)
2. Cimpoi, M., Maji, S., Vedaldi, A.: Deep filter banks for texture recognition and segmentation. In: CVPR (2015)
3. Codella, N., Cai, J., Abedini, M., Garnavi, R., Halpern, A., Smith, J.R.: Deep learning, sparse coding, and SVM for melanoma recognition in dermoscopy images. In: Zhou, L., Wang, L., Wang, Q., Shi, Y. (eds.) MLMI 2015. LNCS, vol. 9352, pp. 118–126. Springer, Cham (2015). doi:10.1007/978-3-319-24888-2_15
4. Codella, N., Nguyen, Q.-B., Pankanti, S., Gutman, D., Helba, B., Halpern, A., Smith, J.R.: Deep learning ensembles for melanoma recognition in dermoscopy images. arXiv preprint arXiv:1610.04662 (2016)
5. Gòng, Y., Wang, L., Guo, R., Lazebnik, S.: Multi-scale orderless pooling of deep convolutional activation features. In: Fleet, D., Pajdla, T., Schiele, B., Tuytelaars, T. (eds.) ECCV 2014. LNCS, vol. 8695, pp. 392–407. Springer, Cham (2014). doi:10.1007/978-3-319-10584-0_26
6. Gutman, D., Codella, N.C., Celebi, E., Helba, B., Marchetti, M., Mishra, N., Halpern, A.: Skin lesion analysis toward melanoma detection: a challenge at the International Symposium on Biomedical Imaging (ISBI) 2016, hosted by the International Skin Imaging Collaboration (ISIC). arXiv preprint arXiv:1605.01397 (2016)
7. He, K., Zhang, X., Ren, S., Sun, J.: Deep residual learning for image recognition. In: CVPR (2016)
8. Kawahara, J., Bentaieb, A., Hamarneh, G.: Deep features to classify skin lesions. In: ISBI (2016)
9. Konstantin, K., Rafael, G.: Computerized analysis of pigmented skin lesions: a review. Artif. Intell. Med. 2(56), 69–90 (2012)
10. Krizhevsky, A., Sutskever, I., Hinton, G.E.: Imagenet classification with deep convolutional neural networks. In: NIPS (2012)
11. Sánchez, J., Perronnin, F., Mensink, T., Verbeek, J.: Image classification with the Fisher vector: theory and practice. Int. J. Comput. Vision 3(105), 222–245 (2013)
12. Sharif, R.A., Azizpour, H., Sullivan, J., Carlsson, S.: CNN features off-the-shelf: an astounding baseline for recognition. In: CVPR Workshop (2014)
13. Simonyan, K., Zisserman, A.: Very deep convolutional networks for large-scale image recognition. arXiv preprint arXiv:1409.1556 (2014)

14. Uricchio, T., Bertini, M., Seidenari, L., Bimbo, A.D.: Fisher encoded convolutional bag-of-windows for efficient image retrieval and social image tagging. In: ICCV Workshop (2015)
15. Yoo, D., Park, S., Lee, J.-Y., So Kweon, I.: Multi-scale pyramid pooling for deep convolutional representation. In: CVPR Workshop (2015)
16. Yu, L., Chen, H., Dou, Q., Qin, J., Heng, P.A.: Automated melanoma recognition in dermoscopy images via very deep residual networks. IEEE Trans. Med. Imag. 4(36), 994–1004 (2017)
17. Yue-Hei Ng, J., Yang, F., Davis, L.S.: Exploiting local features from deep networks for image retrieval. In: CVPR Workshop (2015)

Localizing Cardiac Structures in Fetal Heart Ultrasound Video

Christopher P. Bridge[1](✉), Christos Ioannou[2], and J. Alison Noble[1]

[1] Institute of Biomedical Engineering, University of Oxford, Oxford, UK
christopher.bridge@eng.ac.uk
[2] Fetal Medicine Unit, John Radcliffe Hospital, Oxford, UK

Abstract. Recently, a particle-filtering based framework was proposed to extract 'global' information from 2D ultrasound screening videos of the fetal heart, including the heart's visibility, position, orientation, view classification and cardiac phase. In this paper, we consider how to augment that framework to describe the positions and visibility of important cardiac structures, including several valves and vessels, that are key to clinical diagnoses of congenital heart conditions in the developing heart. We propose a partitioned particle filtering architecture to address the problem of the high dimensionality of the resulting state space. The state space is partitioned into several sequential stages, which enables efficient use of a small number of particles. We present experimental results for tracking structures across several view planes in a real world clinical video dataset, and compare to expert annotations.

1 Introduction

Prenatal screening for congenital heart disease (CHD) is typically performed using a two-dimensional (2D) ultrasound examination in the second trimester to check for various structural and functional anomalies. However, because this is specialist work requiring detailed knowledge of fetal cardiac anatomy, detection rates are highly dependent on the sonographer's experience [6].

In this work, we develop automated methods to localize key anatomical structures in freehand video footage gathered from a screening session. This could be used, for instance, to feed back live information to a sonographer performing the scan, used to develop training tools, or used as the basis of further automated processes for diagnosis and quantification of CHD.

A few recent works have looked at automatically extracting information from fetal screening ultrasound video streams [1–3]. Chen et al. [3] used a combination of a convolutional neural network (CNN) and a temporal recurrent neural network to detect standard planes from fetal scans. Baumgartner et al. [1] also used a CNN to detect various views of the fetus and coarsely localize a variety of structures with a bounding box. In previous work focused on the fetal heart [2],

---

Electronic supplementary material The online version of this chapter (doi:10.1007/978-3-319-67389-9_29) contains supplementary material, which is available to authorized users.

Q. Wang et al. (Eds.): MLMI 2017, LNCS 10541, pp. 247–255, 2017.
DOI: 10.1007/978-3-319-67389-9_29

Table 1. Structures of interest

Four Chamber View (4C)	Left Ventricular Outflow Tract view (LVOT)	Three Vessels View (3V)
4C	LVOT	3V
1. Apex. 2. Mitral Valve End. 3. Mitral Valve Center. 4. Crux Cordis. 5. Tricuspid Valve Center. 6. Tricuspid Valve End. 7. Base. 8. Descending Aorta (Center). 9. Spine.	1. Apex. 2. Aortic Valve. 3. Mitral Valve End. 4. Descending Aorta (Center). 5. Spine.	1. Pulmonary Valve. 2. Ascending Aorta (Center). 3. Superior Vena Cava (Center). 4. Descending Aorta (Center). 5. Spine. 6. Trachea (Center).

we used a particle filtering approach in order to capture the temporal structure of the footage when estimating key variables in a robust, probabilistic manner. In this paper, we build on the method presented in [2] and extend the particle filtering framework to track a number of important cardiac structures.

Though the approach is general, to place the current work in context we focus on the same three views of the heart as [2]: the *four chamber* view (4C) showing the two atria and two ventricles, the *left ventricular outflow tract* view (LVOT), showing the aorta leaving the left ventricle, and the *three vessels* view (3V) showing the pulmonary artery, aorta and superior vena cava. Within these views, we have selected a number of anatomical structures of interest (Table 1).

2   Partitioned Particle Filters

We first review the framework of [2] and then describe how we have extended it. The particle filtering architecture in [2] tracks a *state* that captures 'global' characteristics of the heart at each frame t, specifically the heart's visibility $h_t \in \{0, 1\}$, image location of the heart center $\mathbf{x}_t \in \mathbb{R}^2$, heart orientation $\theta_t \in [0, 2\pi)$, viewing plane classification $v_t \in \{4C, LVOT, 3V\}$, a circular variable $\phi_t \in [0, 2\pi)$ tracking the progress of the cardiac cycle, and $\dot{\phi}_t$ the rate of change of this cardiac phase variable with respect to t.

This set of variables of heterogeneous types is grouped into the *state tuple*, s_t. It is also assumed that the scale of the heart, represented by the radius r, is known approximately at test time.

The *filtering distribution*, $p\left(s_t \mid z_{0:t}\right)$, over these variables at each frame, conditioned on image evidence z_t, is represented by a finite number, N, of particles, $s_t^{(i)}$, $i = 0, 1, \ldots, N-1$ with corresponding weights $w_t^{(i)}$. At each time step, a new state value for each particle is sampled from a *prediction potential* $\psi(s_t \mid s_{t-1})$, which is a distribution over the state value at time $t + 1$ given the state at time t. Then each sample is reweighted according to an *observation potential* $\omega(s_t, z_t)$ that reflects the compatibility of the state hypothesis represented by the particle with the observed image, and can be any non-negative function of its arguments. The observation potentials are learned using the random forests algorithm to perform classification and regression based on rotation-invariant features (RIFs) calculated from the image [4].

To extend [2] to structure tracking we extend the state tuple to contain variables relating to the locations of specific structures of interest. As a result, the localization procedure for the structures is able to use and influence the predictions of the global variables. However, this results in a very high dimensional state space. Particle filters typically do not perform well in such high dimensional spaces because a very large number of particles is needed to adequately cover the space and maintain a good approximation to the true filtering distribution [5].

This problem can be overcome by grouping the state variables into *partitions*, which can then be operated on in sequence [5]. We refer to MacCormick and Isard [5] for a rigorous explanation, but intuitively a state vector/tuple can be partitioned if both the following conditions apply:

1. The prediction potential for the variables in a given partition is (or may be assumed to be) independent of variables in *later* partitions (but may be conditioned on values for variables in *earlier* partitions). This means that the prediction step may take place for each partition before the updated values for variables in later partitions are known.
2. The observation potential for the variables in a given partition is (or may be assumed to be) independent of the variables in *later* partitions (but may consider the variables in *earlier* partitions). Therefore the particles may be reweighted and resampled according to each observation potential in turn.

The key insight into the advantage of the partitioned particle filter is that by operating on the partitions in sequence, the particles are guided into the peaks in the filtering distribution of each partition in turn. Consequently, a partitioned particle filter may make more efficient use of a small number of particles and operate in high dimensional spaces with a reasonable number of particles.

Although the two criteria are quite restrictive, the particle filter in [2] may be naturally broken into three partitions: one containing the visibility h_t, location x_t, and view v_t; a second partition containing the cardiac phase ϕ_t and phase rate $\dot{\phi}_t$; and a third containing the orientation θ_t. The independence assumptions made in [2] mean that the two criteria are satisfied with no alterations to the

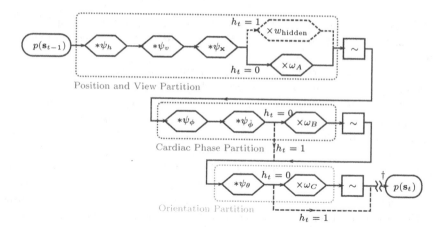

Fig. 1. Partitioned reformulation of filter architecture for tracking 'global' heart variables. The form of this diagram follows the convention used by [5] and shows the sequence of operations performed on the particle set within a single timestep. The round edged boxes represent distributions in the form of particle sets. The hexagonal boxes represent operations on each particle in the particle set: the '∗' represents convolving the particle set with the prediction potential and the '×' represents multiplying the particle weights by the observation potential. The square box containing the '∼' represents the resampling operation across the entire particle set. The black dotted lines indicate routes taken only by 'hidden' particles (those with $h = 1$) and the colored dotted boxes contain the operations within a single partition (one color per partition). The break at the † symbol marks the location where extra stages are added for structure tracking in Sect. 4. (Color figure online)

observations or prediction potentials. The classification forests are independent of the cardiac phase variable by virtue of their training on a dataset containing heart examples from across the cycle. Furthermore both the classification forests and phase regression forests are orientation invariant as a result of using RIFs.

The filter presented in [2] may therefore be reformulated into three partitions to give the filtering architecture in Fig. 1. We introduce the shorthand subscript notation $\psi_h(\cdot)$, $\psi_v(\cdot)$, $\psi_{\mathbf{x}}(\cdot)$, $\psi_\theta(\cdot)$, $\psi_\phi(\cdot)$, $\psi_{\dot\phi}(\cdot)$ for the prediction potentials relating to the six variables, which are as defined in [2]. The observation potentials $\omega_A(\cdot)$, $\omega_B(\cdot)$, and $\omega_C(\cdot)$ are identical to $\psi_a(\cdot)$, $\psi_b(\cdot)$, and $\psi_c(\cdot)$ respectively from [2], and are based on random forests using RIFs. In Sect. 4, we will extend this architecture to use an additional partition for each structure of interest.

3   A Fourier Model for Structure Trajectories

Due to the nature of the cardiac cycle, over a short time interval the positions of the structures are likely to be close to periodic. Furthermore, an estimate of the cardiac phase variable, ϕ_t is available from the output of the global variable prediction. Rather than estimate a structure's position over the cardiac cycle in each frame independently, a Fourier model is used to capture this behavior.

In this model, the position of structure $a \in \mathbb{N}_0$ (where a is an index variable indexing the various structures (Table 1)) in the image at time t is described by the 2D column vector $\mathbf{q}_{a,t} \in \mathbb{R}^2$ containing the x and y components, i.e. $\mathbf{q}_{a,t} = [q_{a,t,1}, q_{a,t,2}]^T$, where $q_{a,t,1} \in \mathbb{R}$ is the x-component and $q_{a,t,2} \in \mathbb{R}$ is the y-component. Firstly, this is expressed relative to the heart center position, $\mathbf{x}_t$, orientation, θ_t, and scale, r, to give the *relative position vector* $\mathbf{p}_{a,t} \in \mathbb{R}^2$, where the two are related by:

$$\mathbf{q}_{a,t} = r\mathbf{R}_{[\theta_t]}\mathbf{p}_{a,t} + \mathbf{x}_t \tag{1}$$

where $\mathbf{R}_{[\theta_t]} \in \mathbb{R}^{2 \times 2}$ is the 2D rotation matrix through angle θ_t.

The relative position vector $\mathbf{p}_{a,t}$ is calculated from the current value of the cardiac phase variable, ϕ_t, by assuming a truncated Fourier series approximation:

$$\mathbf{p}_{a,t} = \begin{bmatrix} c_{a,1,1} & c_{a,2,1} \\ c_{a,1,2} & c_{a,2,2} \\ c_{a,1,3} & c_{a,2,3} \\ c_{a,1,4} & c_{a,2,4} \\ c_{a,1,5} & c_{a,2,5} \\ \vdots & \vdots \end{bmatrix}^T \cdot \begin{bmatrix} 1 \\ \cos \phi_t \\ \sin \phi_t \\ \cos 2\phi_t \\ \sin 2\phi_t \\ \vdots \end{bmatrix} \tag{2}$$

$$= \begin{bmatrix} \mathbf{c}_{a,1} & \mathbf{c}_{a,2} \end{bmatrix}^T \cdot \boldsymbol{\phi}_t \tag{3}$$

Given a short sequence of frames (covering a few cardiac cycles), the coefficients in the column vectors $\mathbf{c}_{a,1}$ and $\mathbf{c}_{a,2}$ may be found using a simple regularized least squares approach, where a prior variance λ is placed on the values of the coefficients with the exception of the zero order coefficients ($c_{a,1,1}$, and $c_{a,2,1}$), which together encode the mean position of structure over the whole cycle.

4   A Filtering Architecture for Structure Localization

We now show how the partitioned architecture in Fig. 1 can be extended to track structures. The basic idea is to include one new partition in the particle filter for each structure, with the partitions for the structures belonging to each of the three views grouped into one 'path' through the filter. This is shown in Fig. 2.

Each partition is identified by the index, a, of the corresponding structure. The Fourier model from Sect. 3 is used and the structure's position is assumed to be fixed given the coefficient vectors $\mathbf{c}_{a,1,t}$ and $\mathbf{c}_{a,2,t}$. However, these coefficient vectors are allowed to vary gradually over time. For notational convenience, the vectors are combined into a single coefficient vector $\tilde{\mathbf{c}}_{a,t} \in \mathbb{R}^{d_a}$. Additionally, there is a binary visibility variable $g_{a,t}$ for the structure that indicates whether the structure is visible or hidden due to the being obscured by an imaging artifact or being located off the edge of the image. The $g_{a,t}$ and $\tilde{\mathbf{c}}_{a,t}$ variables for each structure are incorporated into the state tuple s_t. We now define the prediction and observation potentials in Fig. 2.

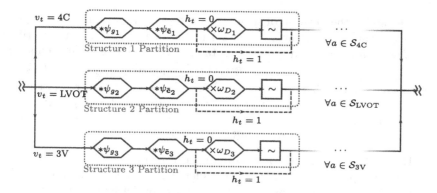

Fig. 2. Filter architecture extension for tracking structures. This is added to the architecture in Fig. 1 by inserting it at the dagger '†' symbol. The three paths through the filter relate to the three views (4C, LVOT, and 3V) of the heart. Structures with indices 1, 2 and 3 are shown as belonging to the three different views, but this is just an illustrative example and may not be the case in practice. $\mathcal{S}_{4C}$, $\mathcal{S}_{LVOT}$, and $\mathcal{S}_{3V}$ are the sets of structure indices in the three views (Table 1).

4.1 Structure Visibility Prediction Potential, $\psi_{g_a}(s_t \mid s_{t-1})$

The visibility prediction potential for each structure's visibility variable operates in exactly the same way as that for the heart visibility in [2]. There is a fixed probability $p_{h \to v}$ of moving from hidden to visible and vice versa $p_{v \to h}$. These are chosen to give a certain fraction of hidden particles at equilibrium.

4.2 Structure Position Prediction Potential, $\psi_{\tilde{c}_a}(s_t \mid s_{t-1})$

At training time, a mean vector $\tilde{\mu}_a \in \mathbb{R}^{d_a}$ and covariance matrix $\tilde{\Sigma}_a \in \mathbb{R}^{d_a \times d_a}$ is calculated for the coefficient vector $\tilde{c}_{a,t}$, assuming a multivariate Gaussian distribution. The prediction potential is assumed to be a linear transition followed by additive Gaussian noise on the centered coefficient vector to allow the coefficients to vary smoothly during the video, i.e. of the form

$$(\tilde{c}_{a,t+1} - \tilde{\mu}_a) = \mathbf{A}(\tilde{c}_{a,t} - \tilde{\mu}_a) + \mathbf{G}n_t \tag{4}$$

In order to ensure that the limiting distribution of the resulting Markov chain is the same as the prior distribution, the update matrix is set $\mathbf{A} = \alpha \mathbf{I}$ where $\alpha \in [0,1]$, the covariance of the noise vector n_t is set to be $\mathbf{Q} = \tilde{\Sigma}_a$, and the noise scaling is set to be $\mathbf{G} = \gamma \mathbf{I}$, where $\gamma \in [0,1]$ and $1 = \alpha^2 + \gamma^2$.

4.3 Observation Potential, $\omega_{D_a}(s_t, z_t)$

The observation potential finds a score for the likelihood of structure a appearing at location $q_{a,t}$ in the image. This uses a random forest classifier trained on the chosen structures and a background class, using the same rotation invariant features as the view classification forest, and the observation potential for a given structure is the posterior probability classification score for that structure at the relevant location. Hidden particles are given a small fixed score Ω_{hidden}.

5   Experiments and Results

We validated the proposed approach on the clinical dataset of fetal heart scanning videos used in [2], containing 91 videos from 12 subjects. We followed a similar leave-one-subject-out cross-validation in which all learned parameters are trained over 11 subjects, and the model is evaluated on the 12th subject. We used the manual annotations of the 'global' variables of interest from [2], and extended these to include structure locations. Pre-trained models from [2] were used for the observation and prediction potentials for the 'global' variables.

The additional models to train for each cross-validation fold included the μ_a and Σ_a parameters for each structure and the structure forest, $\omega_{D_a}(\cdot)$. The μ_a and Σ_a parameters were fitted to sequences of one cardiac cycle in length cut from the videos. All possible such sequences in the training set were used. The structure forests ($\omega_{D_a}(\cdot)$) were trained using 5000 patches containing each structure, and an equivalent number of randomly-selected background patches. The image features shared by all forest models form an RIF feature set with $J = 4$ radial profiles, maximum rotation order $K = 2$, and Fourier expansion order $M = 2$ (see [4] for more details). Only features from the central two radial profiles were used in the structures model, so that the effective patch size of the structures detection forest is half the heart radius, $r/2$.

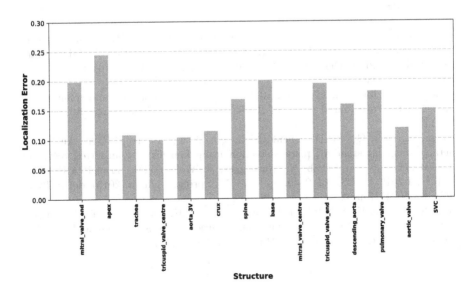

Fig. 3. Mean distance errors between estimated location and ground truth locations for each structure over all videos. The distance is normalized by the heart radius r.

For testing, we used the following parameter values: $p_{h \to v} = 0.35$, $p_{v \to h} = 0.15$ (giving an equilibrium with 0.3 of the total number of particles hidden), $\Omega_{\text{hidden}} = 0.05$, $\gamma = 0.3$, $\lambda = 1$. All random forest classification, phase regression, and structure localization models used 16 trees with a maximum depth of 10. The order of the Fourier models (Sect. 3) was set to 3.

Figure 3 shows the localization error for the structures when point estimates of position are found from the particle set via mean-shift. Those structures whose location is clearly defined by image features (such as the valve centers and vessels) are generally well localized, whereas the most poorly localized structures are those whose location in the image is ambiguous (e.g. the ends of the valves, the base and the apex). We observed that errors in the heart orientation significantly increased the average localization error. The average computation time per frame was 39.5 ms (25 frames per second) on a desktop PC (Intel i7-3770 3.40 GHz, 8 threads, 32 GB RAM), suggesting that this approach is well-suited for real-time applications[1]. Examples can be found in the supplementary video.

6   Conclusions

In this paper we have presented a fast method for fully automated tracking of anatomical structures in ultrasound videos of the fetal heart and presented results on a clinical dataset. Future work will include understanding behavior in the presence of heart abnormalities and the application of this work in support of sonographers in scanning and automated diagnosis.

References

1. Baumgartner, C.F., Kamnitsas, K., Matthew, J., Fletcher, T.P., Smith, S., Koch, L.M., Kainz, B., Rueckert, D.: Real-time detection and localisation of fetal standard scan planes in 2D freehand ultrasound. arXiv abs/1612.05601 (2016). http://arxiv.org/abs/1612.05601
2. Bridge, C.P., Ioannou, C., Noble, J.A.: Automated annotation and quantitative description of ultrasound videos of the fetal heart. Med. Image Anal. **36**, 147–161 (2017)
3. Chen, H., Dou, Q., Ni, D., Cheng, J.-Z., Qin, J., Li, S., Heng, P.-A.: Automatic fetal ultrasound standard plane detection using knowledge transferred recurrent neural networks. In: Navab, N., Hornegger, J., Wells, W.M., Frangi, A.F. (eds.) MICCAI 2015. LNCS, vol. 9349, pp. 507–514. Springer, Cham (2015). doi:10.1007/978-3-319-24553-9_62
4. Liu, K., Skibbe, H., Schmidt, T., Blein, T., Palme, K., Brox, T., Ronneberger, O.: Rotation-invariant HOG descriptors using fourier analysis in polar and spherical coordinates. Int. J. Comput. Vis. **106**(3), 342–364 (2014)

---

[1] Our C++ implementation is available at https://github.com/CPBridge/fetal_heart_analysis.

5. MacCormick, J., Isard, M.: Partitioned sampling, articulated objects, and interface-quality hand tracking. In: Vernon, D. (ed.) ECCV 2000. LNCS, vol. 1843, pp. 3–19. Springer, Heidelberg (2000). doi:10.1007/3-540-45053-X_1
6. Pézard, P., et al.: Influence of ultrasonographers' training on prenatal diagnosis of congenital heart diseases: a 12-year population-based study. Prenat. Diagn. **28**(11), 1016–1022 (2008)

Deformable Registration Through Learning of Context-Specific Metric Aggregation

Enzo Ferrante[1,2(✉)], Puneet K. Dokania[1,4], Rafael Marini[1,3], and Nikos Paragios[1,3]

[1] Center for Visual Computing, CentraleSupelec, INRIA,
Universite Paris-Saclay, Paris, France
[2] Biomedical Image Analysis (BioMedIA) Group,
Imperial College London, London, UK
ferrante.enzo@gmail.com
[3] TheraPanacea, Paris, France
[4] University of Oxford, Oxford, UK

Abstract. We propose a novel weakly supervised discriminative algorithm for learning context specific registration metrics as a linear combination of conventional similarity measures. Conventional metrics have been extensively used over the past two decades and therefore both their strengths and limitations are known. The challenge is to find the optimal relative weighting (or parameters) of different metrics forming the similarity measure of the registration algorithm. Hand-tuning these parameters would result in sub optimal solutions and quickly become infeasible as the number of metrics increases. Furthermore, such hand-crafted combination can only happen at global scale (entire volume) and therefore will not be able to account for the different tissue properties. We propose a learning algorithm for estimating these parameters locally, conditioned to the data semantic classes. The objective function of our formulation is a special case of non-convex function, difference of convex function, which we optimize using the concave convex procedure. As a proof of concept, we show the impact of our approach on three challenging datasets for different anatomical structures and modalities.

1 Introduction

Deformable image registration is a highly challenging problem frequently encountered in medical image analysis. It involves the definition of a similarity criterion (data term) that, once endowed with a deformation model and a smoothness constraint, determines the optimal transformation to align two given images. We adopt a popular graphical model framework [5] to cast deformable registration as a discrete inference problem. The definition of the data term is among the

---

E. Ferrante and P.K. Dokania—Equal contribution.

Electronic supplementary material The online version of this chapter (doi:10. 1007/978-3-319-67389-9_30) contains supplementary material, which is available to authorized users.

most critical components of the registration process. It refers to a function that measures the (dis)similarity between images such as mutual information (MI) or sum of absolute differences (SAD). Metric learning in the context of image registration [2,8,9,11,18] is an alternative that aims to determine the most efficient means of image comparison (similarity measure) from labeled visual correspondences. Our approach can be considered as a specific case of metric learning where the idea is to efficiently combine the well studied mono/multi-modal metrics depending on the local context. We aim to learn the relative weighting from a given training dataset using a learning framework conditioned on prior semantic knowledge. We propose a novel *weakly supervised* discriminative learning framework, based structured support vector machines (SSVM) [13,15] and its extension to latent models LSSVM [16], to learn the relative weights of context specific metric aggregations.

Metric Learning. Various metric learning methods have been proposed in the context of image registration. Lee et al. [8] introduced a multi-modal registration algorithm where the similarity measure is learned such that the target and the correctly deformed source image receive high similarity scores. The training data consisted of pre-aligned images and the learning is performed at the patch level with an assumption that the similarity measure decompose over the patches. [2,9] proposed the use of sensitive hashing to learn a multi-modal metric. Similar to [8], they adopted a patch-wise approach. The dataset consisted of pairs of perfectly aligned images and a collection of positive/negative pairs of patches. Another patch-based alternative was presented by [14] where the training set consisted of non-aligned images with manually annotated patch pairs (landmarks). More recently, approaches based on convolutional neural networks started to gain popularity. Zagoruyko et al. [18] discussed CNN architectures to learn patch based similarity measures. One of them was then adopted in [11] to perform image registration. These methods require ground truth data in the form of correspondences (patches, landmarks or dense deformation fields), which is extremely difficult to obtain in real clinical data. Instead, our method is only based on segmentation masks.

Metric Aggregation. In contrast to the above approaches, our method aggregates standard metrics using contextual information. [3] showed, in fact, that using a multichannel registration method where a set of features is globally considered instead of a single similarity measure, produced robust registration compared to using individual features. However, they did not discuss how these features can be weighted. Following this, [4] proposed to estimate different deformation fields from each feature independently, and then compose them into final diffeomorphic transformation. Such strategy produces multiple deformation models (equal to number of metrics) which might be locally inconsistent. Thus, their combination may not be anatomically meaningful. Our method is most similar to Tang et al. [12], which generates a vector weight map that determines, at each spatial location, the relative importance of each constituent of the overall metric. However, the proposed learning strategy still requires ground truth data in the form of correspondences (pre-registered images) which is not necessary in our case.

Contribution. We tackle the scenario where the ground truth deformations are not known a priori. We consider these deformation fields as latent variables, and devise an algorithm within the LSSVM framework [16]. We model the latent variable imputation problem as the deformable registration problem with additional constraints. In the end, we incorporate the learned aggregated metrics in a context-specific registration framework, where different weights are used depending on the structures being registered.

2   The Deformable Registration Problem

Let us assume a source three dimensional ($3D$) image I, a source $3D$ segmentation mask S^I and a target $3D$ image J. The segmentation mask is formed by labels $s_k \in \mathcal{C}$, where $\mathcal{C}$ is the set of classes. We focus on the 3D to 3D deformable registration problem. Let us also adopt without loss of generality a graphical model [5] for the deformable registration problem. A deformation field is sparsely represented by a regular grid graph $G = (V, E)$, where V is the set of nodes and E is the set of edges. Each node $i \in V$ corresponds to a control point p_i. Each control point p_i is allowed to move in the $3D$ space, therefore, can be assigned a label $\boldsymbol{d_i}$ from the set of $3D$ displacement vectors $\mathcal{L}$. Notice that each $3D$ displacement vector is a tuple defined as $\boldsymbol{d_i} = \{dx_i, dy_i, dz_i\}$, where dx, dy, and dz are the displacements in the x, y, and z directions, respectively. The deformation (labeling of the graph G) denoted as $D \in \mathcal{L}^{|V|}$ is associated to a set of nodes V, where each node is assigned a displacement vector $\boldsymbol{d_i}$ from the set $\mathcal{L}$. The new control point obtained when the displacement $\boldsymbol{d_i}$ is applied to the original control point p_i is denoted as $\bar{p}_i$. Let us define a patch $\bar{\Omega}_i^I$ on the source image I centered at the displaced control point $\bar{p}_i$. Similarly, we define Ω_i^J as the patch on the target image J centered at the original control point p_i, and $\bar{\Omega}_i^{S^I}$ as the patch on the input segmentation mask centered at the displaced control point $\bar{p}_i$. Using the above notations, we define the unary feature vector corresponding to the ith node for a given displacement vector $\boldsymbol{d_i}$ as $\mathcal{U}_i(\boldsymbol{d_i}, I, J) = (u_1(\bar{\Omega}_i^I, \Omega_i^J), \cdots, u_n(\bar{\Omega}_i^I, \Omega_i^J)) \in \mathbb{R}^n$, where n is the number of metrics (or similarity measures) and $u_j(\bar{\Omega}_i^I, \Omega_i^J)$ is the unary feature corresponding to the jth metric on the patches $\bar{\Omega}_i^I$ and Ω_i^J. In case of single metric, we define $n = 1$. Therefore, given a weight matrix $W \in \mathbb{R}^{n \times |\mathcal{C}|}$, where $W(i, j)$ denote the weight of the ith metric corresponding to the class j, the unary potential of the ith node for a given displacement vector $\boldsymbol{d_i}$ is computed as:

$$\bar{\mathcal{U}}_i(\boldsymbol{d_i}, I, J, S^I; W) = \mathbf{w}(\bar{c})^\top \mathcal{U}_i(\boldsymbol{d_i}, I, J) \in \mathbb{R}. \tag{1}$$

where, $\mathbf{w}(\bar{c}) \in \mathbb{R}^n$ is the $\bar{c}^{th}$ column of the weight matrix W and $\bar{c}$ is the most dominant class in the patch on the source segmentation mask $\bar{\Omega}_i^{S^I}$ obtained as $\bar{c} = \text{argmax}_{c \in \mathcal{C}} f(\bar{\Omega}_i^{S^I}, c)$, with $f(\bar{\Omega}_i^{S^I}, c)$ being the number of voxels of class c in the patch $\bar{\Omega}_i^{S^I}$. Other criterion could be used to find the dominant class.

The pairwise clique potential between the control points p_i and p_j is defined as $\mathcal{V}(d_i, d_j)$, where $\mathcal{V}(.,.)$ is the L_1 norm between the two input arguments. Thus, the multi-class energy function is:

$$\mathcal{E}(I, J, S^I, D; W) = \sum_{i \in V} \bar{\mathcal{U}}_i(d_i, I, J, S^I; W) + \sum_{(i,j) \in E} \mathcal{V}(d_i, d_j) \qquad (2)$$

Then, the optimal deformation is obtained as $\hat{D} = \text{argmin}_{D \in \mathcal{L}^{|V|}}$ $\mathcal{E}(I, J, S^I, D; W)$. This problem is NP-HARD in general. Similar to [5], we adopt a pyramidal approach to solve the problem efficiently. We use FastPD [7] for the inference at every level of the pyramid. Notice that the energy function (2) is defined over the nodes of the sparse graph G. Once we obtain the optimal deformation $\hat{D}$, we estimate the dense deformation field using a free form deformation (FFD) model [10] in order to warp the input image.

3   Learning the Parameters

Knowing the weight matrix W a priori is non-trivial and hand tuning it quickly becomes infeasible as the number of metrics and classes increases. We propose an algorithm to learn W conditioned on the semantic labels assuming that in the training phase semantic masks are available for the source and the target images. Instead of learning the complete weight matrix at once, we learn the weights (or parameters) for each class $c \in \mathcal{C}$ individually. Now onwards, the weight vector $\mathbf{w}_c$ denotes a particular column of the weight matrix W, representing the weights corresponding to the cth class.

Training Data. Consider a dataset $\mathcal{D} = \{(\mathbf{x}_i, \mathbf{y}_i)\}_{i=1,\cdots,N}$, where $\mathbf{x}_i = (I_i, J_i)$, I_i is the source image and J_i is the target. Similarly, $\mathbf{y}_i = (S_i^I, S_i^J)$, where S_i^I and S_i^J are the segmentation masks for the source and target images. The size of each segmentation mask is the same as that of the corresponding images. As stated earlier, the segmentation mask is formed by the elements (or voxels) $s_k \in \mathcal{C}$, where $\mathcal{C}$ is the set of classes.

Loss Function. The loss function $\Delta(S^I, S^J) \in \mathbb{R}_{\geq 0}$ evaluates the similarity between the segmentation masks S^I and S^J. Higher $\Delta(.,.)$ implies higher dissimilarity. We use a dice based loss function as this is our evaluation criteria:

$$\Delta(S^I, S^J) = 1 - DICE(S^I, S^J) = 1 - (2 \sum_{i \in V} \frac{|\phi(p_i^I) \cap \phi(p_i^J)|}{|\phi(p_i^I)| + |\phi(p_i^J)|}), \qquad (3)$$

where, $\phi(p_i^I)$ and $\phi(p_i^J)$ are the patches at the control point p_i on the segmentation masks S^I and S^J, respectively, and $|.|$ represents cardinality. This approximation makes the dice decomposable over the nodes of G enabling a very efficient training.

Joint Feature Map. Given $\mathbf{w}_c$ for the c-th class, the deformation D and input $\mathbf{x}$, the multi-class function (2) can be trivially converted into class-based energy

---
Algorithm 1. The CCCP Algorithm.

1: $\mathcal{D}$, $\mathbf{w}_0$, C, α, η, the tolerance ϵ.
2: $t = 0$, $\mathbf{w}_t = \mathbf{w}_0$.
3: **repeat**
4:     For a given $\mathbf{w}_t$, impute latent variables $\hat{D}_i$ for each sample by solving (9).
5:     Update parameters $\mathbf{w}_{t+1}$ by optimizing the convex optimization problem (10).
6:     $t = t + 1$
7: **until** The objective function of the problem (7) does not decrease more than ϵ.

---

function as:

$$\mathcal{E}_c(\mathbf{x}, D; \mathbf{w}) = \mathbf{w}_c^\top \sum_{i \in V} \mathcal{U}_i(\boldsymbol{d_i}, \mathbf{x}) + w_p \sum_{(i,j) \in E} \mathcal{V}(\boldsymbol{d_i}, \boldsymbol{d_j}), \tag{4}$$

where $w_p \in \mathbb{R}_{\geq 0}$ is the parameter for the pairwise term. The final parameter vector $\mathbf{w} \in \mathbb{R}^{n+1}$ is the concatenation of $\mathbf{w}_c$ and w_p. Thus, the function (4) can be written as:

$$\mathcal{E}_c(\mathbf{x}, D; \mathbf{w}) = \mathbf{w}^\top \Psi(\mathbf{x}, D), \tag{5}$$

where $\Psi(\mathbf{x}, D) \in \mathbb{R}^{n+1}$ is the joint feature map defined as:

$$\Psi(\mathbf{x}, D) = \begin{pmatrix} \sum_{i \in V} \mathcal{U}_i^1(\boldsymbol{d_i}, \mathbf{x}) \\ \vdots \\ \sum_{i \in V} \mathcal{U}_i^n(\boldsymbol{d_i}, \mathbf{x}) \\ \sum_{(i,j) \in E} \mathcal{V}(\boldsymbol{d_i}, \boldsymbol{d_j}) \end{pmatrix} \tag{6}$$

Notice that the energy function (4) does not depend on the source segmentation mask S^I. The only use of the source segmentation mask in the energy function (2) is to obtain the dominant class which in this case is not required. However, we will shortly see that the source segmentation mask S^I plays a crucial role in the learning algorithm.

Latent Variables. Ideally, the dataset $\mathcal{D}$ must contain the ground truth deformations D corresponding to the source image I in order to compute the energy term defined in the Eq. (4). Since annotating the dataset with the ground truth deformation is non-trivial, we use them as the latent variables in our algorithm.

The Objective Function. Given $\mathcal{D}$, we learn the parameter $\mathbf{w}$ such that minimizing the energy function (4) leads to a deformation field which when applied to the source segmentation mask gives minimum loss with respect to the target segmentation mask. We denote $g(S, D)$ as the deformed segmentation when the dense deformation field obtained from D is applied to the segmentation mask S. Similarly to the latent SSVM [16], we optimize a regularized upper bound on the loss:

$$\min_{\mathbf{w},\{\xi_i\}} \frac{1}{2}||\mathbf{w}||^2 + \alpha||\mathbf{w} - \mathbf{w}_0||^2 + \frac{C}{N}\sum_i \xi_i,$$

$$s.t. \min_{D, \Delta(g(S_i^I, D), S_i^J)=0} \mathbf{w}^\top \Psi(\mathbf{x}_i, D) \leq \mathbf{w}^\top \Psi(\mathbf{x}_i, \bar{D}) - \Delta(g(S_i^I, \bar{D}), S_i^J) + \xi_i,$$

$$\forall \bar{D}, w_p \geq 0, \xi_i \geq 0, \forall i. \tag{7}$$

where, $\bar{D} = \operatorname{argmin}_D \mathcal{E}(\mathbf{x}_i, D; \mathbf{w})$. The above objective function minimizes an upper bound on the given loss, called slack (ξ_i). The effect of the regularization term is controlled by the hyper-parameter C. The second term is the proximity term to ensure that the learned $\mathbf{w}$ is close to the initialization $\mathbf{w}_0$. The effect of the proximity term is controlled by the hyperparameter α. Intuitively, for a given input-output pair, the constraints of the above objective function enforce that the energy corresponding to the best possible deformation field, in terms of both energy and loss (in order to be semantically meaningful), must always be less than or equal to the energy corresponding to any other deformation field with a margin proportional to the loss and some non negative slack.

The Learning Algorithm. The objective function (7) turns out to be a special case of non-convex functions (difference of convex), thus can be locally optimized using the well known CCCP algorithm [17]. The CCCP algorithm consist of three steps – (1) upperbounding the concave part at a given $\mathbf{w}$, which leads to an affine function in $\mathbf{w}$; (2) optimizing the resultant convex function (sum of convex and affine functions is convex); (3) repeating the above steps until the objective can not be further decreased beyond a given tolerance of ϵ. The complete CCCP algorithm for the optimization of (7) is shown Algorithm 1. The first step of upperbounding the concave functions (Line 4) is the same as the latent imputation step, which we call the *segmentation consistent registration* problem. The second step is the optimization of the resultant convex problem (Line 5), which is the optimization of the SSVM for which we use the well known cutting plane algorithm [6]. In what follows, we discuss these steps in detail.

Segmentation Consistent Registration. This step involves generating the best possible ground truth deformation field (unknown a priori) at a given $\mathbf{w}$, known as the latent imputation step. Since we optimize the dice loss, we formulate this step as an inference problem with additional constraints to ensure that the imputed deformation warps the image minimizing the loss between the deformed source and the target. Mathematically, for a given parameter vector $\mathbf{w}$, the latent deformation is imputed by solving:

$$\hat{D}_i = \operatorname*{argmin}_{D \in \mathcal{L}^{|V|}, \Delta(g(S_i^I, D), S_i^J)=0} \mathbf{w}^\top \Psi(\mathbf{x}_i, D). \tag{8}$$

We relax the above problem as it is difficult and may not have a unique solution:

$$\hat{D}_i = \operatorname*{argmin}_{D \in \mathcal{L}^{|V|}} \left(\mathbf{w}^\top \Psi(\mathbf{x}_i, D) + \eta \Delta(g(S_i^I, D), S_i^J) \right), \tag{9}$$

where, $\eta \geq 0$ controls the relaxation trade-off. Since the loss function used is decomposable, the above problem can be optimized using FastPD inference for the deformable registration with trivial modifications on the unary potentials.

Parameters Update. Given the imputed latent variables, the resultant objective is:

$$\min_{\mathbf{w},\{\xi_i\}} \frac{1}{2}||\mathbf{w}||^2 + \alpha||\mathbf{w} - \mathbf{w}_0||^2 + \frac{C}{N}\sum_i \xi_i,$$

$$s.t.\, \mathbf{w}^\top \Psi(\mathbf{x}_i, \hat{D}_i) \leq \mathbf{w}^\top \Psi(\mathbf{x}_i, \bar{D}) - \Delta(g(S_i^I, \bar{D}), S_i^J) + \xi_i, \forall \bar{D}, w_p, \xi_i \geq 0, \forall i. \quad (10)$$

where, $\hat{D}_i$ is the latent deformation field imputed by solving the problem (9). Intuitively, the above objective function tries to learn the parameters $\mathbf{w}$ such that the energy corresponding to the imputed deformation field is always less than the energy for any other deformation field with a margin proportional to the loss function. The above objective function has exponential number of constraints, one for each possible deformation field $\bar{D} \in \mathcal{L}^{|V|}$. In order to alleviate this problem we use cutting plane algorithm [6]. Briefly, for a given $\mathbf{w}$, each deformation field $\bar{D}$ gives a slack. Instead of minimizing all the slacks for a particular sample at once, we find the deformation field that leads to the maximum value of the slack and store this in a set known as the working set. This is known as *finding the most violated constraint.* Thus, instead of using exponentially many constraints, the algorithm uses the constraints stored in the working set and this process is repeated until no constraints can be further added. Rearranging the terms in the constraints of the objective function (10) and ignoring the constant term $\mathbf{w}^\top \Psi(\mathbf{x}_i, \hat{D}_i)$, the most violated constraint can be obtained by solving:

$$\bar{D}_i = \operatorname*{argmin}_{D \in \mathcal{L}^{|V|}} \left(\mathbf{w}^\top \Psi(\mathbf{x}_i, \bar{D}) - \Delta(g(S_i^I, \bar{D}), S_i^J) \right). \quad (11)$$

Since the loss is decomposable, this problem can be solved using FastPD inference for the deformable registration with trivial modifications on the unary terms.

Prediction. Once we obtain the learned parameters $\mathbf{w}_c$ for each class $c \in \mathcal{C}$ using the Algorithm 1, we form the matrix W where each column of the matrix represents the learned parameter for a specific class. This W is then used to solve the registration problem (Eq. 2) using the approximate inference discussed in Sect. 2.

4   Results and Discussion

As a proof of concept, we evaluate the effect of the aggregated metric on three different medical datasets – (1) RT Parotids, (2) RT Abdominal, and a down-sampled version of (3) IBSR [1], involving several anatomical structures, different image modalities, and inter/intra patient images We used four different metrics: (1) sum of absolute differences (SAD), (2) mutual information (MI), (3) normalized cross correlation (NCC), and (4) discrete wavelet coefficients (DWT). The datasets consists of 8 CT (RT Parotids, head images of $56 \times 62 \times 53$ voxels), 5 CT (RT Abdominal, abdominal images of $90 \times 60 \times 80$ voxels) and 18 MRI images (a downsampled version of IBSR dataset, including brain images $64 \times 64 \times 64$

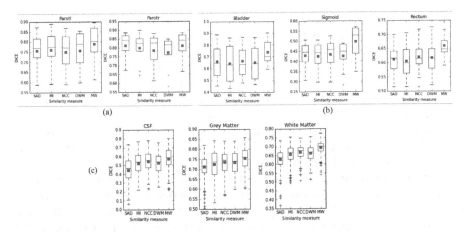

Fig. 1. Results for RT parotids (a), RT abdominal (b) and IBSR (c) datasets. We show dice between the deformed source and the target segmentation masks after registration, for the single-metric registration (SAD, MI, NCC, DWT) and the learned multi-metric registration (MW). In (a), 'Parotl' and 'Parotr' are the left and the right parotids. In (b), 'Bladder', 'Sigmoid', and 'Rectum' are the three organs in the dataset. In (c), annotations correspond to Cerebrospinal fluid (CSF), grey (GM) and white (WM) matter. The red square is the mean and the red bar is median. (Color figure online)

voxels). We performed multi-fold cross validation in every dataset, considering pairs with different patients in training and testing. For a complete description of the datasets and the experimental setting, please refer to the supplementary material. The results on the test sets are shown in Fig. 1. As it can be observed in Fig. 1, the linear combination of similarity measures weighted using the learned coefficients systematically outperforms (or is as good as) single metric based registration, with max improvements of 8% in terms of dice (see Fig. 2).

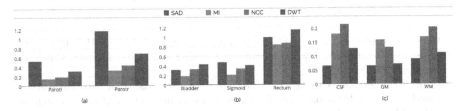

Fig. 2. Example of learned weights for RT Parotids (a), RT Abdominal (b) and IBSR (c) datasets. Since the structures of interest in every dataset present different intensity distributions, different metric aggregations are learned. Note that in case of the RT Parotids, given that both parotid glands present the same intensity distribution, similar weightings are learned for both structures, with SAD dominating the other similarity measures. However, in IBSR dataset, NCC dominates in case of CSF and WM, while MI receives the higher value for gray matter (GM).

Discussion and Conclusions. We have showed that associating different similarity criteria to every anatomical region yields results superior to the classic single metric approach. In order to learn this mapping where ground truth is generally given in the form of segmentation masks, we defined deformation fields as latent variables and proposed a LSSVM based framework. The main limitation of our method is the need of segmentation masks for the source images in testing time. However, different real scenarios like radiation therapy or atlas-based segmentation methods fulfill this condition. Note that, at prediction (testing) time, the segmentation mask is used to determine the metrics weights combination per control node (finding the dominant class). The segmentation labels are not used at testing time to guide the registration process which is purely image based. In our multi-metric registration approach, segmentation masks are only required (at testing time) for the source image and used to choose the best learned metric aggregation. The idea could be further extended to unlabeled data (as it concerns the source image at testing time) where the dominant label class per control node is the output of a classification/learning method. From a theoretical viewpoint, we showed how the three main components of LSSVM: (1) latent imputation (Eq. 9); (2) prediction (optimizing Eq. 2) and (3) finding most violated constraint (Eq. (11)), can be formulated as the exact same problem. The difference among these problems is the unary potentials used. This is extremely important given that further improvements in inference algorithms will directly increase the quality of the results. As future work, the integration of alternative accuracy measures, other than dice, such as the Hausdorff distance between surfaces or real geometric distances for anatomical landmarks could further enhance the performance of the method.

References

1. IBSR: Internet Brain Segmentation Repository. http://www.cma.mgh.harvard.edu/ibsr/
2. Bronstein, M.M., Bronstein, A.M., Michel, F., Paragios, N.: Data fusion through cross-modality metric learning using similarity-sensitive hashing. In: CVPR 2010, pp. 3594–3601. IEEE (2010)
3. Cifor, A., Risser, L., Chung, D., Anderson, E.M., Schnabel, J.A.: Hybrid feature-based Log-Demons registration for tumour tracking in 2-D liver ultrasound images. In: ISBI (2012)
4. Cifor, A., Risser, L., Chung, D., Anderson, E.M., Schnabel, J.A.: Hybrid feature-based diffeomorphic registration for tumor tracking in 2-D liver ultrasound images. IEEE TMI **32**, 1647–1656 (2013)
5. Glocker, B., Komodakis, N., Tziritas, G., Navab, N., Paragios, N.: Dense image registration through MRFs and efficient linear programming. Med. Image Anal. **12**(6), 731–741 (2008)
6. Joachims, T., Finley, T., Yu, C.: Cutting-plane training of structural SVMs. Mach. Learn. **77**, 27–59 (2009)
7. Komodakis, N., Tziritas, G., Paragios, N.: Fast, approximately optimal solutions for single and dynamic MRFs. In: CVPR (2007)

8. Lee, D., Hofmann, M., Steinke, F., Altun, Y., Cahill, N.D., Scholkopf, B.: Learning similarity measure for multi-modal 3D image registration. In: CVPR 2009, IEEE Conference on Computer Vision and Pattern Recognition, pp. 186–193. IEEE (2009)

9. Michel, F., Bronstein, M., Bronstein, A., Paragios, N.: Boosted metric learning for 3D multi-modal deformable registration. In: ISBI (2011)

10. Rueckert, D., Sonoda, L.I., et al.: Nonrigid registration using free-form deformations: application to breast MR images. IEEE TMI **18**, 712–721 (1999)

11. Simonovsky, M., Gutiérrez-Becker, B., Mateus, D., Navab, N., Komodakis, N.: A deep metric for multimodal registration. In: Ourselin, S., Joskowicz, L., Sabuncu, M.R., Unal, G., Wells, W. (eds.) MICCAI 2016. LNCS, vol. 9902, pp. 10–18. Springer, Cham (2016). doi:10.1007/978-3-319-46726-9_2

12. Tang, L., Hero, A., Hamarneh, G.: Locally-adaptive similarity metric for deformable medical image registration. In: ISBI. IEEE (2012)

13. Taskar, B., Guestrin, C., Koller, D.: Max-margin Markov networks. In: NIPS (2003)

14. Toga, A.W.: Learning based coarse-to-fine image registration. In: CVPR (2008)

15. Tsochantaridis, I., Hofmann, T., Joachims, T., Altun, Y.: Support vector machine learning for interdependent and structured output spaces. In: ICML (2004)

16. Yu, C.N., Joachims, T.: Learning structural SVMs with latent variables. In: ICML (2009)

17. Yuille, A., Rangarajan, A.: The concave-convex procedure. Neural Comput. **15**, 915–936 (2003)

18. Zagoruyko, S., Komodakis, N.: Learning to compare image patches via convolutional neural networks

Segmentation of Craniomaxillofacial Bony Structures from MRI with a 3D Deep-Learning Based Cascade Framework

Dong Nie[1,2], Li Wang[1], Roger Trullo[1], Jianfu Li[3], Peng Yuan[3], James Xia[3], and Dinggang Shen[1(✉)]

[1] Department of Radiology and BRIC,
University of North Carolina at Chapel Hill, Chapel Hill, USA
dgshen@med.unc.edu
[2] Department of Computer Science,
University of North Carolina at Chapel Hill, Chapel Hill, USA
[3] Houston Methodist Hospital, Houston, TX, USA

Abstract. Computed tomography (CT) is commonly used as a diagnostic and treatment planning imaging modality in craniomaxillofacial (CMF) surgery to correct patient's bony defects. A major disadvantage of CT is that it emits harmful ionizing radiation to patients during the exam. Magnetic resonance imaging (MRI) is considered to be much safer and noninvasive, and often used to study CMF soft tissues (e.g., temporomandibular joint and brain). However, it is extremely difficult to accurately segment CMF bony structures from MRI since both bone and air appear to be black in MRI, along with low signal-to-noise ratio and partial volume effect. To this end, we proposed a 3D deep-learning based cascade framework to solve these issues. Specifically, a 3D fully convolutional network (FCN) architecture is first adopted to coarsely segment the bony structures. As the coarsely segmented bony structures by FCN tend to be thicker, convolutional neural network (CNN) is further utilized for fine-grained segmentation. To enhance the discriminative ability of the CNN, we particularly concatenate the predicted probability maps from FCN and the original MRI, and feed them together into the CNN to provide more context information for segmentation. Experimental results demonstrate a good performance and also the clinical feasibility of our proposed 3D deep-learning based cascade framework.

1 Introduction

A significant number of patients require craniomaxillofacial (CMF) surgery every year for the correction of congenital and acquired condition of head and face [5]. Comparing to computed tomography (CT) that emits harmful ionizing radiation, magnetic resonance imaging (MRI) provides a safer and non-invasive way to assess CMF anatomy. However, it is extremely difficult to accurately segment CMF bony structures from MRI due to unclear boundaries between the bones and air (both appearing to be black) in MRI, low signal-to-noise ratio, and partial

© Springer International Publishing AG 2017
Q. Wang et al. (Eds.): MLMI 2017, LNCS 10541, pp. 266–273, 2017.
DOI: 10.1007/978-3-319-67389-9_31

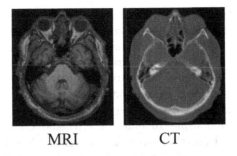

MRI   CT

Fig. 1. The comparison of MRI and its corresponding CT. Bony structures have unclear bone-to-air boundaries and low signal-to-noise in MRI, comparing to CT.

volume effect (Fig. 1). Due to these difficulties, even with the time-consuming and labor-intense manual segmentation, the results are often still inaccurate.

To date, there are only limited reports on effectively segmenting bony structures from MRI, mainly based on multi-atlas-based approaches [10] and learning-based approaches [9]. In multi-atlas-based approaches, multiple atlas images are rigidly or non-rigidly aligned onto a target image. Based on the derived deformation fields, the corresponding label image from each atlas image is warped into the target image space and then fused (based on a certain image-to-image similarity metric) to obtain the segmentation of the target image. In traditional learning-based approaches, the segmentation task is generally formulated as an optimization problem by selecting the best features from a pool of human-engineered features. However, both type of methods need to pre-define image-to-image similarities or image features, which often require a very careful and time-consuming design.

Recently, there are major breakthroughs in learning-based approaches. Convolutional neural networks (CNN), especially its variant - fully convolutional neural network (FCN), has significantly improved performances in various medical image segmentation tasks [2, 7, 8]. FCN consists of two types of operations: down-sampling and up-sampling [6]. The down-sampling operation streams (i.e., convolution and pooling) usually result in coarse and global predictions based on the entire input image to the network, while the up-sampling streams (i.e., deconvolution) can generate dense prediction through finer inference. However, in FCN, the input intensity images are heavily compressed to be highly semantic. This will certainly cause serious information loss and subsequently decrease the localization accuracy, even after utilizing the up-sampling streams trying to recover the full image information. Ronneberger et al. [8] partially alleviated this problem by using U-net to aggregate the lower layer feature maps to the higher layer, for compensating the loss of resolution by the pooling operations. Although a more precise localization may be achieved by U-net, it is still extremely challenging to segment those thin and fine bony structures from MRI (Fig. 1).

To address the aforementioned challenges, we propose a 3D deep-learning cascade framework to automatically segment CMF bony structures from the head MRI. First, we train a 3D U-net model in an end-to-end and voxel-to-voxel fashion to coarsely segment the bony structures. Second, we use a CNN to further refine those coarsely segmented bony structures to acquire more accurate segmentation for the thin bony structures. Also, inspired by the auto-context model [12], we feed the original intensity MR image along with coarsely segmented bony structures as a joint input to the CNN for better guiding the model training during the fine-grained segmentation stage. Our proposed framework has been validated using 16 pairs of MRI and CT images. It is worth indicating the technical contribution of our novel 3D deep-learning based cascade framework, i.e., it can efficiently and accurately segment bony structures from MRI in a coarse-to-fine fashion.

2   Methods

Our proposed deep-learning based cascade framework is mainly designed to solve problem of segmenting CMF bony structures from MR images. The framework includes two stages: (1) coarse segmentation and (2) fine-grained segmentation (Fig. 2).

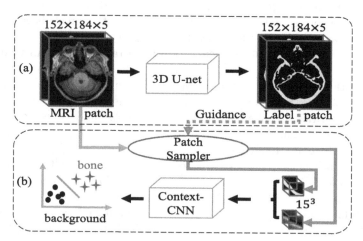

Fig. 2. Architecture for our proposed deep-learning based cascade framework. (a) shows the sub-architecture for coarse segmentation by the 3D U-net, which adopts 5 consecutive slices as input; (b) shows another sub-architecture, context-guided CNN, for fine-grained segmentation, based on the patches sampled on the detected bone locations by (a).

2.1   Data Acquisition and Preprocessing

Dataset consists of 16 pairs of MRI and CT scans from Alzheimer's Disease Neuroimaging Initiative (ADNI) database (see www.adni-info.org for details) were used. The MR scans were acquired using a Siemens Triotim scanner, with the scanning matrix of 126×154, voxel size of $1.2 \times 1.2 \times 1\,mm^3$, TE $2.95\,ms$, TR $2300\,ms$, and flip angle $9°$, while the CT scans were acquired on a Siemens Somatom scanner, with a scanning matrix of 300×400, and a voxel size of $0.59 \times 0.59 \times 3\,mm^3$. Due to high contrast for the bony structure, CT scans herein were employed to extract ground truth for MRI. During image preprocessing, both MRI and CT were initially resampled to $1 \times 1 \times 1\,mm^3$ with final image size of $152 \times 184 \times 149$. Then, each CT image was linearly aligned onto its corresponding MR image. Afterward, the bony structures were segmented from each aligned CT image using thresholding and further refined by an expert. These CT segmentation results provide training labels for the network.

2.2   Coarse Segmentation with Anatomical Constraint

We first segment the CMF bony structure from MRI by using U-net, as it has been successfully applied in various medical image segmentations tasks. The original U-net in [8] was proposed for 2D image segmentation. In order to extend it for 3D segmentation, it is natural to change its 2D filters (e.g., 3×3) to 3D ones (e.g., $3 \times 3 \times 3$), like [1]. The 3D filters are then applied to each training sample, i.e., an entire 3D image. However, in real clinical situation, it is very difficult to obtain unlimited number of MRI dataset, which degrades the final performance. To address this problem, we extract 3D patches as the training samples from each MR image for training, instead of using the entire 3D image as one training sample. This strategy makes the number of patches virtually unlimited. On the other hand, for considering the anatomical shapes of bony structures, we decide to feed a large patch into the network, expecting to form certain anatomical constraint for the network. Specifically, we utilize a patch size of $152 \times 184 \times 5$ to cover the whole bony structure on each slice, by also balancing the number of patches and receptive field. That is, the receptive field is large in the first two dimensions (i.e., 152×184), and still reasonable in the 3rd dimension (i.e., covering 5 consecutive slices) which can alleviate the possible inconsistent segmentations across slices. Accordingly, we set up the similar filters in the first two dimensions as the original U-net, while keep the feature map size unchanged through the whole network for the 3rd dimension. We denote this designed network as "3D U-net" (Fig. 2(a)) in the following text.

2.3   Fine-Grained Segmentation

We further utilize the initial probability maps from 3D U-net (in Sect. 2.2) to extract context information for refining the segmentation. Note that the context information can provide important semantic information for segmenting bony structure. In addition, based on the initial probability maps, we densely extract training patches only in the regions with ambiguous probabilities, which allows us to focus on only the potential problematic regions and also save the computational time.

Prior-guided Patch Sampling: Considering the fact that the initial segmentation probability maps already provide sufficient prior information about the locations of bony structures, we propose to use the initial segmentation probability maps to guide the sampling of training patches to the second deep learning architecture, CNN. Specifically, we randomly sample patches around those predicted bone regions. Moreover, since the probability maps also indicate certain information for the locations of difficult-to-segment bony structure (e.g., fine or small bones), we further densely extract the training patches around voxels with ambiguous probabilities.

Context-guided CNN Training: We first train a CNN [11] with a patch size of $15 \times 15 \times 15$ to determine voxels with ambiguous probabilities. Considering large number of training patches, we form our network based on a 3D VGG [11] by removing two pooling layers together with its surrounding convolutional layers (i.e., (we remove the 2nd and 3rd pooling layer groups)), and setting the class number as 2 (bone or not), as shown in Fig. 2(b). Different from the original auto-context model, our context information is from the U-net, instead of the current CNN. This indicates that our proposed method is not iterative, which may significantly shorten the training time. More importantly, since the 3D U-net is performed on full slices, the initial segmentation by the 3D U-net could thus benefit from the long information range dependency, which indicates a voxel in the segmented maps contain information from the full slice of MRI. This can better serve as context information for the CNN (after the 3D U-net). We denote it as "context-CNN" in the text below.

2.4   Implementation Details

We adopt Caffe [4] to implement the proposed deep learning architecture shown in Fig. 2. Cross-entropy loss is utilized as the general loss of the network. Stochastic gradient decrease algorithm is adopted as the optimizer. To train the network, the hyper-parameters need to be appropriately determined. Specifically, the network weights are initialized by xavier algorithm [3], and the weight decay is set as $1e - 4$. For the network bias, we initialize it to be 0. The initial learning rate is set as 0.01 for both networks, followed by decreasing the learning rate during the training. To augment the dataset, we flip the images along the 3rd dimension (Note, we only do augmentation for training dataset). We extract approximately 5000 training patches for the first sub-architecture (3D U-net), and 320, 000 patches for the second sub-architecture (context-guided CNN) around the regions that are segmented as bone by the first sub-architecture (3D U-net). The platform we use for training is a Titan X GPU.

3   Experiments and Results

We evaluated the proposed deep-learning based cascade framework on 16 MRI subjects in a leave-one-out fashion. Note that the data used in algorithm development were not used in the evaluation experiment. Dice similarity coefficient (DSC) was used to quantitatively measure the overlap between automated segmentation and the ground truth.

Comparison between coarse and fine-grained segmentation: We performed experiments to compare coarse and fine-grained segmentation. The results showed that the initial segmentation method (3D-Unet) achieved an average DSC of 0.8410(0.0315). With the fine-grained segmentation method (context-CNN), the average DSC was improved to 0.9412(0.0316). Figure 3 shows the segmentation results for a randomly selected subject. It clearly demonstrated that the bony structures resulted from fine-grained segmentation became thinner and smoother than the ones resulted from the coarse segmentation. This proves the effectiveness of our proposed cascade model.

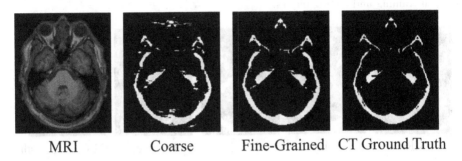

MRI   Coarse   Fine-Grained   CT Ground Truth

Fig. 3. Demonstration of coarse and fine-grained segmentation results by 3D-Unet and context-CNN, along with the original MRI (left) and ground-truth bony structures from CT (right).

Impact of context-CNN: We also validated the impact of the context-CNN. Figure 4 shows the convergence curve for the traditional CNN and the context-CNN, which clearly indicates that the context-CNN converges much faster than the traditional CNN. This is because the context-CNN is provided with the context information, which can quickly guide the segmentation. DSC achieved with the traditional CNN is 0.9307(0.0350), which is improved to 0.9412(0.0316) by the context-CNN. This further demonstrates that the context information can not only speed up the convergence process, but also improve the discriminative ability of the network.

Comparison with Other Methods: We also compared our method with two widely-used methods, i.e., multi-atlas based [10] (denoted as Atlas) and random forest-based [13] (denoted as LINKS, one of the widely-used learning-based methods), to further demonstrate the advantages of segmentation accuracy by our proposed method. The experimental results are shown in Fig. 5. The result achieved with Atlas method is the worst due to registration errors and difficulty of designing image-to-image similarity. The result achieved with LINKS is better because of the carefully designed features. Compared to LINKS, the result achieved with our proposed method is much more consistent with the CT ground truth. This better result is contributed from the better feature representation and joint optimization for the feature engineering and segmentation. The DSC

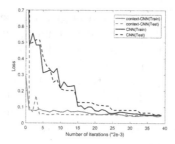

Fig. 4. Comparison of convergence curves of the traditional CNN and the context-CNN in both training and testing phases.

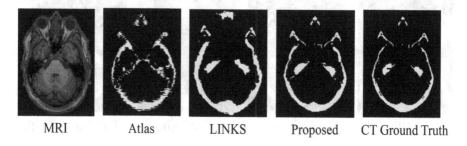

| MRI | Atlas | LINKS | Proposed | CT Ground Truth |

Fig. 5. Comparison of segmentation results by three different methods.

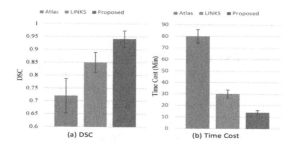

Fig. 6. Quantitative comparison of three segmentation methods in terms of (a) DSC and (b) time cost.

achieved by the three methods are shown in Fig. 6. The quantitative results are consistent with qualitative results as shown in Fig. 5, which further confirms the superiority of our proposed method over other methods. Furthermore, the time cost of our proposed method is the least among all the three methods. It is mainly due to the use of cascade architecture that can allow fast determination for the categories of most voxels by the coarse segmentation, and thus save a significant computational load for the fine-grained segmentation.

4   Discussion and Conclusions

In this paper, we proposed a deep-learning based cascade framework to segment CMF bones from brain MR images. The 3D-Unet is used to perform an initial bone segmentation from MRI. With those initial segmented maps, we then focus on the coarsely predicted bone regions. This can not only provide prior information to support the training patches sampling, but also supply the context information for the context-CNN. With these strategies, our proposed method can work better and fast in segmentation. The experimental results also prove that our proposed method outperforms the other widely used state-of-the-art methods in both segmentation accuracy and computational efficiency.

References

1. Çiçek, Ö., Abdulkadir, A., Lienkamp, S.S., Brox, T., Ronneberger, O.: 3D U-net: learning dense volumetric segmentation from sparse annotation. In: Ourselin, S., Joskowicz, L., Sabuncu, M.R., Unal, G., Wells, W. (eds.) MICCAI 2016. LNCS, vol. 9901, pp. 424–432. Springer, Cham (2016). doi:10.1007/978-3-319-46723-8_49
2. Dou, Q., Chen, H., Jin, Y., Yu, L., Qin, J., Heng, P.-A.: 3D deeply supervised network for automatic liver segmentation from CT volumes. In: Ourselin, S., Joskowicz, L., Sabuncu, M.R., Unal, G., Wells, W. (eds.) MICCAI 2016. LNCS, vol. 9901, pp. 149–157. Springer, Cham (2016). doi:10.1007/978-3-319-46723-8_18
3. Glorot, X., Bengio, Y.: Understanding the difficulty of training deep feedforward neural networks. In: AISTATS, pp. 249–256 (2010)
4. Jia, Y., et al.: Caffe: convolutional architecture for fast feature embedding. In: ACM Multimedia, pp. 675–678. ACM (2014)
5. Kraft, A., et al.: Craniomaxillofacial trauma: synopsis of 14,654 cases with 35,129 injuries in 15 years. Craniomaxillofacial Trauma Reconstr. 5(01), 041–050 (2012)
6. Long, J., et al.: Fully convolutional networks for semantic segmentation. In: CVPR, pp. 3431–3440 (2015)
7. Nie, D., et al.: Fully convolutional networks for multi-modality isointense infant brain image segmentation. In: ISBI, pp. 1342–1345. IEEE (2016)
8. Ronneberger, O., Fischer, P., Brox, T.: U-net: convolutional networks for biomedical image segmentation. In: Navab, N., Hornegger, J., Wells, W.M., Frangi, A.F. (eds.) MICCAI 2015. LNCS, vol. 9351, pp. 234–241. Springer, Cham (2015). doi:10.1007/978-3-319-24574-4_28
9. Seim, H., et al.: Model-based auto-segmentation of knee bones and cartilage in MRI data
10. Shan, L., et al.: Automatic multi-atlas-based cartilage segmentation from knee MR images. In: ISBI, pp. 1028–1031. IEEE (2012)
11. Simonyan, K., Zisserman, A.: Very deep convolutional networks for large-scale image recognition. arXiv preprint arXiv:1409.1556 (2014)
12. Zhuowen, T., Bai, X.: Auto-context and its application to high-level vision tasks and 3d brain image segmentation. IEEE TPAMI 32(10), 1744–1757 (2010)
13. Wang, L., et al.: Links: learning-based multi-source integration framework for segmentation of infant brain images. NeuroImage 108, 160–172 (2015)

3D U-net with Multi-level Deep Supervision: Fully Automatic Segmentation of Proximal Femur in 3D MR Images

Guodong Zeng[1], Xin Yang[2], Jing Li[1], Lequan Yu[2], Pheng-Ann Heng[2],
and Guoyan Zheng[1(✉)]

[1] Institute for Surgical Technology and Biomechanics,
University of Bern, Bern, Switzerland
guoyan.Zheng@istb.unibe.ch
[2] Department of Computer Science and Engineering,
The Chinese University of Hong Kong, Sha Tin, Hong Kong

Abstract. This paper addresses the problem of segmentation of proximal femur in 3D MR images. We propose a deeply supervised 3D U-net-like fully convolutional network for segmentation of proximal femur in 3D MR images. After training, our network can directly map a whole volumetric data to its volume-wise labels. Inspired by previous work, multi-level deep supervision is designed to alleviate the potential gradient vanishing problem during training. It is also used together with partial transfer learning to boost the training efficiency when only small set of labeled training data are available. The present method was validated on 20 3D MR images of femoroacetabular impingement patients. The experimental results demonstrate the efficacy of the present method.

Keywords: Deep learning · Proximal femur · MR images · Segmentation

1 Introduction

Femoroacetabular Impingement (FAI) is a cause of hip pain in adults and has been recognized recently as one of the key risk factors that may lead to the development of early cartilage and labral damage [1] and a possible precursor of hip osteoarthritis [2]. Several studies [2,3] have shown that the prevalence of FAI in young populations with hip complaints is high. Although there exist a number of imaging modalities that can be used to diagnose and assess FAI, MR imaging does not induce any dosage of radiation at all and is regarded as the standard tool for FAI diagnosis [4]. While manual analysis of a series of 2D MR images is feasible, automated segmentation of proximal femur in MR images will greatly facilitate the applications of MR images for FAI surgical planning and simulation.

The topic of automated MR image segmentation of the hip joint has been addressed by a few studies which relied on atlas-based segmentation [5], graph-cut [6], active model [7,8] or statistical shape models [9]. While these methods

© Springer International Publishing AG 2017
Q. Wang et al. (Eds.): MLMI 2017, LNCS 10541, pp. 274–282, 2017.
DOI: 10.1007/978-3-319-67389-9_32

reported encouraging results for bone segmentation, further improvements are needed. For example, Arezoomand et al. [8] recently developed a 3D active model framework for segmentation of proximal femur in MR images and they reported an average recall of 0.88.

Recently, machine-learning based methods, especially those based on convolutional neural networks (CNNs) have witnessed successful applications in natural image processing [10,11] as well as in medical image analysis [12–15]. For example, Prasoon et al. [12] developed a method to use a triplanar CNN that can autonomously learn features from images for knee cartilage segmentation. More recently, 3D volume-to-volume segmentation networks were introduced, including 3D U-Net [13], 3D V-Net [14] and a 3D deeply supervised network [15].

In this paper, we propose a deeply supervised 3D U-net-like fully convolutional network (FCN) for segmentation of proximal femur in 3D MR images. After training, our network can directly map a whole volumetric data to its volume-wise label. Inspired by previous work [13,15], multi-level deep supervision is designed to alleviate the potential gradient vanishing problem during training. It is also used together with partial transfer learning to boost the training efficiency when only small set of labeled training data are available.

2 Method

Figure 1 illustrates the architecture of our proposed deeply-supervised 3D U-net-like network. Our proposed neural network is inspired by the 3D U-net [13]. Similar to 3D U-net, our network also consists of two parts, i.e., the encoder part(contracting path) and the decoder part(expansive path). The encoder part focuses on analysis and feature representation learning from the input data while the decoder part generates segmentation results, relying on the learned features

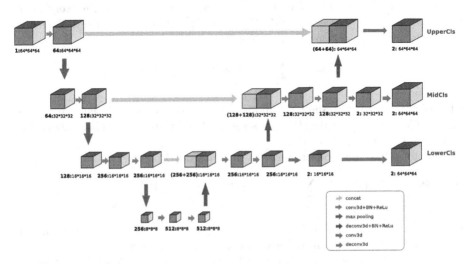

Fig. 1. Illustration of our proposed network architecture

from the encoder part. Shortcut connections are established between layers of equal resolution in the encoder and decoder paths. The difference between our network and the 3D U-net is the introduction of multi-level deep supervision, which gives more feedback to help training during back propagation process.

Previous studies show small convolutional kernels are more beneficial for training and performance. In our deeply supervised network, all convolutional layers use kernel size of $3 \times 3 \times 3$ and strides of 1 and all max pooling layers uses kernel size of $2 \times 2 \times 2$ and strides of 2. In the convolutional and deconvolutional blocks of our network, Batch normalization (BN) [16] and Rectified linear unit (ReLU) are adopted to speed up the training and to enhance the gradient back propagation.

2.1   Multi-level Deep Supervision

Training a deep neural network is challenging. As the matter of gradient vanishing, final loss cannot be efficiently back propagated to shallow layers, which is more difficult for 3D cases when only a small set of annotated data is available. To address this issue, we inject two branch classifiers into network in addition to the classifier of the main network. Specifically, we divide the decoder path of our network into three different levels: lower layers, middle layers and upper layers. Deconvolutional blocks are injected into lower and middle layers such that the low-level and middle-level features are upscaled to generate segmentation predictions with the same resolution as the input data. As a result, besides the classifier from the upper final layer ('UpperCls' in Fig. 1), we also have two branch classifiers in lower and middle layers ('LowerCls' and 'MidCls' in Fig. 1, respectively). With the losses calculated by the predictions from classifiers of different layers, more effective gradients back propagation can be achieved by direct supervision on the hidden layers.

Let W be the weights of main network and w^l, w^m, w^u be the weights of the three classifiers 'LowerCls', 'MidCls' and 'UpperCls', respectively. Then the cross-entropy loss function of a classifier is:

$$\mathcal{L}_c(\chi; W, w^c) = \sum_{x_i \in \chi} -\log p(y_i = t(x_i)|x_i; W, w^c)) \tag{1}$$

where $c \in \{l, m, u\}$ represents the index of the classifiers; χ represents the training samples; $p(y_i = t(x_i)|x_i; W, w^c)$ is the probability of target class label $t(x_i)$ corresponding to sample $x_i \in \chi$.

The total loss function of our deep-supervised 3D network is:

$$\mathcal{L}(\chi; W, w^l, w^m, w^u) = \sum_{c \in \{l,m,u\}} \alpha_c \mathcal{L}_c(\chi; W, w^c) + \lambda(\psi(W) + \sum_{c \in \{l,m,u\}} \psi(w^c)) \tag{2}$$

where $\psi()$ is the regularization term (L_2 norm in our experiment) with hyper parameter λ; $\alpha_l, \alpha_m, \alpha_u$ are the weights of the associated classifiers.

By doing this, classifiers in different layers can also take advantages of multi-scale context, which has been demonstrated in previous work on segmentation of

3D liver CT and 3D heart MR images [15]. This is based on the observation that lower layers have smaller receptive fields while upper layers have larger receptive fields. As a result, multi-scale context information can be learned by our network which will then facilitate the target segmentation in the test stage.

2.2   Partial Transfer Learning

It is difficult to train a deep neural network from scratch because of limited annotated data. Training deep neural network requires large amount of annotated data, which are not always available, although data augmentation can partially address the problem. Furthermore, randomly initialized parameters make it more difficult to search for an optimal solution in high dimensional space. Transfer learning from an existing network, which has been trained on a large set of data, is a common way to alleviate the difficulty. Usually the new dataset should be similar or related to the dataset and tasks used in the pre-training stage. But for medical image applications, it is difficult to find an off-the-shelf 3D model trained on a large set of related data of related tasks.

Previous studies [17] demonstrated that weights of lower layers in deep neural network is generic while higher layers are more related to specific tasks. Thus, the encoder path of our neural network can be transferred from models pre-trained on a totally different dataset. In the field of computer vision, lots of models are trained on very large dataset, e.g., ImageNet [18], VGG16 [19], Googlenet [20], etc. Unfortunately, most of these models were trained on 2D images. 3D pre-trained models that can be freely accessed are rare in both computer vision and medical image analysis fields.

C3D [21] is one of the few 3D models that has been trained on a very large dataset in the field of computer vision. More specifically, C3D is trained on the Sports-1M dataset to learn spatiotemporal features for action recognition. The Sports-1M dataset consists of 1.1 million sports videos, and each video belongs to one of 487 sports categories.

In our experiment, C3D pre-trained model was adopted as the pre-trained model for the encoder part of our neural network. For the decoder parts of our neural network, they were randomly initialized.

2.3   Implementation Details

The proposed network was implemented in python using TensorFlow framework and trained on a desktop with a 3.6 GHz Intel(R) i7 CPU and a GTX 1080 Ti graphics card with 11 GB GPU memory. The source code is publicly available at github[1].

---

[1] https://github.com/zengguodong/FemurSegmentation3DFCN.

3   Experiments and Results

3.1   Dataset and Pre-processing

We evaluated our method on a set of unilateral hip joint data containing 20 T1-weighted MR images of FAI patients. We randomly split the dataset into two parts, ten images are for training and the other ten images are for testing. Data augmentation was used to enlarge the training samples by rotating each image (90, 180, 270) degrees around the z axis of the image and flipped horizontally (y axis). After that, we got in total 80 images for training.

3.2   Training Patches Preparation

All sub-volume patches to our neural network are in the size of $64 \times 64 \times 64$. We randomly cropped sub-volume patches from training samples whose size are about $300 \times 200 \times 100$. In the phase of training, during every epoch, 80 training volumetric images were randomly shuffled. We then randomly sampled patches with batch size 2 from each volumetric image for n times ($n = 5$). Each sampled patch was normalized as zero mean and unit variance before fed into network.

3.3   Training

We trained two different models, one with partial transfer learning and the other without. More specifically, to train the model with partial transfer learning, we initialized the weights of the encoder part of the network from the pre-trained C3D [21] model and the weights of other parts from a Gaussian distribution ($\mu = 0, \sigma = 0.01$). In contrast, for the model without partial transfer learning, all weights were initialized from Gaussian distribution ($\mu = 0, \sigma = 0.01$).

Each time, the model was trained for 14,000 iterations and the weights were updated by the stochastic gradient descent (SGD) algorithm (momentum = 0.9, weight decay = 0.005). The initial learning rate was 1×10^{-3} and halved by 3000 every training iterations. The hyper parameters were chosen as follows: $\lambda = 0.005$, $\alpha_l = 0.33$, $\alpha_m = 0.67$, and $\alpha_u = 1.0$.

3.4   Test and Evaluation

Our trained models can estimate labels of an arbitrary-sized volumetric image. Given a test volumetric image, we extracted overlapped sub-volume patches with the size of $64 \times 64 \times 64$, and fed them to the trained network to get prediction probability maps. For the overlapped voxels, the final probability maps would be the average of the probability maps of the overlapped patches, which were then used to derive the final segmentation results. After that, we conducted morphological operations to remove isolated small volumes and internal holes as there is only one femur in each test data. When implemented with Python using TensorFlow framework, our network took about 2 min to process one volume with size of $300 \times 200 \times 100$.

The segmented results were compared with the associated ground truth segmentation which was obtained via a semi-automatic segmentation using the commercial software package called Amira[2]. Amira was also used to extract surface models from the automatic segmentation results and the ground truth segmentation. For each test image, we then evaluated the distance between the surface models extracted from different segmentation as well as the volume overlap measurements including DICE overlap coefficient [22], Jaccard coefficient [22], precision and recall.

Table 1. Quantitative evaluation results on testing datasets

ID	Surface distance (mm)			Volume overlap measurement			
	Mean	STD	Hausdorff distance	DICE	Jaccard	Precision	Recall
Pat01	0.17	0.31	3.8	0.989	0.978	0.992	0.985
Pat02	0.27	0.46	5.3	0.986	0.973	0.985	0.987
Pat03	0.19	0.35	4.1	0.987	0.975	0.995	0.979
Pat04	0.23	0.67	13.0	0.987	0.974	0.992	0.982
Pat05	0.12	0.21	4.3	0.989	0.979	0.991	0.988
Pat06	0.14	0.26	4.5	0.990	0.980	0.995	0.985
Pat07	0.41	0.95	7.0	0.978	0.958	0.984	0.973
Pat08	0.39	0.93	5.2	0.981	0.963	0.994	0.968
Pat09	0.12	0.17	11.0	0.990	0.981	0.990	0.990
Pat10	0.15	0.28	5.3	0.988	0.976	0.991	0.984
Average	0.22	–	6.4	0.987	0.974	0.991	0.982

3.5   Results

Table 1 shows the segmentation results using the model trained with partial transfer learning. In comparison with manually annotated ground truth data, our model achieved an average surface distance of 0.22 mm, an average DICE coefficient of 0.987, an average Jaccard index of 0.974, an average precision of 0.991 and an average recall of 0.982. Figure 2 shows a segmentation example and the color-coded error distribution of the segmented surface model.

We also compared the results achieved by using the model with partial transfer learning with the one without partial transfer learning. The results are presented in Table 2, which clearly demonstrate the effectiveness of the partial transfer learning.

---

[2] http://www.amira.com/.

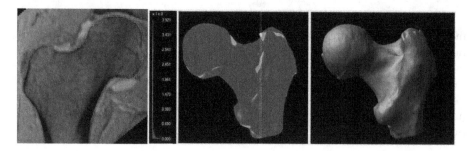

Fig. 2. A segmentation example (left) and the color-coded error distribution of the surface errors (right).

Table 2. Comparison of the average results of the proposed network on the same test dataset when trained with and without transfer learning

Learning method	Surface distance (mm)			Volume overlap measurement			
	Mean	STD	Hausdorff distance	DICE	Jaccard	Precision	Recall
Without transfer learning	0.67	–	12.4	0.975	0.950	0.985	0.964
With transfer learning	0.22	–	6.4	0.987	0.974	0.991	0.982

4   Conclusion

We have introduced a 3D U-net-like fully convolutional network with multi-level deep supervision and successfully applied it to the challenging task of automatic segmentation of proximal femur in MR images. Multi-level deep supervision and partial transfer learning were used in our network to boost the training efficiency when only small set of labeled 3D training data were available. The experimental results demonstrated the efficacy of the proposed network.

Acknowledgment. This study was partially supported by the Swiss National Science Foundation via project 205321_163224/1.

References

1. Laborie, L., Lehmann, T., Engesæter, I., et al.: Prevalence of radiographic findings thought to be associated with femoroacetabular impingement in a population-based cohort of 2081 healthy young adults. Radiology **260**, 494–502 (2011)
2. Leunig, M., Beaulé, P., Ganz, R.: The concept of femoroacetabular impingement: current status and future perspectives. Clin. Orthop. Relat. Res. **467**, 616–622 (2009)
3. Clohisy, J., Knaus, E., Hunt, D.M., et al.: Clinical presentation of patients with symptomatic anterior hip impingement. Clin. Orthop. Relat. Res. **467**, 638–644 (2009)

4. Perdikakis, E., Karachalios, T., Katonis, P., Karantanas, A.: Comparison of MR-arthrography and MDCT-arthrography for detection of labral and articular cartilage hip pathology. Skeletal Radiol. **40**, 1441–1447 (2011)

5. Xia, Y., Fripp, J., Chandra, S., Schwarz, R., Engstrom, C., Crozier, S.: Automated bone segmentation from large field of view 3D MR images of the hip joint. Phys. Med. Biol. **21**, 7375–7390 (2013)

6. Xia, Y., Chandra, S., Engstrom, C., Strudwick, M., Crozier, S., Fripp, J.: Automatic hip cartilage segmentation from 3D MR images using arc-weighted graph searching. Phys. Med. Biol. **59**, 7245–66 (2014)

7. Gilles, B., Magnenat-Thalmann, N.: Musculoskeletal MRI segmentation using multi-resolution simplex meshes with medial representations. Med. Image Anal. **14**, 291–302 (2010)

8. Arezoomand, S., Lee, W.S., Rakhra, K., Beaule, P.: A 3D active model framework for segmentation of proximal femur in MR images. Int. J. CARS **10**, 55–66 (2015)

9. Chandra, S., Xia, Y., Engstrom, C., et al.: Focused shape models for hip joint segmentation in 3D magnetic resonance images. Med. Image Anal. **18**, 567–578 (2014)

10. Krizhevsky, A., Sutskever, I., Hinton, G.: Imagenet classification with deep convolutional neural networks. In: Pereira, F., Burges, C.J.C., Bottou, L., Weinberger, K.Q. (eds.) Advances in Neural Information Processing Systems 25, pp. 1097–1105. Curran Associates, Inc. (2012)

11. Long, J., Shelhamer, E., Darrell, T.: Fully convolutional networks for semantic segmentation. In: Proceedings of the IEEE Conference on Computer Vision and Pattern Recognition (CVPR), pp. 3431–3440 (2015)

12. Prasoon, A., Petersen, K., Igel, C., Lauze, F., Dam, E., Nielsen, M.: Deep Feature Learning for Knee Cartilage Segmentation Using a Triplanar Convolutional Neural Network. In: Mori, K., Sakuma, I., Sato, Y., Barillot, C., Navab, N. (eds.) MICCAI 2013. LNCS, vol. 8150, pp. 246–253. Springer, Heidelberg (2013). doi:10.1007/978-3-642-40763-5_31

13. Çiçek, Ö., Abdulkadir, A., Lienkamp, S.S., Brox, T., Ronneberger, O.: 3D U-Net: Learning Dense Volumetric Segmentation from Sparse Annotation. In: Ourselin, S., Joskowicz, L., Sabuncu, M.R., Unal, G., Wells, W. (eds.) MICCAI 2016. LNCS, vol. 9901, pp. 424–432. Springer, Cham (2016). doi:10.1007/978-3-319-46723-8_49

14. Milletari, F., Navab, N., Ahmadi, S.A.: V-net: fully convolutional neural networks for volumetric medical image segmentation. In: Proceedings of 2016 International Conferece on 3D Vision (3DV), pp. 565–571. IEEE (2016)

15. Dou, Q., Yu, L., Chen, H., Jin, Y., Yang, X., Qin, J., Heng, P.A.: 3D deeply supervised network for automated segmentation of volumetric medical images. Med. Image Anal. **41**, 40–54 (2017)

16. Ioffe, S., Szegedy, C.: Batch normalization: accelerating deep network training by reducing internal covariate shift. In: Proceedings of ICML (2015)

17. Yosinski, J., Clune, J., Bengio, Y., Lipson, H.: How transferable are features in deep neural networks? In: Advances in Neural Information Processing Systems, pp. 3320–3328 (2014)

18. Deng, J., Dong, W., Socher, R., Li, L.J., Li, K., Fei-Fei, L.: ImageNet: a large-scale hierarchical image database. In: CVPR 2009 (2009)

19. Simonyan, K., Zisserman, A.: Very deep convolutional networks for large-scale image recognition. CoRR (2014)

20. Szegedy, C., Liu, W., Jia, Y., et al.: Going deeper with convolutions. In: CVPR 2015, pp. 1–9. IEEE (2015)

21. Tran, D., Bourdev, L., Fergus, R., Torresani, L., Paluri, M.: Learning spatiotem-poral features with 3D convolutional networks. In: Proceedings of the IEEE Inter-national Conference on Computer Vision (CVPR), pp. 4489–4497 (2015)
22. Karasawa, K., Oda, M., Kitasakab, T., et al.: Multi-atlas pancreas segmentation: Atlas selection based on vessel structure. Med. Image Anal. **39**, 18–28 (2017)

Indecisive Trees for Classification and Prediction of Knee Osteoarthritis

Luca Minciullo[1]([✉]), Paul A. Bromiley[1], David T. Felson[2],
and Timothy F. Cootes[1]

[1] The University of Manchester, Manchester, UK
luca.minciullo@manchester.ac.uk
[2] ARUK Epidemiology Unit, The University of Manchester, Manchester, UK

Abstract. Random forests are widely used for classification and regression tasks in medical image analysis. Each tree in the forest contains binary decision nodes that choose whether a sample should be passed to one of two child nodes. We demonstrate that replacing this with something less decisive, where some samples may go to both child nodes, can improve performance for both individual trees and whole forests. Introducing a soft decision at each node means that a sample may propagate to multiple leaves. The tree output should thus be a weighted sum of the individual leaf values. We show how the leaves can be optimised to improve performance and how backpropagation can be used to optimise the parameters of the decision functions at each node. Finally, we show that the new method outperforms an equivalent random forest on a disease classification and prediction task.

Keywords: Random forests · Decision trees · Optimisation

1 Introduction

Decision trees, particularly in the form of Random Forests, are widely used in medical image analysis for tasks such as landmark localisation [5], segmentation [8] and classification [6,7]. In most cases each tree uses hard decision nodes, a threshold on a feature response derived from the input, in which a sample is channelled either to the left or right child node. Thus one input sample ends up at exactly one leaf, which holds the output for the tree.

A natural extension is to replace this binary decision with something softer, so that a sample can go down both branches, but with different weights or probabilities depending on the feature response at the node. An early example of this approach was "Fuzzy Decision Trees" [9] in which a sigmoidal function was used to assign a weight to be passed down each child branch. The approach was extended in [4], where a forest of such trees was integrated into a deep network allowing end-to-end training. However, one problem with using a sigmoidal transfer function is that every input effectively ends up at every leaf of the tree with a non-zero weight, though at most leaves the weight may be very close to zero. This is potentially very inefficient for deep trees.

© Springer International Publishing AG 2017
Q. Wang et al. (Eds.): MLMI 2017, LNCS 10541, pp. 283–290, 2017.
DOI: 10.1007/978-3-319-67389-9_33

In this paper we introduce trees in which only samples near the decision boundary are propagated to both children; most samples only go to one child. This is equivalent to using a simple, sloped step function to compute the weights. Each input is then propagated to a relatively small number of leaves. This allows the use of deep trees whilst retaining most of the efficiency of binary decision trees. We describe the approach in detail, including a greedy method for training a tree. As with fuzzy trees, both the values stored at the leaf nodes and the parameters of the transfer functions can be optimised using either closed form or gradient descent approaches, leading to better performance than that from the greedy training. We demonstrate that replacing random forests with these more indecisive trees leads to improvements in overall performance on a classification task. We show the improvement in performance of our methodology on Osteoarthritis (OA) classification and prediction tasks. OA is the most common form of arthritis, affecting millions of people around the world, the chance of developing the disease being particularly high in older people. The most common signs of OA are osteophytes, bony spurs that grow on the bones of the spine or around the joints, joint space narrowing (JSN), and calcium deposits. We train our trees to use features that measure the shape and appearance of the knee in radiographs, to classify OA status and predict who is at risk of developing the disease.

2   Background

Random Forests are a very successful machine learning ensemble model, where each of the sub-models is a binary decision tree. The randomness comes from two main sources. First, each of the decision trees is trained on a different sample of the original dataset, obtained by generating multiple bootstrap samples. Second, the optimal split is found by considering only a random subset of the features appearing in the data.

Ren et al. [8] showed how the leaves of a forest could be mutually optimised to give better performance than that of a forest with independent trees. Fuzzy decision trees, which can be optimised by a backpropagation-like algorithm, were introduced in [9]. They proposed training a tree in the normal way, then replacing the binary decision threshold with a sigmoidal function to indicate branch membership, the parameters of which could then be optimised. Kontschieder et al. [4] extended this idea to full decision forests, using a sigmoidal decision function. They too used a stochastic gradient descent approach to optimise the parameters of the decision nodes and the leaves. The decisions at each node were based on the output of one node of a deep convolutional network, making the entire system amenable to end-to-end training.

When using a sigmoidal function for branch membership, every sample ends up being propagated to every leaf of the tree, even though at some leaves the membership value may be very small. This may lead to inefficiencies for deep trees. To overcome this we use a ramp function for the membership propagation

$$\pi(\mathbf{x}; t_0, t_1) = \begin{cases} 0 & \text{if} & f(\mathbf{x}) \leq t_0 \\ \frac{(f(\mathbf{x}) - t_0)}{(t_1 - t_0)} & \text{if} & t_0 < f(\mathbf{x}) < t_1 \\ 1 & \text{if} & f(\mathbf{x}) \geq t_1 \end{cases} \tag{1}$$

where $f(\mathbf{x})$ is a feature derived from the input $\mathbf{x}$ and $t_0 < t_1$ are two thresholds defining the ramp function. Thus, if the membership for either branch is zero, we do not need to propagate down that branch. During training we choose the thresholds so that a given proportion of the training samples are in the ambiguous region (see below).

2.1 Evaluating the Result from a Tree

An indecisive tree is a collection of decision nodes and leaf nodes. Each decision node has two child nodes (left and right), a function that computes a scalar feature value from the input $f(\mathbf{x})$, and two threshold values defining the transfer function, t_0, t_1. Each leaf node contains an output value. When an input, $\mathbf{x}$, is evaluated with the tree, the output is a set of leaf values and associated weights, $\mathcal{S} = \{(\mathbf{v}_i, w_i)\}$. Starting at the root node, we propagate an input through the nodes, exploring only the branches with non-zero weights. Each node either adds its value (if it is a leaf) to a set of outputs, or it propagates the input and weight to one or both of its child nodes. This can be computed with a recursive function, starting at the root node with a unit weight: $\mathcal{S} = \text{EVALUATE}(\text{root}, (\mathbf{x}, 1.0), \{\})$. The function is defined as follows:

```
 1: function EVALUATE(node, (x, w), S)
 2:     if node.isLeaf then
 3:         S ← {S, (node.value, w)}
 4:     else
 5:         μ = π(node.f(x), node.t₀, node.t₁)
 6:         wL = (1 − μ)w
 7:         wR = μw
 8:         if wL < wR then
 9:             if (wL < wt) then wL ← 0, wR ← w
10:         else
11:             if (wR < wt) then wR ← 0, wL ← w
12:         end if
13:         if (wL > 0) S ←EVALUATE(node.leftChild, (x, wL), S)
14:         if (wR > 0) S ←EVALUATE(node.rightChild, (x, wR), S)
15:     end if
16: return S
17: end function
```

The tests in lines 8–12 allow a threshold (w_t) to be enforced on the smallest allowable weight. If a split would cause the weight propagated to one child node to fall below the threshold, then that child node is ignored and all the weight is passed to the other child. Setting $w_t > 0$ ensures that no leaf is reached with a weight lower than w_t, and focuses processing on the branches with higher weights. It thus also limits the maximum number of leaves that can be returned to w_t^{-1}. The output of the tree can then be computed from S as the weighted sum of the leaf outputs, $\mathbf{v} = \sum_i w_i \mathbf{v}_i$.

3   Training and Optimising Indecisive Trees

In a similar way to training a normal decision tree, an indecisive tree is trained using a greedy recursive algorithm in which each node finds a feature and threshold to split the data arriving at it so as to minimise a cost function. During training a sample consists of a triplet, $(\mathbf{x}, \mathbf{y}, w)$, containing the input vector, the target output and a weight. To train a node, we consider the set of n samples $\mathcal{D}$ arriving from the parent node. To evaluate a particular choice of feature, $f(\mathbf{x})$, and thresholds t_0, t_1, we compute the sets of data $\mathcal{D}_L$ and $\mathcal{D}_R$ that would be propagated to the child nodes, and the cost function

$$C(f, t_0, t_1) = C(\mathcal{D}_L) + C(\mathcal{D}_R) \tag{2}$$

The cost $C(\mathcal{D})$ depends on the task. For instance, for regression, it can be the sum-of-squared differences. A random selection of features and possible thresholds is evaluated, and those giving the lowest cost retained.

Since finding the optimal pair of thresholds can be computationally expensive, we use the following approach. For each input $(\mathbf{x}_i, \mathbf{y}_i, w_i)$ we compute the feature value $f_i = f(\mathbf{x}_i)$, then rank the samples using this value. Let $(\mathbf{x}_j, \mathbf{y}_j, w_j)$ be the jth sample in this ranked list. By computing running sums through this ranked data we can efficiently locate the index, k, for the hard split leading to the lowest total cost (all samples $j \leq k$ are sent to one child, all $j > k$ to the other). We then introduce an ambiguous region to include a proportion of approximately $r \in [0, 1]$ of the samples by setting $j0 = \max(1, k - 0.5rn)$, $j1 = \min(n, k + 0.5rn)$, and selecting $t_0 = f_{j0}, t_1 = f_{j1}$.

Since the samples in the ambiguous region will go to both children, the total number of samples propagated from nodes at depth d will be approximately $n_0 \cdot (1 + r)^d$, where n_0 is the original number of training examples, though it should be remembered that the total weight for each of the original samples will always sum to unity. In order to avoid propagating large numbers of samples with small weights, we use the same technique as described above (Sect. 2.1). If a sample weight would fall below w_t when propagated to one child node, we ignore that child and propagate all the sample weight to the other child. Decision nodes are added in a recursive manner until a suitable stopping condition (a maximum depth, minimum number of samples or measure of spread) is reached. The values at the leaf nodes can then be set to the weighted mean of the samples reaching that node, for instance for regression, the value

$$\mathbf{t} = \left(\sum w_i \mathbf{y}_i \right) / \left(\sum w_i \right) \tag{3}$$

3.1 Optimising the Leaf Values

A tree with vector output can be expressed as a function of input $\mathbf{x}$

$$\mathbf{y} = \mathbf{V}\mathbf{w}(\mathbf{x}) \tag{4}$$

where $\mathbf{V}$ is a matrix whose columns are all the leaf vectors, and $\mathbf{w}(\mathbf{x})$ is the sparse vector of weights returned by the tree, which selects the leaves to which $\mathbf{x}$ in propagated. Thus the outputs corresponding to the training inputs can be expressed as

$$\mathbf{Y} = \mathbf{V}\mathbf{W} \tag{5}$$

where $\mathbf{Y} = (\mathbf{y}_1|...|\mathbf{y}_n)$ and $\mathbf{W} = (\mathbf{w}(\mathbf{x}_1)|...|\mathbf{w}(\mathbf{x}_n))$ is a sparse matrix.

For regression, as in [8], the leaf values can be found by minimising

$$Q(\mathbf{V}) = ||\mathbf{V}\mathbf{W} - \mathbf{Y}||_2 + \alpha||\mathbf{V}||_2 \tag{6}$$

where α is an optional ridge regression regularisation function. Since $\mathbf{W}$ is sparse the solution can be found efficiently with conjugate gradient descent.

3.2 Optimising the Decision Nodes

If the leaf values are fixed, each decision node only affects the final output through the way it changes the weights on the samples passing through it. As in [4,9] we can use a gradient descent-based backpropagation algorithm to optimise the parameters. However, in our case, since each sample only passes through a small subset of nodes, this can be significantly more efficient, as we only have to compute values at the nodes visited. The cost function to be minimised is of the form

$$Q_T(\theta; \{(\mathbf{x}_i, \mathbf{y}_i)\}) = \sum_i Q(\mathbf{V}\mathbf{w}(\mathbf{x}_i, \theta), \mathbf{y}_i) \tag{7}$$

where θ are the parameters affecting the weights and $Q(\mathbf{t}, \mathbf{y})$ is the cost function comparing the output of the tree, $\mathbf{t} = \mathbf{V}\mathbf{w}(\mathbf{x}, \theta)$ with the target output $\mathbf{y}$.

Gradient at leaf nodes: The contribution to the output from a single leaf node is given by $w\mathbf{v}$, where w is the weight of the sample arriving at the leaf. For one leaf (see Fig. 1),

$$\frac{dQ}{dw} = \frac{dQ}{dt}\frac{dt}{dw} = \mathbf{v}^T\frac{dQ}{dt} \tag{8}$$

Gradient at decision nodes: At a decision node, the weights passed to the output nodes are given by

$$\begin{pmatrix} w_L \\ w_R \end{pmatrix} = w \begin{pmatrix} 1 - \pi(f, t_0, t_1) \\ \pi(f, t_0, t_1) \end{pmatrix} \tag{9}$$

If the parameters at the decision nodes are θ, then

$$\begin{aligned} \frac{dQ}{d\theta} &= \frac{dw_R}{d\theta}\frac{dQ}{dw_R} + \frac{dw_L}{d\theta}\frac{dQ}{dw_L} \\ &= w\frac{d\pi}{d\theta}\frac{dQ}{dw_R} - w\frac{d\pi}{d\theta}\frac{dQ}{dw_L} \\ &= w\frac{d\pi}{d\theta}\left(\frac{dQ}{dw_R} - \frac{dQ}{dw_L}\right) \end{aligned} \tag{10}$$

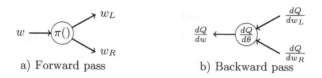

a) Forward pass   b) Backward pass

Fig. 1. During the forward pass (root to leaves), weights are calculated. During the backward pass (leaves to root), gradients are calculated.

Similarly

$$\frac{dQ}{dw} = \pi(\theta)\frac{dQ}{dw_R} + (1 - \pi(\theta))\frac{dQ}{dw_L} \tag{11}$$

During the backward pass we use (10) to compute the gradient w.r.t. the thresholds t_0 and t_1. In the experiments below we keep the features fixed, but it would also be possible to compute gradients of any parameters of the features.

We use the following algorithm to update the parameters of each node (t_0, t_1):

1: **function** UPDATENODES($\mathcal{X} = \{(\mathbf{x}_i, \mathbf{y}_i)\}$)
2:     **for all x in** $\mathcal{X}$ **do**
3:         Feed **x** forward through tree to calculate weights
4:         Visit each node in reverse depth order - compute gradients
5:         Update estimate of mean gradient over batch
6:     **end for**
7:     Update parameters using mean gradient
8: **end function**

In the following the parameter update is made using a momentum term, but something more sophisticated could be used.

4   Experiments

Here we focus on two classification tasks related to knee osteoarthritis. The features used were shape, texture and appearance parameters extracted from lateral knee radiographic images (Fig. 2). Those features were obtained by first building a statistical appearance model [1] of the knee. This model was a PCA-based combination of statistical shape and texture models and was built on fully automated annotations found using a 3-stage Constrained Local Model [2].

Data. The images were taken from the Multicentre Osteoarthritis Study (MOST) dataset [3]. MOST is a longitudinal prospective study that collected data from 3026 participants with a 7-year follow-up. Lateral radiographs have been collected at each time-point for both knees and a KL (Kellgren-Lawrence) grade assessing the severity of the disease was assigned to each knee. For our binary classification tasks the grades were split into two groups: non-OA, KL (0,1), and the OA group, KL(2–4). The first task was OA classification, where the goal was to distinguish patients from the two groups, and used 8606 OA ($KL \geq 2$) and 10604 non-OA images. In the second task we considered 3478

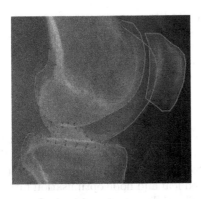
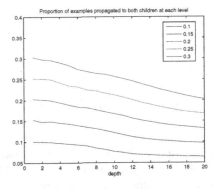

Fig. 2. An example of the landmark points used to build the appearance model (Left). Proportion of examples within the indecisive window at each level for different choices for window width (Right).

baseline images with no OA ($KL \leq 1$) and aimed to discriminate those that would develop OA within 84 months from those that would not.

Knee OA classification tasks. We compared the performance of our Indecisive Forest (IF) with a standard Random Forest (RF) in 5-fold CV experiments. A parameter sweep suggested that a good choice for the parameter responsible for the width of indecision window was $r = 0.3$. In addition, we applied the tuning algorithm described above to optimise the IF, and evaluated the performance. We report the area under the ROC curve to evaluate each of the models in Table 1. This shows that for both classification tasks the IF performed better than a standard Random Forest, with an improvement of at least 2% for both classification and prediction. The optimisation improved the results for the OA classification task, while the OA prediction performance did not change significantly. Our results on both tasks achieved the state-of-the-art on the MOST dataset using only lateral knee radiographs (compared to [7]).

Figure 2 (Right) shows that the proportion of examples within the indecisive region increases when the window width increases and decreases linearly as examples go deeper in the trees.

Table 1. AUC for the two knee OA tasks: comparing a standard Random Forest with both an Indecisive Forest (IF) and an Optimised Indecisive Forest (OIF).

	OA classification	OA prediction
Baseline forest	86.35 ± 0.99	59.03 ± 1.20
IF	87.61 ± 0.94	$\mathbf{61.11 \pm 1.79}$
OIF	$\mathbf{88.15 \pm 0.91}$	59.11 ± 2.01

Timings. The average time to train a standard tree on the prediction dataset was 9.3 s, compared to 94.9 s for each indecisive tree. The average tree optimisation time depended on the dataset and the parameter choice, ranging from 3 s to 2 min. There was little difference in time taken when applying the trees.

5   Discussion and Conclusions

We have presented an improvement on the standard random forest that uses a ramp function with an ambiguous region to train and test decision trees. We showed improved performance, compared to a standard Random Forest, on two OA-related classification tasks. The combined leaf and node optimisation further improved the results on one of the tasks. The indecisive forests take longer to train and optimise. Pilot experiments on regression tasks have shown small but encouraging improvements, something that we will explore in future work.

Acknowledgments. The research leading to this results has received funding from EPSRC Centre for Doctoral Training grant 1512584. This publication also presents independent research supported by the Health Innovation Challenge Fund (grant no. HICF-R7-414/WT100936), a parallel funding partnership between the Department of Health and Wellcome Trust, and by the NIHR Invention for Innovation (i4i) programme (grant no. II-LB_0216-20009). The views expressed are those of the authors and not necessarily those of the NHS, NIHR, the Department of Health or Wellcome Trust.

References

1. Cootes, T.F., Taylor, C.J., et al.: Statistical models of appearance for computer vision (2004)
2. Cristinacce, D., Cootes, T.F.: Feature detection and tracking with constrained local models. In: BMVC (2006)
3. Felson, D., Niu, J., Neogi, T., Goggins, J., Nevitt, M., Roemer, F., Torner, J., Lewis, C., Guermazi, A., Group, M.I.: Synovitis and the risk of knee osteoarthritis: the MOST study. Osteoarthritis Cartilage **24**(3), 458–464 (2016)
4. Kontschieder, P., Fiterau, M., Criminisi, A., Bulo, S.: Deep neural decision forests. In: International Conference on Computer Vision (2015)
5. Lindner, C., Bromiley, P., Ionita, M., Cootes, T.: Robust and accurate shape model matching using random forest regression-voting. IEEE Trans. Pattern Anal. Mach. Intell. **37**(9), 1862–1874 (2015)
6. Minciullo, L., Cootes, T.F.: Fully automated shape analysis for detection of osteoarthritis from lateral knee radiographs. In: ICPR (2016)
7. Minciullo, L., Thomson, J., Cootes, T.F.: Combination of lateral and PA view radiographs to study development of knee OA and associated pain. In: SPIE Medical Imaging, p. 1013411. International Society for Optics and Photonics (2017)
8. Ren, S., Cao, X., Wei, Y., Sun, J.: Global refinement of random forest. In: Computer Vision and Pattern Recognition (2015)
9. Suarez, A., Lutsko, J.: Globally optimal fuzzy decision trees for classification and regression. IEEE Trans. Pattern Anal. Mach. Intell. **21**(12), 1297–1311 (1999)

Whole Brain Segmentation and Labeling from CT Using Synthetic MR Images

Can Zhao[1]([✉]), Aaron Carass[1], Junghoon Lee[2], Yufan He[1], and Jerry L. Prince[1]

[1] Department of Electrical and Computer Engineering,
The Johns Hopkins University, Baltimore, MD 21218, USA
czhao20@jhu.edu
[2] Department of Radiation Oncology, The Johns Hopkins School of Medicine,
Baltimore, MD 21287, USA

Abstract. To achieve whole-brain segmentation—i.e., classifying tissues within and immediately around the brain as gray matter (GM), white matter (WM), and cerebrospinal fluid—magnetic resonance (MR) imaging is nearly always used. However, there are many clinical scenarios where computed tomography (CT) is the only modality that is acquired and yet whole brain segmentation (and labeling) is desired. This is a very challenging task, primarily because CT has poor soft tissue contrast; very few segmentation methods have been reported to date and there are no reports on automatic labeling. This paper presents a whole brain segmentation and labeling method for non-contrast CT images that first uses a fully convolutional network (FCN) to synthesize an MR image from a CT image and then uses the synthetic MR image in a standard pipeline for whole brain segmentation and labeling. The FCN was trained on image patches derived from ten co-registered MR and CT images and the segmentation and labeling method was tested on sixteen CT scans in which co-registered MR images are available for performance evaluation. Results show excellent MR image synthesis from CT images and improved soft tissue segmentation and labeling over a multi-atlas segmentation approach.

Keywords: Synthesis · MR · CT · Deep learning · CNN · FCN U-net · Segmentation

1 Introduction

Computed tomography (CT) imaging of the head has many clinical and scientific uses including visualization and assessment of head injuries, intracranial bleeding, aneurysms, tumors, headaches, and dizziness as well as for use in surgical planning. Yet due to the poor soft tissue contrast in CT images, magnetic resonance imaging (MRI) is almost exclusively used for localizing, characterizing, and labeling gray matter (GM) and white matter (WM) structures in the brain. Unfortunately, there are many scenarios in which only CT images are available—e.g., emergency situations, lack of an MR scanner, patient implants

© Springer International Publishing AG 2017
Q. Wang et al. (Eds.): MLMI 2017, LNCS 10541, pp. 291–298, 2017.
DOI: 10.1007/978-3-319-67389-9_34

or claustrophobia, and cost of obtaining an MR scan—and there is no approach to provide whole brain segmentation and labeling from these data.

There has been very limited work on GM/WM segmentation from CT images. A whole brain segmentation method for 4D contrast-enhanced CT based on a nonlinear support vector machine was recently published [12]. The authors point out that a key part of their method is the formation of a 3D image derived from all of the temporal acquisitions. The segmentation result is impressive, but it is not clear that their method will work on conventional 3D CT data. As well, their method only provides classification of GM, WM, and CSF and does not label the sub-cortical GM or cortical gyri. The authors of [12] provide an excellent summary of much of the previous work on GM/WM segmentation from non-contrast CT (cf. [6,8,10,15]), and also point out the limitations of past approaches. It is clearly an area of investigation that deserves more research. In contrast to the situation in CT, GM/WM segmentation and labeling from MRI has been well studied and several excellent approaches exist (cf. [5,9,14,18]). Thus, it is natural to wonder whether images that are synthesized from CT to look like MR images could be used for automatic segmentation and labeling; this is precisely what we propose.

Image synthesis methods provide intensity transformations between two image contrasts or modalities (cf. [1–3,11,17]). Previously reported image synthesis work has synthesized CT from MRI [1], T_2-weighted (T_2-w) from T_1-weighted (T_1-w) [3], and positron emission tomography (PET) from MRI [11]. In very recent work, Cao et al. [2] synthesized pelvic T_1-w images from CT using a random forest and showed improvement in cross-modal registration. Some researchers have applied convolutional neural networks (CNNs) to synthesis (cf. [11]) yet Cao et al. [2] claimed that robust and accurate synthesis of MR from CT using a CNN is not feasible. We believe that because CNNs are resilient to intensity variations [4] and they can model highly nonlinear mappings, they are ideal for CT-to-MR synthesis. In fact, we demonstrate in this paper that such synthesis is indeed possible and that whole brain segmentation and labeling from these synthetic images is very effective.

2   Methods

Training and Testing Data. Twenty six patients had (T_1-w) MR images acquired using a Siemens Magnetom Espree 1.5 T scanner (Siemens Medical Solutions, Malvern, PA) with geometric distortions corrected within the Siemens Syngo console workstation. The MR images were processed with N4 to remove any bias field and subsequently had their intensity scales adjusted to align their WM peaks. Contemporaneous CT images were obtained on a Philips Brilliance Big Bore scanner (Philips Medical Systems, Netherlands) under a routine clinical protocol for brain cancer patients treated with either stereotactic-body radiation therapy (SBRT) or radiosurgery (SRS). The CT images were resampled to have the same digital resolution as the MR images, which is $0.7 \times 0.7 \times 1$ mm. Then the MR images were rigidly registered to the CT images.

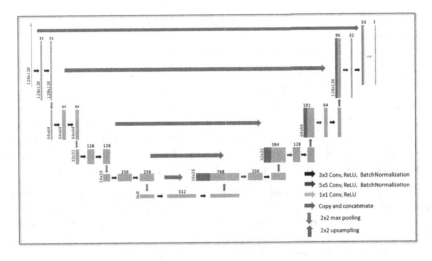

Fig. 1. Our modified U-net with four levels of contraction and expansion.

We use ten patient image pairs as training data for our CNN (see below). For each axial slice in the image domain, twenty-five 128 × 128 paired (CT and MR) image patches are extracted. The 128 × 128 patches can be thought of as subdividing the slice into a 5 × 5 grid with overlap between the image patches. These patch pairs are used to train an FCN based on a modified U-net [16] that will synthesize MR patches from CT patches. The synthetic MR patches are then used to construct an axial slice of the synthetic MR image. Our FCN, with 128 × 128 CT patches as input and 128 × 128 synthetic MR patches as output, is shown in Fig. 1.

FCN Algorithm for CT-to-MR Synthesis. The mapping between CT and MR is too nonlinear to be modeled accurately by the shallow features used in a random forest, which is why we explore a CNN based approach. As the mapping between CT and MR is dependent on anatomical structures, it makes intuitive sense that any CNN synthesis model should incorporate the ideas of semantic segmentation, for which fully convolutional networks (FCNs) were designed. Additionally, having already sacrificed some resolution in bringing the CT into alignment with MR, we want to be careful to not further degrade the image quality. Thus, we have selected as the basis of our FCN the U-net [16], which can achieve state-of-the-art performance for semantic segmentation and preserve high resolution information throughout the contraction-expansion layers of the network.

The encoder follows the typical architecture of a CNN. Each step contains two 3 × 3 convolutional layers, activated by a rectified linear unit (ReLU), and a 2 × 2 max pooling operation for downsampling. In the decoder, each step contains a 2 × 2 upsampling layer followed by a 5 × 5 convolutional layer and a

3×3 convolutional layer. The two convolutional layers are activated by ReLU. And the final layer is a 1×1 convolutional layer.

This FCN has four differences from the standard U-net.

Modification 1: the U-net decoder has two 3×3 layers, whereas we use one 5×5 layer and one 3×3 layer. We do this because the upsampling layer is simply repeating values in a 2×2 window. Thus, a 3×3 layer in the encoder can involve its eight connected neighbors, whereas a 3×3 layer after an upsampling layer only includes three-connected neighbors. By replacing this with a 5×5 layer, we can still involve all eight connected neighbors. There is a slight increase in the number of parameters to estimate, but the result has better accuracy.

Modification 2: CNN vision tasks benefit from increasing model depth; however, deeper models can have vanishing or exploding gradients [7]. In the original U-net, the decoder contains an upsampling layer, a convolutional layer, a layer merging it with high resolution representations, and another convolutional layer. Thus, the upsampled layer is convolved twice while the high resolution representation is convolved only once. We therefore exchange the order of the first convolutional layer and the merging layer so that both are convolved twice. With this change, we retain the same number of layers but our FCN can model greater non-linearity without introducing additional obstacles for back-propagation.

Modification 3: Every convolution loses border pixels; thus, the border of the predicted patch may not be as reliable as the center. The standard U-net crops each patch after each convolutional layer so that the predicted patch is smaller than the input patch. Our FCN keeps the boundary pixels instead of cropping them. However, when reconstructing a slice we use only the central 90×90 region of the image patches (except at the boundaries of the image, where we retain the side of the patch that touches the boundary).

Modification 4: U-net was used for solving segmentation, while synthesis is a regression task. That is, U-net only needed labels to distinguish edges, while we need to predict intensity values. Thus the batch normalization layers which are throughout U-net are a concern; there is no effect on image contrast but absolute intensity values are lost and CT numbers have a physical meaning. In order to include this information, we merge the original CT patches before the last convolutional layer. Also, U-net used softmax to activate the last layer for segmentation, while we use ReLU for regression.

Automatic Whole-Brain Segmentation and Labeling. We use MALP-EM [9] to provide whole-brain segmentation and labeling from the synthetic MR images. Since the synthetic MR images are naturally registered with the CT images, the result is a segmentation and labeling of the CT images. MALP-EM uses an atlas cohort of 30 subjects having both MR images and labels from the OASIS database [13]. These atlases are deformably registered to the target and the labels are combined using joint label fusion (JLF) [18]. Finally, these labels are adjusted using an intensity based EM method to provide additional robustness to pathology, especially traumatic brain injury. We used the code that has been made freely available by the original authors of the method.

3   Experiments and Results

Image Synthesis. Our FCN was trained on 45,575 128 × 128 image patch pairs derived from ten of the co-registered MR and CT images. It took two days to train and 1 min to synthesize one MR image from the input CT on a NVIDIA GPU GTX1070SC. Figures 2(a)–(c) show an example input CT image, the resulting synthetic T1-w, and the ground truth T1-w, respectively.

Experiment 1: MALP-EM Segmentation. We applied MALP-EM on both synthetic and ground truth T1-w images. Figure 2(e) shows the segmentation result from the synthetic T1-w in Fig. 2(b), while Fig. 2(f) shows the result from the ground truth T1-w in Fig. 2(c). There are differences between the two results, but this is the first result showing such a detailed labeling of CT brain images. We compute Dice coefficients between segmentation results obtained using synthetic T1-w and those obtained using the true T1-w. Here are mean Dice coefficients for a few brain structures. For hippocampus, they are 0.62 (right) and 0.59 (left); for precentral gyrus, they are 0.52 (right) and 0.55 (left); for postcentral gyrus, they are 0.51 (right) and 0.52 (left); and for caudate, they are

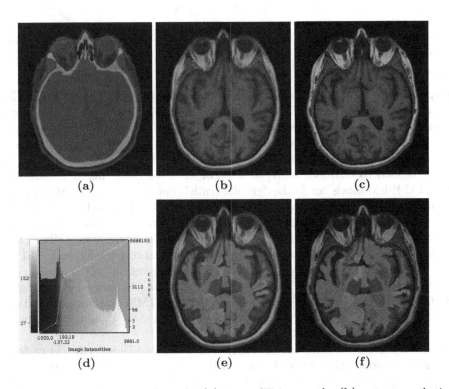

Fig. 2. For one subject, we show the (**a**) input CT image, the (**b**) output synthetic T1-w, and the (**c**) ground truth T1-w image. (**d**) is the dynamic range of (**a**). Shown in (**e**) and (**f**) are the MALP-EM segmentations of the synthetic and ground truth T1-w images, respectively.

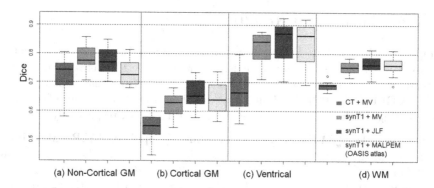

Fig. 3. With MALP-EM processing of the ground truth T1-w as the reference, we compute the Dice coefficient between multi-atlas segmentations using either the subject CT images with MV label fusion (red), or synthetic T1-w with MV (green) or JLF (blue), as the label fusion, and MALP-EM (yellow). Note that MALP-EM uses the OASIS atlas with manually delineated labels, while the other three use the remaining 15 images with MALP-EM computed labels from the true T1-w images as atlases. (Color figure online)

0.70 (right) and 0.73 (left). After merging the labels, box plots of the Dice coefficients for four labels: non-cortical GM, cortical GM, ventricles, and WM, are shown in Fig. 3 (yellow).

Experiment 2: Comparison to Direct Multi-atlas Segmentation. To demonstrate the benefits of our approach, we carried out a set of algorithm comparisons. Ideally, we would like to evaluate how well our CT images could be labeled directly from the OASIS atlases; but there are no CT data associated with OASIS. Instead, we used the 16 subjects (which do not overlap the 10 subjects used to train our FCN) in a set of leave-one-out experiments and let the MALP-EM labels act as the "ground truth". For each of the 16 subjects, we used the remaining 15 (having T1-w and MALP-EM labels) as atlases. To mimic the desired experiment, we first carried out multi-modal registration from each of the 15 T1-w atlases to the target CT using mutual information (MI) as the registration cost metric. Because this is a multi-modal registration task, JLF is not available to combine labels, so we used majority voting (MV) instead. We next computed a synthetic T1-w image from the target CT image and registered each atlas to this target using mean squared error (MSE) as the registration metric. To provide a richer comparison, we combined these 15 labels using both MV and JLF.

Given these three leave-one-out results, we computed Dice coefficient on four labels: non-cortical GM, cortical GM, ventricles, and WM. The results are shown in Fig. 3 (using the red, green, and blue graphics). We can see that use of the synthetic T1-w is significantly better than using the original CT images whether labels are combined with either MV or JLF. JLF seems to provide somewhat better performance.

4   Discussion and Conclusion

The synthetic images that we achieve with FCN are quite good visually as demonstrated by the single (typical) example shown here (Fig. 2(b)), visually much better than those shown in Cao et al. [2] (their Fig. 7). This speaks very well to the potential of the FCN architecture for estimating synthetic cross-modality images. Besides whole-brain segmentation and labeling, there are a host of other potential applications for these images.

A limitation of our evaluation is our lack of manual brain labels in a CT dataset, as it would be interesting to compare our approach with a top multi-atlas segmentation algorithm that would use only CT data. The fact that our method appears to perform worse than the straight multi-atlas results in Fig. 3 is because the MALP-EM result is using manually delineated OASIS labels to estimate automatically generated MALP-EM labels, whereas the other two approaches are estimating MALP-EM labels from MALP-EM atlases. In the future, a more thorough evaluation including a quantitative comparison with Cao et al. [2] is warranted.

Recent research on contrast-enhanced 4D CT brain segmentation achieves slightly higher mean Dice than ours, with 0.81 and 0.79 for WM and GM [12], compared to ours as 0.77 and 0.76. However, because their data was 4D CT, its combined 3D image probably has lower noise and also enables them to use temporal features which we do not have. Furthermore, theirs was a contrast CT study while ours is a non-contrast study.

In summary, we have used a modified U-net to synthesize $T1$-w images from CT, and then directly segmented the synthetic $T1$-w using either MALP-EM or a multi-atlas label fusion scheme. Our results show that using synthetic MR can significantly improve the segmentation over using the CT image directly. This is the first paper to provide GM anatomical labels on a CT neuroimage. Also, despite previous assertions that CT-to-MR synthesis is impossible from CNNs, we show that it is not only possible but it can be done with sufficient quality to open up new clinical and scientific opportunities in neuroimaging.

Acknowledgments. This work was supported by NIH/NIBIB under grant R01 EB017743.

References

1. Burgos, N., Cardoso, M.J., Thielemans, K., Modat, M., Pedemonte, S., Dickson, J., Barnes, A., Ahmed, R., Mahoney, C.J., Schott, J.M., et al.: Attenuation correction synthesis for hybrid PET-MR scanners: application to brain studies. IEEE Trans. Med. Imag. **33**(12), 2332–2341 (2014)
2. Cao, X., Yang, J., Gao, Y., Guo, Y., Wu, G., Shen, D.: Dual-core steered non-rigid registration for multi-modal images via bi-directional image synthesis. Med. Image Anal. (2017, in press)
3. Chen, M., Carass, A., Jog, A., Lee, J., Roy, S., Prince, J.L.: Cross contrast multi-channel image registration using image synthesis for MR brain images. Med. Image Anal. **36**, 2–14 (2017)

4. Dodge, S., Karam, L.: Understanding how image quality affects deep neural networks. In: 2016 Eighth International Conference on Quality of Multimedia Experience (QoMEX), pp. 1–6. IEEE (2016)
5. Fischl, B.: Freesurfer. Neuroimage **62**(2), 774–781 (2012)
6. Gupta, V., Ambrosius, W., Qian, G., Blazejewska, A., Kazmierski, R., Urbanik, A., Nowinski, W.L.: Automatic segmentation of cerebrospinal fluid, white and gray matter in unenhanced computed tomography images. Acad. Radiol. **17**(11), 1350–1358 (2010)
7. He, K., Zhang, X., Ren, S., Sun, J.: Deep residual learning for image recognition. In: Proceedings of the IEEE Conference on Computer Vision and Pattern Recognition, pp. 770–778 (2016)
8. Hu, Q., Qian, G., Aziz, A., Nowinski, W.L.: Segmentation of brain from computed tomography head images. In: 27th Annual International Conference of the Engineering in Medicine and Biology Society, IEEE-EMBS 2005, pp. 3375–3378. IEEE (2006)
9. Kamnitsas, K., Ledig, C., Newcombe, V.F., Simpson, J.P., Kane, A.D., Menon, D.K., Rueckert, D., Glocker, B.: Efficient multi-scale 3D CNN with fully connected CRF for accurate brain lesion segmentation. Med. Image Anal. **36**, 61–78 (2017)
10. Kemmling, A., Wersching, H., Berger, K., Knecht, S., Groden, C., Nölte, I.: Decomposing the hounsfield unit. Clin. Neuroradiol. **22**(1), 79–91 (2012)
11. Li, R., Zhang, W., Suk, H.-I., Wang, L., Li, J., Shen, D., Ji, S.: Deep learning based imaging data completion for improved brain disease diagnosis. In: Golland, P., Hata, N., Barillot, C., Hornegger, J., Howe, R. (eds.) MICCAI 2014. LNCS, vol. 8675, pp. 305–312. Springer, Cham (2014). doi:10.1007/978-3-319-10443-0_39
12. Manniesing, R., Oei, M.T., Oostveen, L.J., Melendez, J., Smit, E.J., Platel, B., Sánchez, C.I., Meijer, F.J., Prokop, M., van Ginneken, B.: White matter and gray matter segmentation in 4D computed tomography. Sci. Rep. **7** (2017)
13. Marcus, D.S., Wang, T.H., Parker, J., Csernansky, J.G., Morris, J.C., Buckner, R.L.: Open access series of imaging studies (OASIS): cross-sectional MRI data in young, middle aged, nondemented, and demented older adults. J. Cogn. Neurosci. **19**(9), 1498–1507 (2007)
14. Moeskops, P., Viergever, M.A., Mendrik, A.M., de Vries, L.S., Benders, M.J., Išgum, I.: Automatic segmentation of MR brain images with a convolutional neural network. IEEE Trans. Med. Imag. **35**(5), 1252–1261 (2016)
15. Ng, C.R., Than, J.C.M., Noor, N.M., Rijal, O.M.: Preliminary brain region segmentation using FCM and graph cut for CT scan images. In: 2015 International Conference on BioSignal Analysis, Processing and Systems (ICBAPS), pp. 52–56. IEEE (2015)
16. Ronneberger, O., Fischer, P., Brox, T.: U-Net: convolutional networks for biomedical image segmentation. In: Navab, N., Hornegger, J., Wells, W.M., Frangi, A.F. (eds.) MICCAI 2015. LNCS, vol. 9351, pp. 234–241. Springer, Cham (2015). doi:10.1007/978-3-319-24574-4_28
17. Roy, S., Wang, W.T., Carass, A., Prince, J.L., Butman, J.A., Pham, D.L.: PET attenuation correction using synthetic CT from ultrashort echo-time MR imaging. J. Nuclear Med. **55**(12), 2071–2077 (2014)
18. Wang, H., Suh, J.W., Das, S.R., Pluta, J.B., Craige, C., Yushkevich, P.A.: Multi-atlas segmentation with joint label fusion. IEEE Trans. Patt. Anal. Mach. Intell. **35**(3), 611–623 (2013)

Structural Connectivity Guided Sparse Effective Connectivity for MCI Identification

Yang Li[1], Jingyu Liu[1], Meilin Luo[1(✉)], Ke Li[2], Pew-Thian Yap[3],
Minjeong Kim[3], Chong-Yaw Wee[4], and Dinggang Shen[3]

[1] School of Automation Sciences and Electrical Engineering,
Beihang University, Beijing, China
together_az@foxmail.com
[2] School of Aeronautic Science and Engineering, Beihang University, Beijing, China
[3] Department of Radiology and BRIC, UNC Chapel Hill, Chapel Hill, NC, USA
[4] Department of Biomedical Engineering, National University of Singapore,
Singapore, Singapore

Abstract. Recent advances in network modelling techniques have enabled the study of neurological disorders at a whole-brain level based on functional connectivity inferred from resting-state magnetic resonance imaging (rs-fMRI) scan possible. However, constructing a directed effective connectivity, which provides a more comprehensive characterization of functional interactions among the brain regions, is still a challenging task particularly when the ultimate goal is to identify disease associated brain functional interaction anomalies. In this paper, we propose a novel method for inferring effective connectivity from multimodal neuroimaging data for brain disease classification. Specifically, we apply a newly devised weighted sparse regression model on rs-fMRI data to determine the network structure of effective connectivity with the guidance from diffusion tensor imaging (DTI) data. We further employ a regression algorithm to estimate the effective connectivity strengths based on the previously identified network structure. We finally utilize a bagging classifier to evaluate the performance of the proposed sparse effective connectivity network through identifying mild cognitive impairment from healthy aging.

1 Introduction

Mild cognitive impairment (MCI), as the intermediate state of cognitive function between normal aging and dementia, has attracted a great deal of attention recently due to its high progression rate to dementia. More than 50% of individuals with MCI progress to dementia within 5 years [5]. MCI is thus an appropriate target for early diagnosis and intervention of Alzheimer's disease (AD). However, its mild symptoms cause most existing computer-aided diagnosis frameworks perform relatively inferior with low sensitivity [7].

Recently, neuroimaging-based techniques have been shown to be a powerful tool for predicting the progression of MCI to AD [12]. For example, functional connectivity inferred from resting-state magnetic resonance image (rs-fMRI) data can reflect temporal interactions between distinct region-of-interest

© Springer International Publishing AG 2017
Q. Wang et al. (Eds.): MLMI 2017, LNCS 10541, pp. 299–306, 2017.
DOI: 10.1007/978-3-319-67389-9_35

(ROI) in the brain [13]. However, functional connectivity conveys only the pairwise correlation [4], ignoring the directed causal influence between ROIs [10]. Such analysis is susceptible to noise due to the low frequency (< 0.1 Hz) spontaneous fluctuation of blood oxygen level dependent (BOLD) signals, thus may not accurately reveal the brain states at rest. This limits the capability of correlation-based functional connectivity to provide an adequate and complete account of the interactions among multiple brain regions. As an alternative, effective connectivity, has been employed to reflect the causal interactions between a pair of ROIs [4].

Most of the biological networks are intrinsically sparse [3]. Sparse modeling methods such as the least absolute shrinkage and selection operator (Lasso) have been applied to construct sparse brain connectivity networks [2]. However, Lasso which is normally applied on a single modality of neuroimaging data (e.g., rs-fMRI), inevitably ignores the important complementary information from other modalities. Additionally, sparse models through penalizing the linear regression are mainly focused on the resulted squared loss, ignoring the relations between the signals of different time points, which are of great importance for revealing the characteristics of dynamic model. To resolve those issues, we proposed, in this paper, an Ultra-Weighted-Lasso approach to construct a more accurate sparse effective connectivity network and used it for MCI classification. Specifically, the proposed approach was a modified version of Lasso to incorporate structural connectivity information derived from diffusion tensor imaging (DTI) data for deriving the brain network structure. The regression loss of the proposed modified Lasso model involves a term that conveys the relation between different time points, *i.e.*, the derivative. In this way, a more accurate effective connectivity structure can be obtained. The connectivity strength of each edge in the identified network can then be inferred using an Ultra-Orthogonal-Forward regression (UOFR) model which also takes into consideration the derivatives of the signal. We seek to evaluate the capability of this new effective connectivity network for improving the MCI classification performance.

2   Materials and Methodology

A dataset with 27 participants (10 MCI and 17 healthy controls) was used in this study. There are no significant differences in terms of age, gender, years of education, and Mini Mental State Examination (MMSE) score between MCI and healthy subjects. Both rs-fMRI and DTI scans were acquired using a 3 Tesla (Signa EXCITE, GE) scanner with following parameters: rs-fMRI: TR/TE = $2000/32$ ms, flip angle = $77°$, imaging matrix = 64×64, FOV = 256×256 mm^2, voxel thickness = 4 mm, 34 slices, and 150 volumes; DTI: b = 0 and 1000 s/mm^2, flip angle = $90°$, TR/TE = $17000/78$ ms, imaging matrix = 128×128, FOV = 256×256 mm^2, voxel thickness = 2 mm, and 72 continuous slices. The same scanner was used to acquire the T1-weighted anatomical MRI images using the following parameters: TE = 2.976 ms, TR = 7.460 ms, flip angle = $12°$. The imaging matrix = 256×224 with a rectangular FOV of (256×256 mm^2), voxel thickness $= 1\,\mathrm{mm}$, and 216 continuous slices. Subjects were instructed to keep eyes open and stare at a fixation cross in the middle of the screen to prevent them falling into sleep and avoid the saccade-related activation due to eyes-closed during scanning.

For DTI data, all images were first parcellated into 90 regions based on the automated anatomical labeling (AAL) template [9] using a deformable DTI registration algorithm. Whole-brain streamline fiber tractography was then performed on each image with minimal seed point fractional anisotropy (FA) of 0.45, stopping FA of 0.25, minimal fiber length of $20\,\mathrm{mm}$, and maximal fiber length of $400\,\mathrm{mm}$. The number of fibers passing through each pair of regions was counted and two regions were considered as anatomically connected if fibers passing through their respective masks were present. For rs-fMRI data, standard preprocessing procedure was carried out using the statistical parametric mapping (SPM8) software, including the removal of the first 10 volumes, slice timing correction, head-motion artifact correction, regression of nuisance signals (ventricle, white matter, and 6 head-motion parameters), signal de-trending, and band-pass filtering (0.0250.1 Hz). All fMRI images were coregistered to their own T1-weighted image before parcellated into 90 regions based on AAL template.

2.1 Effective Connectivity Inference via Ultra-Weighted-Lasso

Suppose we have M ROIs, the mean time series of i-th ROI for the n-th subject, $\mathbf{y}_i$, can be regarded as a response vector that can be estimated as a linear combination of the mean time series of other ROIs as

$$\mathbf{y}_i = \mathbf{A}_i \alpha_i + \mathbf{e}_i, \tag{1}$$

where $\mathbf{e}_i$ is the noise, $\mathbf{y}_i = [y_i(1), y_i(2), \cdots, y_i(N)]^T$ is the time series with N being the number of time points, $\mathbf{A}_i = [\mathbf{y}_1, \mathbf{y}_2, \cdots, \mathbf{y}_{i-1}, \mathbf{y}_{i+1}, \cdots, \mathbf{y}_M]$ is the data matrix of the i-th ROI, and $\alpha_i = [\alpha_1, \cdots, \alpha_{i-1}, \alpha_{i+1}, \cdots, \alpha_M]^T$ is the weight vector. The solution of the l_1-norm regularized optimization problem results in a sparse weight vector, α_i, which can be computed as follows:

$$\alpha_i = \arg\min_{\alpha_i} \frac{1}{2} \parallel \mathbf{y}_i - \mathbf{A}_i \alpha_i \parallel_2^2 + \lambda \parallel \alpha_i \parallel_1, \tag{2}$$

where $\lambda > 0$ is the regularization parameter, controlling the sparsity of the model. Note that the first term in Eq. (2) uses only the least squares loss of the regression result, ignoring the relations between different time points in signal $\mathbf{y}$, $i.e.$, derivative. To resolve the issue, the Eq. (2) can be modified as

$$\alpha_i = \arg\min_{\alpha_i} \frac{1}{2} \parallel \mathbf{y}_i - \mathbf{A}_i \alpha_i \parallel_2^2 + \sum_{l=1}^{K} \parallel D^l \mathbf{y}_i - \sum_{j=1, j \neq i}^{M} \alpha_j D^l \mathbf{y}_j \parallel_2^2 + \lambda \parallel \alpha_i \parallel_1, \tag{3}$$

where $D^l \mathbf{y}$ is a measurement of the l-order weak derivative of the signal $\mathbf{y}$ and satisfies

$$\int_{[0,T]} \mathbf{y}_i D^l \varphi(t) dt = (-1)^l \int_{[0,T]} \varphi(t) D^l \mathbf{y}_i dt, \tag{4}$$

where the test function $\varphi(t) \in C_0^\infty(0, T)$ is smooth and exhibits the properties of compact support within $[0, T]$. Thus, for simplicity, $D^l \mathbf{y}$ in Eq. (4) can be replaced by

$$R_{\mathbf{y}_i}^l(\tau) = \int_{[\tau, T+\tau]} \mathbf{y}_i D^l \varphi(t) dt, \quad \tau \in [0, N - T] \tag{5}$$

where τ is the time shift of the test function. Hence, we can obtain the model as

$$\alpha_i = \arg\min_{\alpha_i} \frac{1}{2} \parallel \mathbf{y}_i - \mathbf{A}_i \alpha_i \parallel_2^2 + \sum_{l=1}^K \parallel R_{\mathbf{y}_i}^l(\tau) - \sum_{j=1, j\neq i}^M \alpha_j R_{\mathbf{y}_j}^l(\tau) \parallel_2^2 + \lambda \parallel \alpha_i \parallel_1. \tag{6}$$

Please refer to [6] for more information about the detail discussion of both weak derivatives and test functions.

Additionally, it is notable that the Lasso model may produce a suboptimal estimation by inflicting the same penalization on every regressor. To resolve this issue, we can, on one hand, rely on the time series for the penalization adjustment of different regressors using adaptive-Lasso [14]. On the other hand, since the structural connectivity is highly correlated with functional connectivity [4], with a stronger structural connectivity indicating a higher opportunity of the functional connectivity, we opt, in this paper, to utilize the structural connectivity derived from DTI to modify the penalization weight for the rs-fMRI time series as

$$\alpha_i = \arg\min_{\alpha_i} \frac{1}{2} \parallel \mathbf{y}_i - \mathbf{A}_i \alpha_i \parallel_2^2 + \sum_{l=1}^K \parallel R_{\mathbf{y}_i}^l(\tau) - \sum_{j=1, j\neq i}^M \alpha_j R_{\mathbf{y}_j}^l(\tau) \parallel_2^2$$

$$+ \lambda \sum_{j=1, j\neq i}^M w_i(j) |\alpha_i(j)|, \tag{7}$$

where $w_i(j)$ is the penalization weight for the j-th regressor. Let $S_{i,j}$ be the structural connectivity between the i-th ROI and the j-th ROI, $w_i(j)$ can then be defined as

$$w_i(j) = \exp\{1 - n_i \cdot f_{i,j}\}, \tag{8}$$

where n_i is the total number of structural connectivity for the i-th ROI, and $f_{i,j} = S_{i,j} / \sum_{j=1, j\neq i}^M S_{i,j}$ is the proportion of structural connectivity between i-th ROI and j-th ROI to the sum of connectivity of i-th ROI. Equation (8) indicates that for a pair of brain regions that with a strong structural connectivity, there is high probability that an effective connectivity exists between them and a small penalization should be imposed. The regression model, which is referred as Ultra-Weighted-Lasso, incorporates the weak derivatives and penalization to derive a more accurate sparse effective connectivity structure based on the resulted α.

2.2   Effective Network Construction via UOFR

The non-zero element $\alpha_i(j)$ in α_i indicates the existence of effective influence the j-th ROI exerting on the i-th ROI. Herein, an algorithm of Ultra

Orthogonal Forward Regression (UOFR) which takes into consideration the derivatives, is used to calculate the effective connectivity strength. For the time series $\mathbf{y}_i$ and $\{\mathbf{y}_j \,|\, \alpha_i(j) > 0;\, j \in [1, 2, \cdots, M]\}$, the series are firstly extended as $\widetilde{\mathbf{y}} = [y(1), y(2), \cdots, y(N), R_{\mathbf{y}}^1(1), R_{\mathbf{y}}^1(2), \cdots, R_{\mathbf{y}}^1(N - T), \cdots, R_{\mathbf{y}}^K(N - T)]^T$, which is referred as ultra time series. Then, a forward orthogonalization is applied to the ultra time series $\{\widetilde{\mathbf{y}}_j \,|\, \alpha_i(j) > 0;\, j \in [1, 2, \cdots, M]\}$ to calculate the in error reduction ratio (ERR) as [6]

$$ERR_i(j) = \frac{< \widetilde{\mathbf{y}}_i, \widetilde{\mathbf{y}}_j >^2}{< \widetilde{\mathbf{y}}_i, \widetilde{\mathbf{y}}_i >< \widetilde{\mathbf{y}}_j, \widetilde{\mathbf{y}}_j >} \tag{9}$$

where $< \cdot >$ is the inner product. For each round of orthogonalization, the maximum ERR_i, i.e., $ERR_i(j)$, which reflects the effect the j-th ROI exerting on the i-th ROI, is referred as the effective connectivity strength of $g_{i,j}$, which reflects the effect the j-th ROI exerting to the i-th ROI. Note that $g_{i,j}$ is non-negative and varies from 0 to 1.

2.3 Feature Extraction

Weighted-clustering coefficient (GC_i) and betweenness centrality (GB_i) are extracted from the constructed sparse effective connectivity network for the MCI classification and are defined as

$$GC_i = \frac{\sum_{j,k \neq i} \left(g_{i,j}^{1/3} + g_{j,i}^{1/3} \right) \left(g_{i,k}^{1/3} + g_{k,i}^{1/3} \right) \left(g_{j,k}^{1/3} + g_{k,j}^{1/3} \right)}{2 \left(|\Delta_i| \left(|\Delta_i| - 1 \right) - 2|\Delta_i^{\leftrightarrow}| \right)}, \tag{10}$$

where $g_{i,j}$ denotes the effective connectivity from the i-th ROI to the j-th ROI, $|\Delta_i|$ denotes the number of ROIs that are adjacent to the i-th ROI, and $|\Delta_i^{\leftrightarrow}|$ is the number of bilateral edges between the i-th ROI and its neighbors, respectively.

$$GB_i = \sum_{j \neq i \neq k} \frac{\sigma_{j,k}(i)}{\sigma_{j,k}}, \tag{11}$$

where $\sigma_{j,k}$ denotes the total number of shortest paths from the j-th ROI to the k-th ROI, and $\sigma_{j,k}(i)$ is the number of those paths that pass through the i-th ROI.

2.4 Classification and Evaluation

Decision tree (DT) with a bagging strategy [1] and leave-one-out cross-validation (LOOCV) is used as classifier for MCI classification. Specifically, for N_s total number of subjects involved, one is first left out for testing, and the remaining $N_s - 1$ are used for feature selection and DT construction, where $N_s - 1$ decision trees (DTs) are constructed using different $N_s - 2$ training subjects and validated using the second left out validation subject. The predicated label of the first left out testing subject is obtained based on the majority voting of the constructed $N_s - 1$ DTs. The process is repeated for N_s times, each time left out different subject as the testing subject. Finally, the overall classification performance is obtained by comparing the predicted labels of all subjects with the ground truth.

3   Experimental Results

The constructed effective connectivity maps of one healthy control (NC) and one MCI patient are shown in Fig. 1(a)−(b), respectively. The constructed effective networks are sparse and asymmetric, indicating that the interaction within a pair of ROIs, *i.e.*, $g_{i,j}$ and $g_{j,i}$ are not restricted to be equal. The sums of ERR for effective connectivity of each ROI for corresponding MCI and NC subjects are shown in Fig. 1(c)−(d). Almost all ROIs show a sum larger than 0.95, indicating that the rs-fMRI time-series of an ROI can be well represented by the time series of other selected. It also assure the convergence of the network.

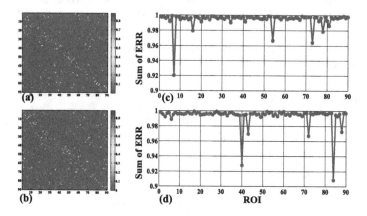

Fig. 1. Effective connectivity maps based on Ultra-Weighted-Lasso and UOFR for one (a) MCI and one (b) NC subjects. Sums of ERR for effective connectivity of each ROI for the corresponding (c) MCI and (d) NC subjects.

In this work, the proposed sparse effective connectivity network based framework is compared with other related works using the same dataset, including the framework that uses single modality data, either DTI or rs-fMRI data, separately [12], and the framework that directly fuses features from multiple modalities at the feature level (Direct) [12]. We further compared the performance of our proposed framework to the results of the Weighted-Lasso with OFR procedure (Weighted-Lasso-OFR) which omits the derivative information, and the results of Ultra-Lasso with UOFR procedure (Ultra-Lasso-UOFR) which without penalization weights from DTI-based structural connectivity. The LOOCV classification results of all compared frameworks are summarized in Table 1. The proposed framework, which combines the information from multimodal neuroimaging data and the Ultra-Weighted-Lasso and the UOFR approaches by yielding a cross-validation accuracy of 96.3%, which is at least 7.4% improvement compared to the second best performed framework (Direct). Furthermore, it also outperforms all other frameworks in terms of the rest of the computed statistical measurements. Particularly, an area of 0.994 under the receiver operating characteristic curve (AUC) demonstrates an excellent generalization power of our proposed

Table 1. Classification performance of the proposed and competing frameworks. (ACC = Accuracy; SEN = Sensitivity; SPE = Specificity; BAC = Balanced Accuracy)

Methods	ACC (%)	AUC	SEN (%)	SPE (%)	BAC (%)
DTI	88.9	0.935	80.0	94.1	87.1
fMRI	70.4	0.788	70.0	70.6	70.3
Direct	88.9	0.912	90.0	88.2	89.1
Weighted-Lasso-OFR	85.2	0.859	80.0	88.2	84.1
Ultra-Lasso-UOFR	81.5	0.824	60.0	94.1	77.1
Proposed	**96.3**	**0.994**	**100.0**	**94.1**	**97.1**

framework.Our method achieved a gain of at least 11% in accuracy while requiring only extra 15% more of computation time if compared to the single-modal Ultra-Lasso-UOFR and multimodal Weighted-Lasso-OFR approaches, implying its efficacy in accurate inference of effective connectivity.

The most discriminant regions selected by our framework are mainly located in the frontal lobe (e.g., superior frontal gyrus [13]), the temporal lobe (e.g., temporal pole [8]), the occipital lobe (e.g., middle occipital gyrus and superior occipital gyrus [8]) and other regions such as cingulum gyri [11,13], hippocampus [8], and thalamus [8], in line with those reported in the AD/MCI literature. The selected most discriminant regions are graphically displayed in Fig. 2.

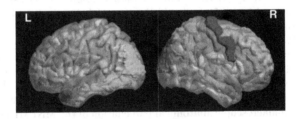

Fig. 2. Most discriminant regions selected during MCI classification

4 Discussions and Conclusion

In this study, we propose an Ultra-Weighted-Lasso-UOFR based effective connectivity network inference method using multimodal DTI and rs-fMRI data, and explore its diagnostic power for distinguishing MCI patients from healthy subjects. In this framework, multimodal integration is achieved via an Ultra Weighted-Lasso method where weighted penalties derived from the DTI data are incorporated into a sparse regression procedure for identifying the topology of effective connectivity network. This method provides a more accurate detection of the high dimensional effective interaction architecture among brain regions via the returned non-zero coefficients. Additionally, effective connectivity strength is estimated using an orthogonal forward regression procedure based on the identified network structure. Experimental results on MCI classification demonstrate the superiority of the constructed sparse effective connectivity network over other competing methods. In conclusion, the proposed approach sheds a light on integrating information from multimodal neuroimaging data to infer sparse effective connectivity for brain disease diagnosis.

References

1. Akhoondzadeh, M.: Decision tree, bagging and random forest methods detect TEC seismo-ionospheric anomalies around the time of the chile, $(m-w = 8.8)$ earthquake of 27 february 2010. Adv. Space Res. **57**(12), 856–867 (2016)
2. Allen, E.A., Damaraju, E., Plis, S.M., Erhardt, E.B., Eichele, T., Calhoun, V.D.: Tracking whole-brain connectivity dynamics in the resting state. Cereb Cortex **24**, 663–676 (2012)
3. Boccaletti, S., Latora, V., Moreno, Y., Chavez, M., Hwang, D.U.: Complex networks: structure and dynamics. Phys. Rep. **424**(4), 175–308 (2006)
4. Friston, K.J.: Functional and effective connectivity: a review. Brain Connect. **1**(1), 13–36 (2011)
5. Gauthier, S., Reisberg, B., Zaudig, M., Petersen, R.C., Ritchie, K., Broich, K., Belleville, S., Brodaty, H., Bennett, D., Chertkow, H.: Mild cognitive impairment. The Lancet **367**(9518), 1262–1270 (2006)
6. Li, Y., Cui, W.G., Guo, Y.Z., Huang, T., Yang, X.F., Wei, H.L.: Time-varying system identification using an ultra-orthogonal forward regression and multiwavelet basis functions with applications to EEG. IEEE Trans. Neural Netw. Learn. Syst. **PP**(99), 1–13 (2017)
7. Liu, F., Wee, C.Y., Chen, H., Shen, D.: Inter-modality relationship constrained multi-modality multi-task feature selection for Alzheimer's disease and mild cognitive impairment identification. Neuroimage **84**, 466–475 (2014)
8. Salvatore, C., Cerasa, A., Battista, P., Gilardi, M.C., Quattrone, A., Castiglioni, I.: Magnetic resonance imaging biomarkers for the early diagnosis of Alzheimer's disease: a machine learning approach. Front. Neurosci. **9**, 307 (2015)
9. Tzourio-Mazoyer, N., Landeau, B., Papathanassiou, D., Crivello, F., Etard, O., Delcroix, N., Mazoyer, B., Joliot, M.: Automated anatomical labeling of activations in SPM using a macroscopic anatomical parcellation of the MNI MRI single-subject brain. Neuroimage **15**(1), 273–289 (2002)
10. Wang, K., Liang, M., Wang, L., Tian, L., Zhang, X., Li, K., Jiang, T.: Altered functional connectivity in early Alzheimer's disease: a restingstate fMRI study. Hum. Brain Mapp. **28**(10), 967–978 (2007)
11. Wang, Z., Nie, B., Li, D., Zhao, Z., Han, Y., Song, H., Xu, J., Shan, B., Lu, J., Li, K.: Effect of acupuncture in mild cognitive impairment and Alzheimer disease: a functional MRI study. PLoS One **7**(8), e42730 (2012)
12. Wee, C.Y., Yap, P.T., Zhang, D., Denny, K., Browndyke, J.N., Potter, G.G., Welsh-Bohmer, K.A., Wang, L., Shen, D.: Identification of MCI individuals using structural and functional connectivity networks. Neuroimage **59**(3), 2045–2056 (2012)
13. Xu, L., Wu, X., Li, R., Chen, K., Long, Z., Zhang, J., Guo, X., Yao, L.: Prediction of progressive mild cognitive impairment by multi-modal neuroimaging biomarkers. J. Alzheimer's Dis. **51**(4), 1045–1056 (2016)
14. Zou, H.: The adaptive lasso and its oracle properties. JASA **101**(476), 1418–1429 (2006)

Fusion of High-Order and Low-Order Effective Connectivity Networks for MCI Classification

Yang Li[1], Jingyu Liu[1(✉)], Ke Li[2], Pew-Thian Yap[3], Minjeong Kim[3], Chong-Yaw Wee[4], and Dinggang Shen[3]

[1] School of Automation Sciences and Electrical Engineering,
Beihang University, Beijing, China
liyang@buaa.edu.cn, junyi@email.unc.edu
[2] School of Aeronautic Science and Engineering,
Beihang University, Beijing, China
[3] Department of Radiology and BRIC, UNC Chapel Hill, Chapel Hill, NC, USA
[4] Department of Biomedical Engineering, National University of Singapore,
Kent Ridge, Singapore

Abstract. Functional connectivity network derived from resting-state fMRI data has been found as effective biomarkers for identifying patients with mild cognitive impairment from healthy elderly. However, the ordinary functional connectivity network is essentially a low-order network with the assumption that the brain is static during the entire scanning period, ignoring the temporal variations among correlations derived from brain region pairs. To overcome this weakness, we proposed a new type of high-order network to more accurately describe the relationship of temporal variations among brain regions. Specifically, instead of the commonly used undirected pairwise Pearson's correlation coefficient, we first estimated the low-order effective connectivity network based on a novel sparse regression algorithm. By using the similar approach, we then constructed the high-order effective connectivity network from low-order connectivity to incorporate signal flow information among the brain regions. We finally combined the low-order and the high-order effective connectivity networks using two decision trees for MCI classification and experimental results obtained demonstrate the superiority of the proposed method over the conventional undirected low-order and high-order functional connectivity networks, as well as the low-order and high-order effective connectivity networks when they were used separately.

1 Introduction

Mild cognitive impairment (MCI) is considered to be a transitional state between normal senility and Alzheimer's disease (AD) [1, 2]. Around 10% to 15% of MCI patients deteriorate to AD every year, and more than half of them develop into AD within 5 years [1, 2]. Due to its serious negative impacts on the healthcare system, economy and society, it is thus crucial to accurately identify MCI at its early stage so that appropriate actions can be taken to minimize the burdens. However, MCI is difficult to diagnose because of its relative subtle symptoms of the cognitive impairment [3]. Functional connectivity, defined as the temporal correlations of brain regions

© Springer International Publishing AG 2017
Q. Wang et al. (Eds.): MLMI 2017, LNCS 10541, pp. 307–315, 2017.
DOI: 10.1007/978-3-319-67389-9_36

[4, 5], is often described through the functional connectivity network using the knowledge of graph theory [6–9].

In conventional modeling approaches [3, 7, 9, 10], the vertices of functional connectivity networks correspond to the brain regions and the edges correspond to the correlation among brain regions. This kind of network is regarded as low-order network and the correlation of low-order network is regarded as low-order correlation [6]. It is noteworthy that the low-order correlation is normally calculated using the whole time series. This correlation is a fixed value with no temporal variations of the correlation are encoded [6]. However, the brain activities are indeed not static across the entire scanning period and the correlations among brain regions varied across time. Therefore, the conventional methods, which ignoring the temporal variations among correlations, may fail to diagnose MCI accurately. Recently, a high-order network modeling method [6] has been proposed to preserve the dynamic correlation information neglected in the conventional methods. Specifically, the vertices of high-order network correspond to the brain region pairs while the edges correspond to the relevance among temporarily correlated time series. However, the existing high-order network modeling approach [6] is based on pairwise Pearson's correlation coefficient, thus inconsistent with the sparse nature and small-world characteristic of most biologically networks [11]. Furthermore, the high-order correlation-based networks are undirected networks that cannot characterize the directed causal influence between the brain regions. To overcome these drawbacks, we enhance the network modeling approach with a novel sparse regression algorithm. Particularly, different from the traditional sparse regression model with a l_1-norm penalization [12] which leads to different network structures at individual level, the proposed sparse model utilizes a $l_{2,1}$-norm penalization to encourage an identical network structure among subjects. Moreover, an ultra-least squares (ULS) criterion is employed to extract more information from fMRI time series, such as the information of the classical dependent relation of the fMRI data and the dependent relation of the associated weak derivatives. While the low-order network ignores the temporal variations of correlation, the high-order network unable to characterize the holistic correlation calculated on the whole time series. Therefore, to incorporate both the low-order correlation and the temporally dynamic information encoded in the high-order correlation for better classification performance, we first constructed a decision tree (DCT) for each type of correlations and then fused their classification scores to provide the final classification decision. The fused DCT model considers not only the integrated correlation calculated on the whole time series but also the temporal variations of correlation. We compared our proposed framework (i.e., fusion of high- and low-order effective connectivity networks) with other related methods on a dataset and experimental results demonstrate the superiority of the proposed framework for MCI classification.

2   Materials

In this study, the fMRI data were collected from 28 MCI individuals and 33 healthy controls. All the subjects were scanned using a standard echo-planar imaging (EPI) sequence on a 3 T Siemens TRIO scanner with following parameters: TR = 3000 ms,

TE = 30 ms, acquisition matrix = 74 × 74, 45 slices, and voxel thickness = 3 mm. One-hundred and eighty resting-state fMRI volumes were acquired. Standard prepro-cessing pipeline of the fMRI images was performed using Statistical Parametric Map-ping 8 (SPM8) software package which includes removal of first 10 fMRI volumes, slice timing correction, head-motion correction, regression of nuisance signals (ventricle, white matter, global signal, and head-motion with Friston's 24-parameter model [9]), signal de-trending, and band-pass filtering (0.01−0.08 Hz). Next, the brain space was parcellated into 90 ROIs based on the automated anatomical labeling (AAL) atlas [6].

3   Methods

3.1   The ULS Criterion

Suppose there is a linear system with k inputs and one output, the ordinary least squares regression problem can be solved via the least squares criterion as follows:

$$J_{LS} = \left\| y - \sum_{i=1}^{k} \theta_i x_i \right\|_2^2, \tag{1}$$

where y, x_i denote the system output and input variables, θ_i is the parameter and e is the system noise, respectively. Supposing $[0, T]$ is the time span of observed data and $\hat{y}(t)$ is prediction function of $y(t)$, it is obvious that the least squares criterion only measures the discrepancy between $y(t)$ and $\hat{y}(t)$ on the whole interval $[0, T]$, ignoring how the discrepancy distributed at every individual time point. Therefore, the least squares criterion cannot accurately describe the similarity of function shape and discards the information of correlations among the data points, thus leading to the common over-fitting problem for the identification of dynamic system [13].

In order to overcome this drawback, a new ULS criterion has been adopted to produce a more accurate evaluation standard about the model fitness, which is defined as the combination of the least squares criterion and the weak derivative:

$$J_{ULS} = \left\| y - \sum_{i=1}^{k} \theta_i x_i \right\|_2^2 + \sum_{l=1}^{L} \left\| D^l y - \sum_{i=1}^{k} \theta_i D^l x_i \right\|_2^2, \tag{2}$$

where D^l denotes the l-th order weak derivative. The new criterion considers not only the discrepancy between two functions at a whole level, but also the discrepancy between weak derivatives of the two functions.

3.2   Effective Network Structure Estimation via Ultra-Group Lasso

Suppose we have M ROIs and N subjects, the objective function of widely used Lasso with a l_1-norm penalization is defined as follows:

$$f(\theta_m^n) = \left\| y_m^n - A_m^n \theta_m^n \right\|_2^2 + \lambda \left\| \theta_m^n \right\|_1, \tag{3}$$

where y_m^n denotes the fMRI time series of m-th ROI for n-th subject, $A_m^n = [y_1^n, \ldots, y_{m-1}^n, y_{m+1}^n, \ldots, y_M^n]$ is data matrix which includes all ROIs time series except the m-th ROI, $\theta_m^n = [\theta_1^n; \ldots; \theta_{m-1}^n; \theta_{m+1}^n; \ldots; \theta_M^n]$ denotes the weight vector and $\lambda > 0$ is the regularization parameter that controls the sparsity level of the regression model. Constructing sparse effective network structure can be considered as an optimization problem, i.e. minimizing the above objective function.

To minimize inter-subject variability, a Group-Lasso algorithm has been used to estimate an identical network structure across subjects by replacing l_1-norm penalization with $l_{2,1}$-norm penalization. The objective function of Group-Lasso is given as

$$f(\theta_m) = \sum_{n=1}^{N} \left\| y_m^n - A_m^n \theta_m^n \right\|_2^2 + \lambda \|\theta_m\|_{2,1}, \tag{4}$$

where $\theta_m = [\theta_m^1, \ldots, \theta_m^{n-1}, \theta_m^{n+1}, \ldots, \theta_m^N]$ denotes the weight matrix. By incorporating the ULS criterion with the Group-Lasso algorithm, we proposed an Ultra-Group Lasso (UG-Lasso) algorithm to estimate a more accurate effective network structure via the following objective function

$$f(\theta_m) = \sum_{n=1}^{N} \left\| y_m^n - A_m^n \theta_m^n \right\|_2^2 + \sum_{n=1}^{N} \sum_{l=1}^{L} \left\| D^l y_m^n - D^l A_m^n \theta_m^n \right\|_2^2 + \lambda \|\theta_m\|_{2,1}. \tag{5}$$

3.3 Effective Connectivity Strength Estimation via UOLS

It is important to note that the estimated coefficient based on Eq. (5) cannot be regarded as the effective connectivity strength, because they are biased as the result of group-constrained sparse penalization. Furthermore, even some of the coefficients are negative, leading to difficulty in interpreting and analyzing the effective connectivity network. Therefore, we proposed to utilize an Ultra-Orthogonal Least Squares (UOLS) algorithm to estimate the effective connectivity strength between the time series of two brain regions [13]. Suppose there are P ROIs have been found correlated to m-th ROI based on the UG-Lasso in Eq. (5), the effective connectivity between m-th ROI and the other P ROIs can be estimated by minimizing the objective function:

$$f(\alpha_m^n) = \left\| y_m^n - \Phi_m^n \alpha_m^n \right\|_2^2 + \sum_{l=1}^{L} \left\| D^l y_m^n - D^l \Phi_m^n \alpha_m^n \right\|_2^2, \tag{6}$$

where $\Phi_m^n = [y_1^n, y_2^n, \ldots, y_P^n]$ is the data matrix including time series of P ROIs and $\alpha_m^n = [\alpha_1^n, \alpha_2^n, \ldots, \alpha_P^n]$ is the weight vector, i.e. the strength of effective connectivity.

3.4 Construction of High-Order UG-Lasso-UOLS-Based Networks

The first step in high-order network construction is applying a sliding window to partition ROIs time series into multiple overlapping segments. Suppose the size of the sliding window is S and the step size between adjacent windows is r. For one ROI time series containing Z temporal image volumes, y_m^n, the total number of time series segments generated using the sliding window can be computed as $K = \lfloor (Z - S)/r \rfloor + 1$. Let $y_m^n(k)$ be the k-th segment generated from y_m^n, for n-th subject, the k-th segments of all M ROIs can be represented in a matrix form as $\boldsymbol{Y}^n(k) = [\boldsymbol{y}_1^n(k), \boldsymbol{y}_2^n(k), \ldots, \boldsymbol{y}_M^n(k)] \in R^{S \times M}$. Further, the set of k-th segments for all subjects and all ROIs can be expressed as $\boldsymbol{Y}(k) \in R^{S \times M \times N}$. Thus, by applying sliding window to fMRI series, we can obtain K sets of time series segments $\boldsymbol{Y}(k)$.

For each set of segments $\boldsymbol{Y}(k)$, we applied an UG-Lasso across subjects to derive the network structure and then applied an UOLS at individual level to estimate the connectivity strength of each derived connection, producing a total of $K \times N$ temporal low-order effective connectivity networks. Taking each ROI with $\{y_m^n(k)\}$ as the vertex and $\left\{ C_{ij}^n(k) \right\}$ as the strength of connection for each pair of vertices, the temporal low-order effective connectivity network can be expressed as $\boldsymbol{G}^n(k) = (\{y_m^n(k)\}, \left\{ C_{ij}^n(k) \right\})(k = 1, 2, \ldots, K)$. A larger value of $\left\{ C_{ij}^n(k) \right\}$ indicates a stronger connection between i-th ROI and j-th ROI in the k-th window [6].

For the n-th subject, the correlation time series of each ROI pair (i,j) $\boldsymbol{C}_{ij}^n = [C_{ij}^n(1), C_{ij}^n(2), \ldots, C_{ij}^n(K)] \in R^K$ can be obtained by concatenating all $C_{ij}^n(k)(k = 1, 2, \ldots, K)$. Different from $\boldsymbol{y}_m^n$ representing the time series of a ROI, $\boldsymbol{C}_{ij}^n$ characterizes the variations of correlation of ROI pair (i,j) across time [6]. Considering the low-order network is directional, the total number of correlation time series $\left\{ C_{ij}^n | 1 \leq i \leq M, 1 \leq j \leq M, i \neq j \right\}$ for the n-th subject is $M(M-1)$. For the set of all correlation time series $\left\{ C_{ij}^n \right\}$, we employed an UG-Lasso to estimate the network structure and then employed an UOLS to estimate the connectivity strength, establishing a total of N high-order networks with identical network structure. By considering each ROI pair (i,j) with $\left\{ C_{ij}^n \right\}$ as vertices and $\left\{ E_{ij,pq}^n \right\}$ as the weights of edges, high-order network can be expressed as $\boldsymbol{G}^n = \left(\left\{ C_{ij}^n \right\}, \left\{ E_{ij,pq}^n \right\} \right)$, where $\left\{ E_{ij,pq}^n \right\}$ represents the correlation for each pair of correlation time series $\left(\left\{ C_{ij}^n \right\}, \left\{ C_{pq}^n \right\} \right)$. Therefore, high-order network is devoted to describe the relationship of temporal correlations among brain regions.

However, there is an obvious deficiency about high-order network, i.e., the scale of high-order network is too large [6]. As mentioned above, the number of vertices $\left\{ C_{ij}^n \right\}$ is $M(M-1)$, thus the number of edges is proportional to M^4. The large-scale of high-order network leads to a large amount of computation and poor generalization performance. To overcome this deficiency, we applied the Ward's hierarchical grouping [14] to group the correlation time series into clusters. Then, the mean correlation time series of each cluster was used as the vertices of high-order network. As a result, the scale of high-order network can be significantly reduced and the generalization capability of the high-order network can be significantly improved.

3.5   Feature Extraction and Selection

In this work, we extract four frequently used network features from low-order and high-order effective connectivity networks, respectively, including the weighted clustering coefficient, betweenness centrality, in-degree and out-degree [15]. For a node i of an effective connectivity network, the weighted clustering coefficient is defined as

$$WC_i = \frac{\sum_{j \neq i} \sum_{h \neq (i,j)} \left(c_{i,j}^{1/3} + c_{j,i}^{1/3} \right) \left(c_{i,h}^{1/3} + c_{h,i}^{1/3} \right) \left(c_{j,h}^{1/3} + c_{h,j}^{1/3} \right)}{2[d_i(d_i - 1) - 2d_i^{\leftrightarrow}]}, \tag{7}$$

where $c_{i,j}$ is the effective connectivity strength from node i to j, d_i represents the number of adjacent points of node i, $d_i^{\leftrightarrow}$ denotes the number of bilateral edges between i and its adjacent nodes.

After feature extraction, we use a filter-based approach which based on the correlation coefficient between the features and the class labels of training samples to select the most discriminative features for classification. The features selected in the first step will form a feature set S_1. Then, for the diversification of the feature selection methods, we apply the Relief algorithm [16] to compute the weights for the features which are not belong to S_1. The features whose weights are larger than the predefined threshold will be selected to form a feature set S_2. Finally, $S = S_1 \cup S_2$ will be the final feature pool for MCI classification.

3.6   Classification via Fusion DCT Model

After completing the feature selection, we performed 10-fold cross-validation for MCI classification to evaluate the performance of our proposed method. For each fold of cross-validation, two DCT submodels were constructed based on the features selected from both the low-order UG-Lasso-UOLS-based network and the high-order UG-Lasso-UOLS-based network, respectively. For a testing subject, each DCT submodel can provide a classification score for each subject, and we get the final classification scores for each subject via combining the classification scores from the two DCT submodels with equal weight. We repeated the cross-validation for 20 times and reported our results as the mean of these 20 repetitions.

4   Results and Discussions

In this work, we compared the proposed fusion UG-Lasso-UOLS-based method with other methods including low-order correlation-based method, high-order correlation-based method [6], fusion correlation-based method [6], low-order UG-Lasso-UOLS-based method (combination of [3, 13]), and high-order UG-Lasso-UOLS-based (combination of [3, 6, 13]) method on the same dataset. To characterize performance comparison between different methods, we used four typical performance measures including accuracy (ACC), sensitivity (SEN), specificity (SPC), and area under curve (AUC). As shown in Table 1, the proposed fusion UG-Lasso-UOLS-based method yields the best accuracy of 85.5%, the best sensitivity of 86.6% and the best

AUC of 0.896, respectively. Although the best specificity of 88.9% belongs to high-order UG-Lasso-UOLS-based method, it also indicates dynamic correlation information is important and should be incorporated for MCI classification. Furthermore, our proposed method performed significantly better than all competing methods in terms of ACC, SPC, and AUC based on two-sample t-test results on 20 repetitions. Table 1 also shows the p-values for the comparison of AUC between the proposed method and other methods.

Table 1. Performance comparison from different network modeling methods

Method	ACC(%)	SEN(%)	SPC(%)	AUC	p-values
Low-order correlation-based	62.4	51.4	71.7	0.600	2.7×10^{-17}
High-order correlation-based	69.3	63.9	73.9	0.711	3.8×10^{-13}
Fusion correlation-based	69.7	63.0	75.3	0.730	1.8×10^{-12}
Low-order UG-Lasso-UOLS	81.5	74.3	87.6	0.756	2.0×10^{-13}
High-order UG-Lasso-UOLS	81.6	72.9	**88.9**	0.755	5.6×10^{-11}
Fusion UG-Lasso-UOLS	**85.5**	**86.6**	84.6	0.896	–

The most discriminative brain regions and clusters are defined as the ones with the highest selected frequency in 20 repetitions of 10-fold cross-validation corresponding to the low-order and the high-order network, respectively [6]. The most discriminative brain regions selected from low-order network includes hippocampus left, orbitofrontal cortex (superior) right, inferior parietal lobule right, inferior frontal gyrus (opercular) right, anterior cingulate gyrus left, and these regions are frequently reported as highly associated with AD/MCI pathology [6, 10]. Direction information of effective connection among the top 20 most discriminative ROIs is provided in Fig. 1. As for high-order networks, the ROI pairs in the most discriminative clusters includes middle occipital gyrus left and middle occipital gyrus right, Heschl gyrus left and Superior temporal gyrus left, etc. It means that the temporal variations of correlation between these ROI pairs are discriminative for MCI classification. Additionally, Fig. 2 shows the difference of correlation among the top 20 most discriminative clusters between MCI and NC subjects.

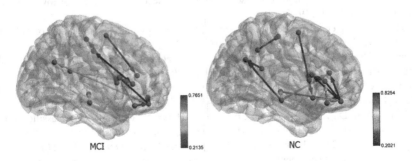

Fig. 1. Comparison of effective connections from low-order effective connectivity networks among the top 20 most discriminative ROIs with a threshold weight of 0.2.

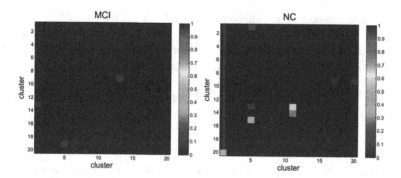

Fig. 2. Comparison of correlation difference from high-order effective connectivity networks among the top 20 most discriminative clusters.

5   Conclusions

In this paper, we proposed a novel fusion approach to infer high- and low-order effective connectivity networks for MCI classification. By using the UG-Lasso and UOLS, our approach can minimize inter-subject variability and extract the temporal information of connections among fMRI data, which can be further used to construct the effective connection for low-order and high-order networks. Additionally, by fusing DCT models constructed using low-order and high-order networks, our proposed approach considers integrated correlation that computed both the entire time series and the temporal variations of correlation, simultaneously. Promising results obtained demonstrate the superiority of our proposed method and the importance of dynamic temporal correlation information for MCI classification.

References

1. Petersen, R.C., et al.: Current concepts in mild cognitive impairment. Arch. Neurol. **58**, 1985–1992 (2001)
2. Gauthier, S., et al.: Mild cognitive impairment. Lancet **367**, 1262–1270 (2006)
3. Wee, C.Y., et al.: Constrained sparse functional connectivity networks for MCI classification. MICCAI, 212–219 (2012)
4. Aertsen, A.M., et al.: Dynamics of neuronal firing correlation: modulation of "effective connectivity". J. Neurophysiol. **61**, 900–917 (1989)
5. van den Heuvel, M.P., et al.: Exploring the brain network: A review on resting-state fMRI functional connectivity. Eur Neuropsychopharm **20**, 519–534 (2010)
6. Chen, X.B., et al.: High-order resting-state functional connectivity network for MCI classification. Hum. Brain Mapp. **37**, 3282–3296 (2016)
7. Jie, B., Shen, D., Zhang, D.: Brain Connectivity Hyper-Network for MCI Classification. In: Golland, P., Hata, N., Barillot, C., Hornegger, J., Howe, R. (eds.) MICCAI 2014. LNCS, vol. 8674, pp. 724–732. Springer, Cham (2014). doi:10.1007/978-3-319-10470-6_90
8. Wee, C.Y., et al.: Sparse temporally dynamic resting-state functional connectivity networks for early MCI identification. Brain Imaging Behav. **10**, 342–356 (2016)

9. Wee, C.Y., et al.: Resting-state multi-spectrum functional connectivity networks for identification of MCI patients. PLoS ONE 7, e37828 (2012)
10. Wee, C.Y.: Identification of MCI individuals using structural and functional connectivity networks. Neuroimage **59**, 2045–2056 (2012)
11. Supekar, K., et al.: Network Analysis of Intrinsic Functional Brain Connectivity in Alzheimer's Disease. PLoS Comput. Biol. **4**, e1000100 (2008)
12. Lee, H., et al.: Sparse brain network recovery under compressed sensing. IEEE Trans. Med. Imaging **30**, 1154–1165 (2011)
13. Li, Y., et al.: Time-varying system identification using an ultra-orthogonal forward regression and multiwavelet basis functions with applications to EEG. IEEE Trans. Neural Netw. Learn. Syst. 1–13 (2017)
14. Ward Jr., J.H.: Hierarchical grouping to optimize an objective function. J. Am. Stat. Assoc. **58**, 236–244 (1963)
15. Rubinov, M., et al.: Complex network measures of brain connectivity: Uses and interpretations. Neuroimage **52**, 1059–1069 (2010)
16. Kira, K., et al.: The feature selection problem: traditional methods and a new algorithm. AAAI 129–134 (1992)

Novel Effective Connectivity Network Inference for MCI Identification

Yang Li[1], Hao Yang[1(✉)], Ke Li[2], Pew-Thian Yap[3], Minjeong Kim[3], Chong-Yaw Wee[4], and Dinggang Shen[3]

[1] School of Automation Sciences and Electrical Engineering,
Beihang University, Beijing, China
hansyang@buaa.edu.cn
[2] School of Aeronautic Science and Engineering,
Beihang University, Beijing, China
[3] Department of Radiology and BRIC,
University of North Carolina at Chapel Hill, Chapel Hill, USA
[4] Department of Biomedical Engineering,
National University of Singapore, Singapore, Singapore

Abstract. Inferring effective brain connectivity network is a challenging task owing to perplexing noise effects, the curse of dimensionality, and inter-subject variability. However, most existing network inference methods are based on correlation analysis and consider the datum points individually, revealing limited information of the neuron interactions and ignoring the relations amongst the derivatives of the data. Hence, we proposed a novel ultra group-constrained sparse linear regression model for effective connectivity inference. This model utilizes not only the discrepancy between observed signals and the model prediction, but also the discrepancy between the associated weak derivatives of the observed and the model signals for a more accurate effective connectivity inference. What's more, a group constraint is applied to minimize the inter-subject variability and the proposed modeling was validated on a mild cognitive impairment dataset with superior results achieved.

1 Introduction

Mild cognitive impairment is considered as the clinical stage between normal aging and dementia. MCI patients suffer from a cognitive decline that does not interfere notably with activities of daily living. Anatomical and physiological researches suggest that cognitive process is greatly associated with the interactions among distributed brain regions [1].

Constructing functional and effective brain connectivity from neuroimaging data holds great promise for understanding the functional interactions between brain activities. Recently, many connectivity modeling approaches based on functional magnetic resonance imaging (fMRI) have been proposed and employed disease for identification, e.g., Alzheimer's disease (AD) and MCI from normal controls (NCs).

Recent works demonstrated that sparse learning techniques provide excellent performances in a series of neuroimaging applications [2, 3]. The use of certain sparsity

© Springer International Publishing AG 2017
Q. Wang et al. (Eds.): MLMI 2017, LNCS 10541, pp. 316–324, 2017.
DOI: 10.1007/978-3-319-67389-9_37

connectivity modeling can elucidate robust connections from a set of noisy connections and increase the discriminative power for disease diagnosis. Lee et al. [2] adopted a least absolute shrinkage and selection operation (Lasso) to construct the functional connectivity network. Wee et al. [3] introduced Group Lasso based connectivity network by adopting a $l_{2,1}$ regularizer to the original Lasso. Both methods achieved a relatively high accuracy in disease classification. However, these methods consider only the datum points (brain regions in our case) individually, ignoring the inter-datum connections which are represented by the derivatives of the signals. The absence of interconnections information may lead to overfitting problems in effective connectivity network modelling.

To address this issue, in this paper, we presented a novel sparse linear regression model to infer effective connectivity network and used it for accurate identification of MCI patients from NCs. Specifically, ultra-fMRI time series were first generated by concatenating the original fMRI signal and its corresponding weak derivatives. The structure of effective connectivity network was then determined using an ultra-group Lasso method. Based on this structure, an ultra-orthogonal forward regression (UOFR) algorithm was employed to estimate the strength of each effective connection. The proposed method was applied for MCI identification and superior classification performance was achieved.

2 Materials and Methodology

2.1 Data Acquisition and Preprocessing

The present study involved 61 participants (28 MCI patients and 32 controls) who were diagnosed based on a battery of general neurological examination, collateral and subject symptom, neuropsychological assessment evaluation, and functional capacity reports. Data acquisition was performed using a 3 T Siemens TRIO scanner. One-hundred and eighty resting-state fMRI volumes of each participant were collected with the following parameters: TR = 3000 ms, TE = 30 ms, acquisition matrix = 74 74, 45 slices, and voxel thickness = 3 mm.

The preprocessing pipeline including slice time correction, head motion correction, spatial smoothing, and template wrapping was performed using Statistical Parametric Mapping 8 (SPM8) software package. It should be noted that nuisance signals were band-pass filtered within frequency interval [$0.01 \leq f \leq 0.08$ Hz]. The mean fMRI time series of each region-of-interest according to AAL atlas was then computed for each subject by averaging the fMRI time series over all voxels in each ROI.

2.2 Network Structure Detection via Ultra-group Lasso

Suppose there are M ROIs and N subjects, the mean time series of m-th ROI for n-th subject can be represented as $y_m^n = [y_m^n(1); y_m^n(2); \ldots; y_m^n(T)]$ with T being the number of time points in the time series. For each ROI, its mean time series y_m^n can be modeled the linear combination of time courses of other ROIs as

$$y_m^n = A_m^n \theta_m^n + e_m^n \tag{1}$$

where $A_m^n = [y_1^n, \ldots, y_{m-1}^n, y_{m+1}^n, \ldots, y_M^n]$ denotes a data matrix that includes all mean time series except for the m-th ROI, θ_m^n and e_m^n denote the weight vector and noise.

For a dynamic system, the datum points are time dependent and are connected between each other through the derivatives of time continuous functions. These interconnections convey many important characteristics of a dynamic system. However, the standard least squares criterion considers the datum points individually, discarding the connections among them. The absence of the information conveyed by these interconnections may lead to overfitting problems of dynamic systems [4]. To address this issue, an ultra-least squares (ULS) criterion was introduced by incorporating the weak derivatives into the least squares criterion. The weak derivatives $D^l y$ is defined in Sobolev space as

$$D^l y(t) = \int_{[0,T]} y(t) D^l \varphi(t) dt = (-1)^l \int_{[0,T]} \varphi(t) D^l y(t) dt \tag{2}$$

for any test function $\varphi(t) \in C_0^\infty([0, T])$, which is smooth and possesses compact support on $[0, T]$ [4]. In this study, the $(m + 1)$-th order B-spline functions were employed as the modulating functions. Then, the derivatives $D^l y$ can be redefined as

$$D^l y(\tau) = \int_{[\tau, T_0 + \tau]} y(t) D^l \varphi(t - \tau) dt, \ \tau \in [0, T - T_0] \tag{3}$$

Based on the description above, the ULS criterion is defined as

$$J_{ULS} = \|y_m^n - A_m^n \theta_m^n\|_2^2 + \sum_{l=1}^k \|D^l y_m^n - (D^l A_m^n) \theta_m^n\|_2^2 \tag{4}$$

where $D^l A_m^n = [D^l y_1^n, \ldots, D^l y_{m-1}^n, D^l y_{m+1}^n, \ldots, D^l y_M^n]$.

By concatenating the original signals and the weak derivatives together as $\tilde{y}_m^n = [y_m^n; D^1 y_m^n; D^2 y_m^n; \cdots; D^k y_m^n]$, $\tilde{A}_m^n = [A_m^n; D^1 A_m^n; D^2 A_m^n; \cdots; D^k A_m^n]$, the ULS criterion can be rewritten as

$$J_{ULS} = \|\tilde{y}_m^n - \tilde{A}_m^n \theta_m^n\|_2^2 \tag{5}$$

which has the same form as the standard least squares criterion.

By applying the ULS criterion to the Lasso algorithm, we introduce the ultra-Lasso as

$$J_{Ultra-Lasso} = \|\tilde{y}_m^n - \tilde{A}_m^n \theta_m^n\|_2^2 + \lambda |\theta_m^n| \tag{6}$$

where $\lambda > 0$ is the regularization parameter controlling the 'sparsity' of the model, $\tilde{y}_m^n$ is the ultra-version of the target signal, $\tilde{A}_m^n$ represents the set of ultra-regressors and θ_m^n is the regression parameter, respectively.

However, since the sparsity constraint in Lasso is applied at an individual level, the nonzero elements in θ_m^n differ across subjects. This inevitably causes inter-subject variability which may influence further group analysis. To minimize the inter-subject variability and gain the same model structure for multiple subjects, a group constraint [3] was imposed into ultra-Lasso as

$$J_{UGL} = \sum_{j=1}^{n} \left\| \tilde{y}_m^j - \tilde{A}_m^j \theta_m^n \right\|_2^2 + \lambda \left\| \theta_m \right\|_{2,1} \tag{7}$$

where $\theta_m = [\theta_m^1, \theta_m^2, \cdots, \theta_m^N]$ and $\|\theta_m\|_{2,1}$ is the summation of l_2-norms of row vectors in θ_m. Specifically, the weights corresponding to certain parameters across different subjects are grouped together. This promotes a common connection topology, while in the meantime allows for variation of coefficient values between subjects. By employing the ultra-group Lasso, a subset of region-of-interests (ROIs) with nonzero weights is selected to be considered connecting with the target ROI.

2.3 Effective Connectivity Construction via UFOR

The coefficients θ_m estimated via the ultra-group Lasso can simply be regarded as the effective connectivity (connection weights) between ROI to construct an effective connectivity network. However, these estimated coefficients are unscaled and biased, and it may lead to difficult interpretation and analysis of the effective network. Thus, an UOFR algorithm [4] was employed to estimate the connectivity strength based on the structure detected by the ultra-group Lasso. Given the ultra-target signal $\tilde{y}_m^n$ and candidate regressor dictionary $D_m^n = \{\tilde{x}_i | \tilde{x}_i \in \tilde{A}_m^n, \theta_m^n(i) \neq 0\}$, where $\tilde{x}_i = [y_i^n; D^1 y_i^n; D^2 y_i^n; \cdots; D^k y_i^n]$ represents ultra-time series of ROIs selected via the ultra-group Lasso, the values of error reduction ratio (ERR) can be computed as

$$ERR_i = \frac{\left\langle \tilde{x}_i, \tilde{y}_m^n \right\rangle^2}{\left\langle \tilde{x}_i, \tilde{x}_i \right\rangle \left\langle \tilde{y}_m^n, \tilde{y}_m^n \right\rangle} \tag{8}$$

Regressor (defined as $\tilde{x}_{max}$) with the greatest ERR was first removed from the dictionary D_m^n, and was regarded as the connection weight between the corresponding ROI and the target ROI. The remaining regressors in D_m^n were then orthogonalized with $\tilde{x}_{max}$ using a Gram-Schmidt algorithm. This process was repeated until the regressor dictionary D_m^n becomes empty. All the maximum ERR values were arranged into an effective connectivity matrix of size $M \times M$ for M-dimensional ROIs, where the matrix contains every possible effective connectivity of ROIs pairs [5].

2.4   Feature Selection and Classification

To characterize the brain networks with a small number of neurobiologically mean-ingful and easily computable measures, topological properties, such as out-degree and in-degree, weighted-clustering, betweenness centrality, were extracted as features from the connectivity matrix following [6]. In order to ensure that all features were within the same scale and to minimize bias in feature selection, the feature vectors are scaled to the range [0, 1] individually across subjects.

After features extraction, a feature selection method based on the importance scores from a standard random forest was adopted. The importance scores have been shown to select a highly reduced subset of discriminative features and was detailed in [7] and we briefly outline it here. At each node τ within the binary trees T of the random forest, the Gini impurity measures how well a potential split is separating the samples of the two classes in this particular node [7]. It is defined and calculated as

$$G(\tau) = 1 - p_1^2 - p_0^2 \tag{9}$$

where $p_k = \frac{n_k}{n}$ denotes the fraction of the n_k samples from class k = $\{0, 1\}$ out of the total n samples at node τ. By splitting and sending the samples to two sub-nodes τ_l and τ_r (with respective samples fractions $p_l = \frac{n_l}{n}$ and $p_r = \frac{n_r}{n}$) with a threshold t_θ on variable θ, the Gini coefficient decreases $\Delta G(\tau)$ is calculated as

$$\Delta G(\tau) = G(\tau) - p_l G(\tau_l) - p_r G(\tau_r) \tag{10}$$

By searching over all variables θ and all possible thresholds t_θ, the maximum $\Delta G(\tau)$ is determined. Individually for all variables θ, the decrease in Gini impurity is recorded and accumulated for all nodes τ and all trees T in the forest:

$$I_G(\theta) = \sum_T \sum_\tau \Delta G_\theta(\tau, T) \tag{11}$$

The Gini importance I_G indicates the frequency a particular feature is selected for a split and the discriminative power of this feature for the classification problem. Based on this criterion, features ranked and selected prior to the training of a classifier. The Gini importance criterion has shown robustness against noise and effectiveness in selecting useful features [7].

Finally, a linear SVM was trained for MCI classification using the features selected based on the Gini importance. A nested leave-one-out cross-validation (LOOCV) scheme was adopted in this study to evaluate the classification performance.

3   Experiment Results

3.1   Classification Performance

We compared our proposed method with several other related methods for connectivity network based MCI classification in Table 1. Experiment results demonstrate that, by the use of ultra least criterion and the group Lasso, the proposed method models the relationship among brain regions more accurately and achieves much improved performance in identifying MCI subjects from NC. It indicates excellent diagnostic power of proposed classification framework and also validates the effectiveness of the modeling method.

Table 1. Comparison of classification performance of different connectivity-networks

Method	ACC(%)	SEN(%)	SPE(%)	BAC(%)	AUC
Pearson correlation	70.49	75.00	66.67	70.83	0.69
Lasso	73.77	67.86	78.79	73.32	0.75
Ultra Lasso	77.05	75.00	78.79	76.89	0.73
Group Lasso	77.05	78.57	75.76	77.16	0.72
Proposed	80.33	75.00	84.85	79.92	0.81

By comparing results of methods with the ultra-least criterion and those without, we find that methods with ultra-least criterion obtained 3.28% accuracy increase. This implies that the ultra-least criterion efficiently increases the noise resistibility and robustness of the method by incorporating the weak derivatives into the least squares criterion and thus helps improve the classification performance afterwards. It should also be noted that the Group Lasso method achieves an accuracy of 77.05% which is 3.28% higher than ordinary Lasso. By grouping together the weights corresponding to certain features across different subjects, the group constraint reduces inter-subject variability and thus enables relatively easier differentiation between MCI subjects and healthy controls [3].

3.2 Brain Regions Involved in Classification

As a LOO strategy is employed to evaluate the proposed method, features selected at each loop might be quite different. To evaluate the importance of brain regions, the frequency that features being selected are counted and features with highest selected times are considered to be significant in the classification of MCI. As each ROI corresponds to several features, the selected times of features corresponding to the same ROI is added up. The top ten ROIs and their locations are listed in Table 2.

It worth noticing that these top 10 regions locate in the frontal lobe (e.g. Superior frontal gyrus, orbital part) and the temporal lobe (e.g. Superior temporal gyrus). And regions such as hippocampus are also found to be associated with MCI/AD diagnosis. These results are exemplified in previous literatures [8–10].

As topological properties are extracted as features, brain regions are evaluated by selected frequency in classification at a nodal level. To further evaluate the significant differences of each connection, a standard two-sample t-test was employed on full dataset. Connections with a p-value smaller than 0.01 are listed in Table 3.

Figure 1 graphically shows the differences of these connections between MCI and NC (the thickness of edges indicates the strength of connections). It is interesting to note that the effective connectivity for most of the optimal connections are much

Table 2. The most selected brain regions in classification

Index	Full name	Location
37	Hippocampus	Limbic lobe
71	Caudate nucleus	Subcortical gray nuclei
6	Superior frontal gyrus, orbital part	Frontal lobe
28	Gyrus rectus	Frontal lobe
31	Anterior cingulate and paracingulate gyri	Limbic lobe
42	Amygdala	Subcortical gray nuclei
52	Middle occipital gyrus	Occipital lobe
54	Inferior occipital gyrus	Occipital lobe
65	Angular gyrus	Parietal lobe
81	Superior temporal gyrus	Temporal lobe

smaller in MCI patients than that of NCs. Moreover, several ROIs (Hippocampus, Superior frontal gyrus, orbital part; Angular gyrus) selected in classification showed significant differences between two groups based on the two-sample t-test, further justify their contribution to MCI pathology.

Table 3. The most discriminative connections. (STG = Superior temporal gyrus; PCG = Posterior cingulate gyrus; TPOmid = Temporal pole, middle temporal gyrus; CUN = Cuneus; HIP = Hippocampus; PHG = Parahippocampal gyrus; ORBsup = Superior frontal gyrus, orbital part; ANG = Angular gyrus; PCL = Paracentral lobule; ROL = Rolandic operculum; ORBmid = Middle frontal gyrus, orbital part; TPO-sup = Temporal pole, superior temporal gyrus; PUT = Lenticular nucleus, putamen; AMYG = Amygdala; ORBinf = Inferior frontal gyrus, orbital part; PreCG = Precentral gyrus; PCL = Paracentral lobule; MFG = Middle frontal gyrus; L = Left; R = Right)

Selected ROIs	Direction of connectivity	Neighbors of selected ROIs	p-values
PHG.R	←	STG.R	0.0054
CUN.R	→	TPOmid.L	0.0061
ANG.R	←	CUN.L	0.0063
PCL.R	←	PUT.L	0.0064
ROL.L	→	CUN.L	0.0068
ORBmid.R	→	ORBinf.R	0.0070
TPOsup.R	←	AMYG.L	0.0070
PCG.R	→	HIP.L	0.0077
ORBsup.R	→	PreCG.R	0.0080
PCL.L	→	MFG.L	0.0094
IPL.R	→	SMG.R	0.0089
AMYG.L	←	Vermis9	0.0099

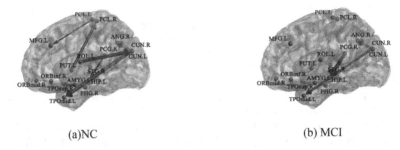

(a)NC   (b) MCI

Fig. 1. Comparison of connectivity strengths based on the most discriminative connections

4 Discussion and Conclusion

In summary, we have proposed a novel sparse effective connectivity network estimation method by imposing a group constraint and an ULS criterion into ordinary Lasso. We use an ultra-group Lasso to detect the network structure and re-estimate the connectivity strength via an UOFR algorithm. The network structure detection process prunes the ROI candidates, thus reducing the parameters of the model to prevent overfitting problems in effective network modelling. Promising experiment results demonstrated the efficacy of the proposed approach for MCI classification.

References

1. Sporns, O.: Towards network substrates of brain disorders. Brain **137**, 2117–2118 (2014). doi:10.1093/brain/awu148
2. Lee, H.L.D., Kang, H., Kim, B.N., Chung, M.K.: Sparse brain network recovery under compressed sensing. IEEE Trans. Med. Imaging **30**(5), 1154–1165 (2011)
3. Wee, C.Y., Yap, P.T., Zhang, D., Wang, L., Shen, D.: Group-constrained sparse fMRI connectivity modeling for mild cognitive impairment identification. Brain Struct. Funct. **219**(2), 641–656 (2014). doi:10.1007/s00429-013-0524-8
4. Li, Y., Cui, W.G., Guo, Y.Z., Huang, T., Yang, X.F., Wei, H.L.: Time-varying system identification using an ultra-orthogonal forward regression and multiwavelet basis functions with applications to EEG. IEEE Trans. Neural Netw. Learn. Syst. **PP**(99), 1–13 (2017). doi:10.1109/TNNLS.2017.2709910
5. Li, Y., Wee, C.Y., Jie, B., Peng, Z.W., Shen, D.G.: Sparse multivariate autoregressive modeling for mild cognitive impairment classification. Neuroinformatics **12**(3), 455–469 (2014). doi:10.1007/s12021-014-9221-x
6. Rubinov, M., Sporns, O.: Complex network measures of brain connectivity: uses and interpretations. Neuroimage **52**(3), 1059–1069 (2010). doi:10.1016/j.neuroimage.2009.10.003
7. Menze, B.H., Kelm, B.M., Masuch, R., Himmelreich, U., Bachert, P., Petrich, W., Hamprecht, F.A.: A comparison of random forest and its Gini importance with standard chemometric methods for the feature selection and classification of spectral data. BMC Bioinformatics **10** (2009)

8. Nir, T.M., Jahanshad, N., Villalon-Reina, J.E., Toga, A.W., Jack, C.R., Weiner, M.W., Thompson, P.M., Alzheimer's Disease Neuroimaging Initiative (ADNI): Effectiveness of regional DTI measures in distinguishing Alzheimer's disease, MCI, and normal aging. Neuroimage Clin **3**, 180–195 (2013). doi:10.1016/j.nicl.2013.07.006

9. Salvatore, C., Cerasa, A., Battista, P., Gilardi, M.C., Quattrone, A., Castiglioni, I., Alzheimer's Disease Neuroimaging Initiative: Magnetic resonance imaging biomarkers for the early diagnosis of Alzheimer's disease: a machine learning approach. Front. Neurosci. **9**, 307 (2015). doi:10.3389/Fnins.2015.00307

10. Jie, B., Zhang, D.Q., Gao, W., Wang, Q., Wee, C.Y., Shen, D.G.: Integration of network topological and connectivity properties for neuroimaging classification. IEEE Trans. Bio Med. Eng. **61**(2), 576–589 (2014). doi:10.1109/Tbme.2013.2284195

Reconstruction of Thin-Slice Medical Images Using Generative Adversarial Network

Zeju Li[1], Yuanyuan Wang[1,2(✉)], and Jinhua Yu[1,2(✉)]

[1] Department of Electronic Engineering, Fudan University, Shanghai, China
{yywang, jhyu}@fudan.edu.cn
[2] Key Laboratory of Medical Imaging Computing and Computer Assisted
Intervention of Shanghai, Shanghai, China

Abstract. Slice thickness is a very important parameter for medical imaging such as magnetic resonance (MR) imaging or computed tomography (CT). Thinner slice imaging obviously provides higher spatial resolution and more diagnostic information, however also involves higher imaging cost both in time and expense. For the sake of efficiency, a relatively thick slice interval is usually used in the daily routine medical imaging. A novel generative adversarial network was proposed in this paper to reconstruct medical images with thinner slice thickness from regular thick slice images. A fully convolutional network with three-dimensional convolutional kernels and residual blocks was firstly applied to generate the slices between the imaging intervals. A novel perceptual loss function was proposed to guarantee both the pixel similarity and the spatial coherence in 3D. Moreover, a discriminator network with a sustained adversarial loss was utilized to push the solution to be more realistic. 43 pairs of MR images were used to validate the performance of the proposed method. The presented method is able to recover preoperative t2flair MR images with slice thickness of 2 mm from routine t2flair MR images with thickness of 6 mm. The reconstruction results on two datasets show the superiority of the presented method over other competitive image reconstruction methods.

Keywords: Image reconstruction · Generative adversarial network · Deep learning

1 Introduction

Tomographic medical imaging techniques such as magnetic resonance (MR) imaging and computed tomography (CT) produce tomographic images of cross-sections of human body. Medical instruments pick slices at regular intervals and generalize three-dimensional (3D) volumetric images from a series of slices collected in a certain direction. Medical images with thinner slices preserve higher spatial resolution in coronal and sagittal axis and provide more clinical information. However, thin-slice medical images are not always available because of economic and efficiency issues. For example, glioma patients who get head MR images with slice thickness of 6 mm with routine MRI examination have to get another preoperative t2flair MR images with thickness of 2 mm to obtain more diagnosis information for further treatment. Nevertheless, the reconstruction is also essential for many medical images related

© Springer International Publishing AG 2017
Q. Wang et al. (Eds.): MLMI 2017, LNCS 10541, pp. 325–333, 2017.
DOI: 10.1007/978-3-319-67389-9_38

researches. Therefore, it is of great clinical value to reconstruct thin-slice tomographic medical images.

The task of tomographic images reconstruction is always considered as the image registration problem [1]. 3D information is reproduced by co-registering thicker slices to thinner slices or maps. Registration methods utilize the mutual information between the resource and target volumes and build up transform projection based on affine, spline or radon transform. Registration based reconstruction algorithms largely base on the limited information provided by the paired samples. The information provided by other paired samples are not well utilized. Furthermore, in these algorithms the estimated slices are generated only using neighbor slices, the global information of tomographic images is therefore not included. The performance of these registration based methods is limited by the two constrains.

In this study, the task of image reconstruction for tomographic medical images is seen as single image super-resolution (SISR) problem in 3D. SISR means generating a high-resolution (HR) image from its low-resolution (LR) image for a single image. Actually, reconstruction of tomographic medical images could be viewed as SISR in the coronal plane. Recently, convolutional neural network (CNN) and generative adversarial network (GAN) have made remarkable breakthroughs in SISR [2]. The impressive SSIR results inspire us the reconstruction of tomographic medical images might have better solutions. In this paper, a state-of-the-art SISR method, called super-resolution GAN (SRGAN), is extended to three-dimensional version (3DSRGAN). Specifically, a fully connected CNN with 3D convolutional kernels and residual blocks was proposed to generate tomographic medical images from fewer slices. A perceptual loss function, which consists of four separate losses, is proposed to encourage the network to produce more realistic and reasonable medical images. Pixel-wise loss is the basis of the loss function to encourage pixel-wise image similarity. A 3D total variation loss is proposed to ensure continuity of the deformation in the coronal plane. Traditional regularization loss is presented to avoid overfitting of the deep network. Furthermore, an adversarial loss is added to provide external adjustments which could make the generated results be closer to the original images in the global context. In the experiment, our method is applied to reconstruct preoperative t2flair head MR images of glioma patients from routine t2flair MR images. Preoperative MR images is acquired with thinner slice and preserve slice spacing of 2 mm. On the other side, routine MR images get slice spacing of 6 mm. By comparing the reconstruction results with the original images of two datasets, it shows that 3DSRGAN is more effective and efficient than other popular methods in the task of tomographic medical images reconstruction.

2   Method

It is widely acknowledged that CNN has made great breakthroughs in the field of computer vision. CNN has proved to be a well-performed deep learning model by the use of hierarchical features and convolutional layers. Lately, an adversarial approach, namely GAN, was proposed to learn deep generative models. The idea of GAN is to raise an adversarial network to discriminate the generated samples from the realistic samples. With the supervision of adversarial network, the generative model is driven to approximate the distribution of the training data and produces more realistic results.

More recently, GAN plays an important role in SISR and recovers photo-realistic textures from heavily down-sampled images. The ultimate results of GAN in SISR motivate us to build a generator network G to generate the information between sampling intervals of tomographic medical images. Concretely, given a tomographic medical images with fewer slices I^{FS} with size $L \times W \times H$, we want to generate the medical images with more slices I^{MS} with size $L \times W \times rH$ of the same examination position.

In CNN, tensor calculation including convolutional kernels is normally in the shape of 2D because natural images are 2D. However, when applied to tomographic medical image, it is more suitable to extend the process to 3D to take fully advantage of the volume data of medical images. 3D convolutional kernels make it possible to calculate the volume as a whole instead of processing slice by slice using 2D convolutional kernels. In this study, SRGAN is extended to 3DSRGAN by the flexible application of 3D convolutional kernels and 3D deconvolutional kernels. The details of the network structures would be described in the following paragraph.

2.1 Generative Adversarial Network

The details of the network structures are described in the following paragraph. The structure of proposed 3DSRGAN is demonstrated in Fig. 1. A 7-layers CNN with 3D convolutional kernels is proposed to generate the reconstructed MRI from MRI with fewer slices (FSMRI). Simultaneously, a discriminator with 6 convolutional layers is trained to discriminate reconstructed MRI from MRI with more slices (MSMRI). The basic block of the discriminator network is convolutional layer + relu + batch normalization rather than convolutional layer + batch normalization + relu to make sure the output of the last layer has negative component. Otherwise, the outputs of relu would be all positive and the classification ability of sigmoid function would be diminished.

FSMRI is up-sampled to be the same size with MSMRI by deconvolutional layers with unbalanced stride of [1,1,3]. In the discriminator network, down-sampling of

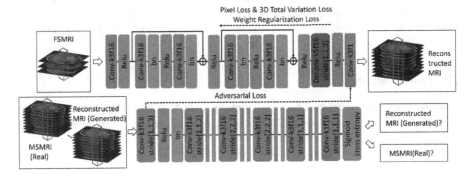

Fig. 1. Flowchart of proposed 3DSRGAN. The size of kernels and the number of filters are illustrated in the blocks. Stride of convolutional kernels is [1,1,1] unless an additional explanation is given.

MSMRI and reconstructed MRI is accomplished by using convolutional kernels with strides instead of pooling, as suggested by DCGAN.

Residual block is a core of the proposed network. The idea of residual blocks was proposed recently to guarantee the integrity of the forward and backward propagated signal. Residual connections help deep network avoid the problems of gradient vanishing and enable the training of networks with very deep structures. Although our generator network is not necessarily deep, it also suffers from gradient vanishing problem for two reasons. First, the use of 3D convolutional kernels would increase the number of trainable network parameters dramatically and make it difficult to pass residual during backward propagation. What's more, a relatively complicated loss function is designed for the generator network and creates difficulties for the global convergence of the network. Residual blocks preserve the flowing signals in the network and would benefit the training of the generator network. Specifically, we add residual blocks between the outputs every two layers. The first convolutional layer is not considered into residual blocks because we want to build to residual network upon high-level features rather than low-level features extracted directly from the images.

In the phase of training, I^{FS} with size $L \times W \times H$ is divided into several volumes with size $15 \times 15 \times H$ to be the input of the network. Similarly, I^{MS} with size $L \times W \times rH$ is divided into several volumes with size $15 \times 15 \times rH$ to be the output of the generator network. In order to quicken the learning speed, both the input and the output volumes are normalized to the range from 0 to 1, separately. Then we normalize the volume blocks on each sequence to have zero mean and unit variance. The outputs of generator network, together with volume of I^{MS}, are concatenated to be the inputs of the discriminator network. The discriminator network is trained to distinguish the volumes from different sources and provide suggestion for improvement back to the generator network. During testing, I^{FS} is input to the generator network with full size with the same preprocessing of zero mean and unit variance. Besides, the mean and variance of batch normalization layers are fixed using the parameters gotten from training.

To demonstrate the effectiveness of our 3D model, a 2D super-resolution CNN (2DSRCNN) is also developed for tomographic medical image reconstruction. 2DSRCNN consists of 12 convolutional layers with small convolutional kernels. 2DSRCNN could be seen as a simplified structure of the 3D generator network and is trained to recover 2D images in the coronal plane. Specifically, for each volume, 2DSRCNN recover L high-resolution images with size $W \times rH$ from L low-resolution images with size $W \times H$.

2.2   Loss Function

In the training phase, we make use of training data to obtain the parameter θ_G of generative convolutional network G_θ. I^{MS} is taken as target and I^{FS} as input:

$$\hat{\theta}_G = \arg\min_{\theta_G} l^G(G_\theta(I^{FS}), I^{MS}) \tag{1}$$

where l^G is the loss function of the generative model. The network is trained by minimizing the loss function l^G which indicated the differences between the generative results and the real images.

In this study, we propose a perceptual loss function designed for the 3D reconstruction problem. The perceptual loss consists of a pixel loss, an adversarial loss, a 3D total variation loss and a weight regulation loss:

$$l^G = \lambda_1 * l^G_{MSE} + \lambda_2 * l^G_{Ad} + \lambda_3 * l^G_{tv} + \lambda_4 * l^G_{\theta} \tag{2}$$

The four components are designed for different optimization purposes and would be discussed in the following paragraphs separately.

Pixel Loss. No one can deny the importance of pixel similarity in the task of reconstruction. l^G_{MSE} is taken as the main body of the present perceptual loss. The pixel-wise MSE loss is calculated as:

$$l^G_{MSE} = \frac{1}{rLWH} \sum_{x=1}^{L} \sum_{y=1}^{W} \sum_{z=1}^{rH} (I^{MS}_{x,y,z} - G(I^{FS})_{x,y,z})^2 \tag{3}$$

Adversarial Loss. Basically, the loss function relied heavily on the mean squared reconstruction error (MSE) in the related study. However, solutions totally based on MSE always appear overly smooth due to the pixel-wise average of all the possible solutions. To address this problem, we proposed a discriminator network to help generator network produce more realistic results.

Typically, the loss function of the discriminator network is calculated as:

$$l^D = \frac{1}{2} \left[l_{bce}\left(D(I^{MS}), 0\right) + l_{bce}\left(D(G(I^{FS})), 1\right) \right] \tag{4}$$

After the discriminator network is settled, generator network would be in turn affected by the feedback from the discriminator:

$$l^G_{Ad} = l_{bce}\left(D(G(I^{FS})), 0\right) \tag{5}$$

This adversarial loss encourages the generator network to confuse the discriminator network. The loss term is large if the discriminator network can discriminate the output of the generator network. The external adjustments brought by the adversarial loss are based on high-order statistics and are accessible by the standard pixel-wise loss function. In our study, the generator network and discriminator network are both updated in each step of a mini batch to provide timely adjustments.

3D Total Variation Loss. Different from the total variation loss which encourages spatial smoothness in output 2D images, we proposed a 3D total variation loss function to encourage spatially coherent solutions in the coronal plane of output 3D blocks. 3D total variation loss is calculated as:

$$l_{tv}^G = \frac{1}{rLWH} \sum_{x=1}^{L} \sum_{y=1}^{W} \sum_{z=1}^{rH-1} (G(I^{FS})_{x,y,z+1} - G(I^{FS})_{x,y,z})^2 \tag{6}$$

The 3D total variation loss is defined based on the sum of MSE between every neighbor slices of the reconstruction images. The variation loss encourages the generator network to estimate the absent data by making use of the neighbor slices. This would strengthen space connectivity of the reconstruction images in 3D and lead to more reasonable results.

Weight Regularization Loss. Structures in different MR images are quite different and networks tend to get poor performance with different dataset. L2 regularization loss is added to prevent overfitting the training data.

3 Experimental Results

Our methods and experiments were all developed by using Tensorflow. Both the generator network and the discriminator network were trained using Adam optimizer with beta1 = 0.9, beta2 = 0.999 and epsilon = 1e−8. The networks were initialized using the Xavier method. The primary learning rates were 1e−2 and 1e−3 for the generator network and discriminator network, separately. The learning rates were decayed in an exponential way with a basis of 0.99. Specifically, we chose the following loss for our experiments:

$$l^G = l_{MSE}^G + 0.1 * l_{Ad}^G + 1e - 8 * l_{tv}^G + 1e - 5 * l_\theta^G \tag{7}$$

In order to illustrate the effectiveness of adversarial loss, the training of 3DSRCNN and 3DSRGAN were all stop at 25 epoch.

3.1 Material

We validated 3DSRGAN on the reconstruction of brain MR images of glioma patients. T2flair MR images of 43 glioma patients were taken from Huashan Hospital, Shanghai, China. All of these 43 glioma patients have preoperative MR images. The preoperative t2flair MR images were acquired using Siemens scanner with voxel size 0.47 × 0.47 × 2 mm, TR = 9000 ms, TE = 96 ms, TI = 2501 ms, flip angle = 150°. 15 of these glioma patients were found to have routine MR images. The time interval between the two MRI examinations is less than 3 months and no obvious changes were observed in patients' conditions. The routine t2flair MR images were also acquired using Siemens scanner with voxel size 0.47 × 0.47 × 6 mm, TR = 9000 ms, TE = 94 mm, TI = 2501 ms, flip angle = 150°. In this study, preoperative t2flair MR images are down-sampled to slice thickness of 6 mm and used as a simulation dataset. Moreover, 15 cases with both preoperative and routine MR images were taken as a real images dataset. We take 30 cases from the simulation dataset and 10 cases from the real images dataset for training, separately. The rest of cases in the two dataset were taken as independent test samples. MRI volumes were spatially normalized to the Montreal Neurological Institute (MNI) reference brain to make sure the images were exactly aligned.

3.2 Reconstruction Results

The presented methods were applied to the two datasets mentioned above, separately. To demonstrate the effectiveness of our proposed method, two popular registration methods were used as comparison, namely nearest neighbor (NN) interpolation and 4th B-spline interpolation. The two methods are based on nonlinear deformation and often applied to the reconstruction of thin-slices MR images [1].

To qualitatively compare the reconstruction results of different methods, the reconstruction results of a slice between the sampling intervals are visualized in Fig. 2. Compared with NN and B-spline, 3DSRGAN could provide more realistic results. The error estimation of the skull and brain structure are reduced. Different from reconstruction methods based on interpolation, 3DSRGAN take advantage of a lot of prior knowledge learned from plenty training data. The large number of CNN parameters allows 3DSRGAN to produce more complex mapping relationship between the resource images and the target images. On the other side, the reconstruction results of 3DSRGAN were generated using the global 3D information of the images from fewer slices. 3DSRGAM is able to take advantage of all the given H slices to generate the images between the sampling intervals. Mapping relationship was established from H slices to rH slices. It would benefit the process of image reconstruction with global context. However, registration based methods reconstruct the images with the

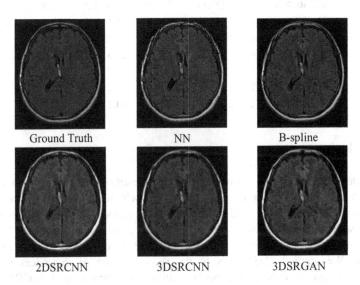

Ground Truth	NN	B-spline
2DSRCNN	3DSRCNN	3DSRGAN

Fig. 2. Visual comparison of original MSMR images and reconstruction result from FSMR images by different methods.

interpolation of neighbor slices. Therefore, the prediction results of 3DSRGAN could be more reasonable. Compared with 2DSRCNN, 3DSRGAN process the images as volumes. Spatially coherent solutions are guaranteed by the use of 3D convolutional kernels. It leads to more accurate and smooth results in the axial plane. Compared with 3DSRCNN, 3DSRGAN benefit a lot from the external adjustment of the discriminator and more details are reproduced. These details make the reconstruction more similar to the original images. It should also be mentioned that the use of residual blocks could make the network converge faster and obtain a better result on both the training data and the test data.

To demonstrate the results of our method in quantitative way, the MSE and peak signal to noise ratio (PSNR) were calculated by taking the images with slice thickness of 2 mm as the ground truth. The global validations are summarized in Table 1. Obviously, the results of 3DSRGAN outperform the results generated by other mentioned methods. In addition, the operation time of 3DSRGAN is shortest because the reconstruction just require one time of the forward propagation of the 3D generator network.

Table 1. Quantitative reconstruction results by different methods. Our methods are validated on two dataset with separate test data.

Dataset	Methods	MSE		PSNR		Operation
		Mean (std.)	Med.	Mean (std.)	Med.	time(s)
Simulation dataset	NN	193.9 (50.7)	182.1	25.4 (1.1)	25.5	322
	B-spline	157.6 (39.4)	149.0	26.3 (1.1)	26.4	202
	2DSRCNN	141.3 (32.7)	140.0	26.7 (1.0)	26.7	4.3
	3DSRCNN	139.5 (36.8)	132.6	26.8 (1.2)	26.9	2.5
	3DSRGAN	**132.4 (34.5)**	**130.5**	**27.1 (1.1)**	**27.0**	**2.5**
Real images dataset	NN	448.8 (140.2)	489.3	21.9 (1.7)	21.2	/
	B-spline	415.8 (132.1)	447.5	22.3 (1.7)	21.6	/
	2DSRCNN	299.8 (90.2)	329.1	23.7 (1.6)	23.0	/
	3DSRCNN	269.5 (84.6)	288.7	24.1 (1.5)	23.5	/
	3DSRGAN	**262.2 (75.9)**	**277.6**	**24.2 (1.4)**	**23.7**	/

4 Conclusion

In this study, we proposed a novel GAN based method for the reconstruction of thin-slice tomographic medical images from images with thick slices. A GAN structure with 3D convolutional kernels and residual blocks is proposed to generate the medical images between the sampling intervals. A novel perceptual loss function which consists of four components is proposed to make the reconstruction results more realistic and reasonable. We applied 3DSRGAN to the reconstruction of thin-slices head MR images of glioma patients. Experiments results demonstrated that 3DSRGAN can provide better reconstruction results than other popular methods.

In the future, other modalities of MR images (such as T1, T2, T1 enhancing) and CT images of the same examination position would be included for the reconstruction of thin-slice t2flair MR images. The effectiveness of enlarging the size of training dataset is also an interesting topic of the future work.

Acknowledgments. This work was supported by the National Basic Research Program of China (2015CB755500), the National Natural Science Foundation of China (11474071).

References

1. Klein, A., Andersson, J., Ardekani, B.A., Ashburner, J., Avants, B., Chiang, M., et al.: Evaluation of 14 nonlinear deformation algorithms applied to human brain MRI registration. NeuroImage **46**(3), 786–802 (2009)
2. Ledig, C., Theis, L., Huszar, F., Caballero, J., Cunningham, A., Acosta, A., et al.: Photo-realistic single image super-resolution using a generative adversarial network. arXiv:1609.04802 (2016)

Neural Network Convolution (NNC) for Converting Ultra-Low-Dose to "Virtual" High-Dose CT Images

Kenji Suzuki[1]([✉]), Junchi Liu[1], Amin Zarshenas[1], Toru Higaki[2],
Wataru Fukumoto[2], and Kazuo Awai[2]

[1] Department of Electrical and Computer Engineering & Medical Imaging
Research Center, Illinois Institute of Technology,
Chicago, IL, USA
ksuzuki@iit.edu
[2] Department of Diagnostic Radiology,
Institute of Biomedical and Health Sciences, Hiroshima University,
Hiroshima, Japan

Abstract. To reduce radiation dose in CT, we developed a novel deep-learning technique, neural network convolution (NNC), for converting ultra-low-dose (ULD) to "virtual" high-dose (HD) CT images with less noise or artifact. NNC is a supervised image-based machine-learning (ML) technique consisting of a neural network regression model. Unlike other typical deep learning, NNC can learn thus output desired images, as opposed to class labels. We trained our NNC with ULDCT (0.1 mSv) and corresponding "teaching" HDCT (5.7 mSv) of an anthropomorphic chest phantom. Once trained, our NNC no longer require HDCT, and it provides "virtual" HDCT where noise and artifact are substantially reduced. To test our NNC, we collected ULDCT (0.1 mSv) of 12 patients with 3 different vendor CT scanners. To determine a dose reduction rate of our NNC, we acquired 6 CT scans of the anthropomorphic chest phantom at 6 different radiation doses (0.1–3.0 mSv). Our NNC reduced noise and streak artifacts in ULDCT substantially, while maintaining anatomic structures and pathologies such as vessels and nodules. With our NNC, the image quality of ULDCT (0.1 mSv) images was improved at the level equivalent to 1.1 mSv CT images, which corresponds to 91% dose reduction.

Keywords: Deep learning · Radiation dose reduction · Image quality improvement · Image-based machine learning · Virtual imaging

1 Introduction

CT has been proven to be useful to detect and diagnose various diseases. For example, CT was proved to be effective in screening for lung cancer [1]. Recent studies [2] showed that CT scans might be responsible for up to 2% of cancers in the U.S., and CT scans performed in each year would cause 29,000 new cancer cases in the future due to ionizing radiation exposures to patients. To address this serious issue, researchers and CT venders developed various iterative reconstruction (IR) techniques [3–5] to enable dose reduction by reconstruction of scan raw data. A recent survey study with more

© Springer International Publishing AG 2017
Q. Wang et al. (Eds.): MLMI 2017, LNCS 10541, pp. 334–343, 2017.
DOI: 10.1007/978-3-319-67389-9_39

than 1,000 hospitals in Australia [6], however, revealed that IR reduced radiation dose by 17–44%, which is not sufficient for screening population. Furthermore, full IR is computationally very expensive; for example, GE Veo took 30–45 min. Per one scan on a specialized massively parallel computer of 112 CPU cores [4]. Therefore, it is crucial to develop a technique that can reduce radiation dose in CT substantially in a reasonable time.

In this study, we invented and developed a novel machine-learning (ML) approach to radiation dose reduction in CT in 2010 and 2012 [7], respectively. We presented our initial results in abstracts at clinical conferences [8–10]. No ML approach was developed for radiation dose reduction in CT. Some investigators developed radiation dose reduction in CT by means of ML in 2017 [11, 12]. Our technology employed our original deep-learning technique called neural network convolution (NNC), which is extensions of our original ML techniques with image input [13–17] back in 1994. Unlike most other deep-learning models such as AlexNet, LeNet, and most other convolutional neural networks (CNNs) that learn output class labels (e.g., cancer or non-cancer), our NNC learns directly "teaching" desired images thus outputs images, which we believe an extremely important concept. Our NNC's property of high computational efficiency would solve the problem of the high computational cost with IR techniques. By means of our NNC, we aimed to accomplish substantial dose reduction for screening population in efficient computation for a routine clinical use. We evaluated our dose-reduction technology with anthropomorphic phantom and patient images acquired with different vender CT scanners for its robustness and performance and to determine its dose reduction rate quantitatively.

2 Radiation Dose Reduction Technology Based on NNC

2.1 Basic Principles of Our Radiation Dose Reduction Technology

The schematic diagrams of our proposed radiation dose reduction technology based on NNC are illustrated in Fig. 1. Our technology has a training step and an application step. In the training step, we acquire pairs of lower-dose (LD) CT images (e.g., 0.1 mSv) reconstructed by the filtered back-projection (FBP) algorithm and corresponding "teaching" (or desired) higher-dose (HD) CT images (e.g., 5.7 mSv) reconstructed by FBP of an anthropomorphic chest phantom. Through the training, the NNC learns the relationship between the input LDCT and teaching HDCT images to convert LDCT images with noise and artifacts due to low radiation exposure into HDCT images. Once trained, the NNC no longer requires HDCT images. In the application step, the trained NNC model is applied to unseen new LDCT images of a patient to produce "high-dose-like" CT images where noise and artifacts are substantially reduced while maintaining lesions and anatomic structures such as lung nodules and lung vessels; thus we term "virtual" HD (VHD) CT.

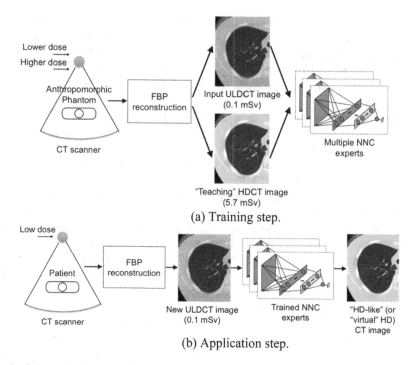

(a) Training step.

(b) Application step.

Fig. 1. Schematic diagrams of our proposed radiation dose reduction technology based on our original deep-learning model, NNC.

2.2 Architecture and Training of NNC

In the field of image processing, Suzuki et al. developed supervised nonlinear filters and edge enhancers based on a neural network (NN), called neural filters [15, 18] and neural edge enhancers [17, 19], respectively. In the field of computer-aided diagnosis (CAD), Suzuki et al. invented a massive-training artificial NN (MTANN) by extending neural filters and edge enhancers to accommodate pattern-recognition and classification tasks [16, 20–23]. In this study, we extended MTANNs and developed a general framework for supervised image processing, which we call it a machine-learning convolution. An NNC consists of a linear-output-layer neural network (NN) regression (LNNR) model [17] that is capable of deep layers. The NNC can be considered as a supervised nonlinear filter that can be trained with input images and the corresponding "teaching" images. The LNNR model, which is capable of operating on image data directly, employs a linear function instead of a sigmoid function in the output layer because the characteristics of an NN were improved significantly when applied to the continuous mapping of values in image processing [17]. The NNC model consists of an input layer, a convolutional layer, multiple fully-connected hidden layers, and an output layer. The input layer of the LNNR receives the pixel values in a 2D subregion (or kernel, image patch), R, extracted from input ULDCT images. The output $O(x,y)$ of the NNC is a continuous value, which corresponds to the center pixel in the subregion (or image patch), represented by

$$\widehat{g}(x,y) = NN\{f(x-i, y-j)|(i,j) \in R\}, \tag{1}$$

where $NN(\cdot)$ is the output of the LNNR model, and $f(x,y)$ is a pixel value of an input CT image. Note that only one unit is employed in the output layer. Other ML model such as support vector regression and nonlinear Gaussian process regression [22] can be used instead of the LNNR model, which forms a ML convolution. The entire CT images are obtained by scanning the LNNR model in a convolutional manner, thus term NNC.

For training to convert input LDCT images with noise and artifacts into desired HDCT images, we define the error function to be minimized, represented by

$$E = \frac{1}{P} \sum_{(x,y)\in R_T} \{g(x,y) - \hat{g}(x,y)\}^2, \tag{2}$$

where R_T is a training region. The NNC is trained by a linear-output-layer back-propagation (BP) algorithm [17], which was derived for the LNNR model in the same way as for the BP algorithm [24]. After training with this training algorithm, the NNC is expected to output the values close to desired pixel values in the teaching images. Thus, the trained NNC would output high-dose-like CT images with less noise or artifacts when new LDCT images are entered.

2.3 Anatomy-Specific NNC with Soft Gating Layers

Noise and artifact properties are different in different anatomies in reconstructed CT images. Although a single NNC can reduce noise and artifacts in the entire CT images, it may not reduce some noise or artifacts in specific anatomic segments sufficiently, because the capability of a single NNC in suppressing a wide variety of patterns is limited. To improve the overall performance, we extended the capability of a single NNC and developed an anatomy-specific multiple-NNC scheme that consisted of multiple NNC models together with gating layers, as shown in Fig. 2. In a training step, gating layers control which NNC among multiple NNC is used for training of which anatomic segments. Each anatomy-specific NNC, denoted as NNC$_s$, is trained independently with training samples extracted from the corresponding anatomic segment by a pair of gating layers. After training, each trained anatomy-specific NNC becomes an expert for the corresponding anatomic segment.

In an application step, three anatomic segments were segmented automatically by using thresholding followed by dilation and erosion operations in mathematical morphology. Gating layers control applications of the trained anatomy-specific NNC to corresponding anatomic segments. The gating layers compose the outputs from multiple anatomy-specific NNC into an entire output CT image by using the segmented anatomic segments. To avoid unnatural sudden changes near the boundaries between anatomic segments, "soft" gating layers, as opposed to "hard" gating layers, blend the outputs from anatomy-specific NNCs near the boundaries by using a weighting

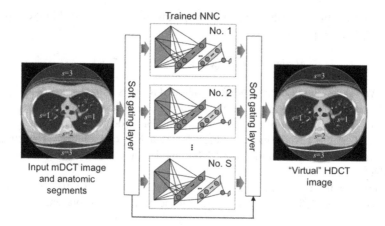

Fig. 2. The architecture of an anatomy-specific multiple NNC scheme that consists of multiple NNC arranged in parallel together with gating layers.

Gaussian function $fw_s(x, y)$. The entire output image is composed of three output anatomic segments of three trained anatomy-specific NNC, represented by

$$\hat{g}(x, y) = \sum_{s=1}^{3} \hat{g}_s(x, y) \cdot fw_s(x, y), \tag{3}$$

where $\hat{g}_s(x, y)$ is the output pixel of the *s-th* trained anatomy-specific NNC.

2.4   Experiments to Validate and Test Our "Virtual" HD Technology

2.4.1   Training with an Anthropomorphic Chest Phantom

To train our NNC, we acquired CT scans of an anthropomorphic chest phantom (Lungman, Kyoto Kagaku, Kyoto, Japan) without motion at LD (0.1 mSv) and HD (5.7 mSv) levels with a CT scanner (LightSpeed VCT with 64 slices, GE, Milwaukee, WI) at Hiroshima University Hospital, Hiroshima, Japan. We changed radiation doses by changing x-ray tube current, while fixing an x-ray tube voltage at 120 kVp. Tube current, tube current time product, and CTDIvol for the LDCT and HDCT were 4 and 570 mA, 4 and 230 mAs, and 0.24 and 13.57 mGy, respectively. CT slices were reconstructed by using FBP reconstruction with the "lung" kernel. Reconstructed CT size was 512×512 pixels, and reconstructed slice thickness was 5 mm. The 5 mm slice thickness was chosen by following the Japanese lung cancer screening guideline. We trained NNC with pairs of the ULDCT (0.1 mSv) slices and corresponding "teaching" (desired) HDCT (5.7 mSv) slices.

2.4.2   Phantom Validation

To validate our radiation dose reduction technology based on our NNC, we acquired CT scans of the anthropomorphic chest phantom at five more different dose levels, namely, 0.25, 0.5, 1.0, 1.5, and 3.0 mSv. Tube current; tube current time product; and

CTDIvol for the CT scans were 25, 50, 100, 150, and 300 mA; 10, 20, 40, 60, and 120 mAs; and 0.60, 1.19, 2.38, 3.57, and 7.14 mGy, respectively. We applied the trained anatomy-specific NNC scheme to reconstructed CT slices. To evaluate the performance of our virtual HD technology, we used the structural similarity (SSIM) index [25], which overcame the limitation of conventional contrast-to-noise-ratio (CNR) with lack of spatial information (e.g., structure) in evaluation, for measuring the image quality of CT. We used the highest dose CT scan (5.7 mSv) as the "gold standard" in the calculation of the SSIM. We used a two-fold cross validation.

2.4.3   Clinical Case Evaluation

To evaluate our technology, we acquired ULD scans of 12 patients with three different vender CT scanners for a robustness test. Tube current, tube current time product, $CTDI_{vol}$, and effective dose for the ULDCT were 10–20 mA, 6.0 ± 3.5 mAs, 0.37 ± 0.22 mGy, and 0.14 ± 0.08 mSv, respectively. X-ray tube voltages were 120–135 kVp. Reconstructed slice thickness was 5 mm. We applied the trained anatomy-specific NNC scheme to the ULDCT studies. We used CNR to evaluate the image quality quantitatively. We were not able to use the SSIM for the quantitative evaluation, because the SSIM required ideal images in the calculation.

3   Results

3.1   Phantom Experiments

It took 46.7 h for the training of each NNC on a PC (Intel i7-4790K CPU, 4.5 GHz) or 1.73 h on a GPU (GeForce GTX TITAN Z, Nvidia, CA). In our VHD image, heavy noise and streak and other artifacts in the input ULDCT image (0.1 mSv) is reduced substantially, while maintaining anatomic structures such as pulmonary vessels. We examined the relationship between the image quality in terms of SSIM and effective dose. An average SSIM of our VHD image of 0.94 was equivalent to the image quality of 1.1 mSv CT images, which corresponds to 91% dose reduction, as shown in Fig. 3.

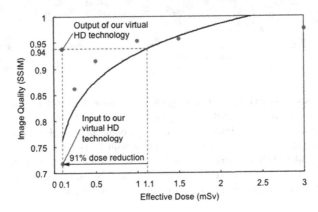

Fig. 3. Estimation for equivalent effective dose from SSIM for our virtual HDCT of CT scans of an anthropomorphic chest phantom.

3.2   Clinical Case Evaluation

To evaluate the performance of our VHD technology, we applied our GE-scanner-, phantom-trained NNC to 12 patient cases. Figure 4 shows comparisons of our VHDCT image for one of 12 patients with a lung nodule (enlarged to show details) acquired with the Toshiba CT scanner with the corresponding "gold-standard" real HD CT image. Noise and artifacts in the input ULDCT image is substantially reduced in our VHDCT image, while the conspicuity of the lung nodule and anatomic structures such as lung vessels is improved. We compared our VHD image with the state-of-the-art IR product (Toshiba AIDR-3D: strong, Toshiba, Tokyo, Japan) and ones of the recent best known denoising algorithms, K-SVD [26] and BM3D [27]. The image quality of our VHCT image is superior to the IR image and the BM3D-denoised image (the result by K-SVD is not shown due to much inferior performance) in terms of the conspicuity of the nodule and artifacts, as shown in Fig. 4. In the IR image, the nodule appears of lower-contrast with fuzzy boundary in the background with emphysema-like artifacts. The fuzzy chest wall is another issue with the IR image. In the BM3D-denoised image, diagnostic information (e.g., nodule and vessels) disappears. The processing time for each CT scan was 70.9 s. on a PC (Intel i7-4790 K at 4.5 GHz). With our preliminary VHD technology, an average CNR of 0.1 mSv ULDCT images of the patients was improved from 6.1 ± 2.1 to 13.5 ± 1.9 (two-tailed t-test; $P \ll 0.05$), as shown in Table 1. This CNR improvement was equivalent to the improvement by increasing radiation dose from 0.1 to 1.1 mSv (i.e., 91% dose reduction).

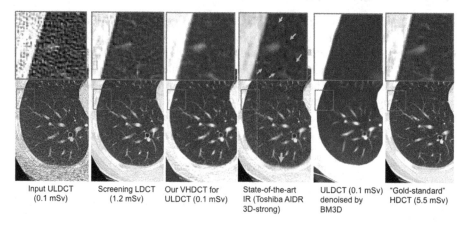

| Input ULDCT (0.1 mSv) | Screening LDCT (1.2 mSv) | Our VHDCT for ULDCT (0.1 mSv) | State-of-the-art IR (Toshiba AIDR 3D-strong) | ULDCT (0.1 mSv) denoised by BM3D | "Gold-standard" HDCT (5.5 mSv) |

Fig. 4. Comparison of our virtual HDCT image for a patient with a small lung nodule (enlarged to show details) with the state-of-the-art IR and "gold-standard" real HDCT image, which demonstrates retained diagnostic information (the lung nodule and vessels) in our virtual HDCT. In the IR image, the nodule appears of lower-contrast with fuzzy boundary in the background with emphysema-like artifacts (dark spots indicated by arrows; which is a common serious problem with all IR's). The fuzzy chest wall (indicated by an arrow) is another issue with the IR image. In the BM3D-denoised image, diagnostic information disappears.

Table 1. Evaluation results of the image quality of our VHDCT for 12 patients with 3 different CT scanners.

	Image	CNR (dB)
Patients	Input ULDCT	6.08 ± 2.07
(n = 12)	Our virtual HDCT	13.51 ± 1.94

4 Conclusion

We developed radiation dose reduction technology in CT based on our original NNC deep-learning technique. Our technology leaned to convert LDCT images to higher-dose-like CT images, thus term a "virtual" HDCT technology. Our virtual HDCT technology converted ULDCT (0.1 mSv) into images equivalent to 1.1 mSv HDCT images: It reduced noise and streak and other artifacts in ULDCT substantially, while maintaining anatomic structures and pathologies such as vessels and nodules. Quantitate evaluation with 12 clinical cases demonstrated that our VHDCT technology could reduce radiation dose by 91%. It took 70.9 s per one case on an ordinary PC to convert to VHDCT images. Substantial reduction of radiation dose in CT with our technology would be beneficial to lung cancer screening population. Low computational cost is an advantage of our technology over IR.

Acknowledgments. The authors are grateful to Y. Liu, Ph.D. at Zhejiang University of Technology, S. Chen, Ph.D., at University of Shanghai for Science and Technology, M.K. Kalra, M.D. at Massachusetts General Hospital, S. Date, M.D. at Hiroshima University Hospital, Y. Funama, Ph.D. at Kumamoto University for discussing the issues and current status of CT and dose reduction techniques.

References

1. National Lung Screening Trial Research, T., Church, T.R., Black, W.C., Aberle, D.R., Berg, C.D., Clingan, K.L., Duan, F., Fagerstrom, R.M., Gareen, I.F., Gierada, D.S., Jones, G.C., Mahon, I., Marcus, P.M., Sicks, J.D., Jain, A., Baum, S.: Results of initial low-dose computed tomographic screening for lung cancer. N. Engl. J. Med. 368, 1980–1991 (2013)
2. Brenner, D.J., Hall, E.J.: Computed tomography–an increasing source of radiation exposure. N. Engl. J. Med. **357**, 2277–2284 (2007)
3. Kalra, M.K., Woisetschlager, M., Dahlstrom, N., Singh, S., Digumarthy, S., Do, S., Pien, H., Quick, P., Schmidt, B., Sedlmair, M., Shepard, J.A., Persson, A.: Sinogram-affirmed iterative reconstruction of low-dose chest CT: effect on image quality and radiation dose. AJR Am. J. Roentgenol. **201**, W235–W244 (2013)
4. Volders, D., Bols, A., Haspeslagh, M., Coenegrachts, K.: Model-based iterative reconstruction and adaptive statistical iterative reconstruction techniques in abdominal CT: comparison of image quality in the detection of colorectal liver metastases. Radiology **269**, 469–474 (2013)
5. Lambert, L., Ourednicek, P., Jahoda, J., Lambertova, A., Danes, J.: Model-based vs hybrid iterative reconstruction technique in ultralow-dose submillisievert CT colonography. Br. J. Radiol. **88**, 20140667 (2015)

6. Thomas, P., Hayton, A., Beveridge, T., Marks, P., Wallace, A.: Evidence of dose saving in routine CT practice using iterative reconstruction derived from a national diagnostic reference level survey. Br. J. Radiol. **88**, 20150380 (2015)

7. Suzuki, K.: Supervised machine learning technique for reduction of radiation dose in computed tomography imaging. United States Patent No. US9332953 (2012)

8. Suzuki, K., Liu, Y., Higaki, T., Funama, Y., Awai, K.: Supervised conversion of ultra-low-dose to higher-dose CT images by using pixel-based machine learning: Phantom and initial patient studies. In: Program of Scientific Assembly and Annual Meeting of Radiological Society of North America (RSNA), Chicago, IL, vol. SST14-06 (2013)

9. Fukumoto, W., Suzuki, K., Higaki, T., Awaya, Y., Fujita, M., Awai, K.: Lung Cancer Screening (LCS) in Ultra-low-dose CT (U-LDCT) by Means of Massive-Training Artificial Neural Network (MTANN) Image-Quality Improvement: An Initial Clinical Trial. In: Program of Scientific Assembly and Annual Meeting of Radiological Society of North America (RSNA), Chicago, IL, vol. SSG14-01, (2015)

10. Suzuki, K., Higaki, T., Fukumoto, W., Awai, K.: "Virtual" high-dose CT: Converting ultra-low-dose (ULD) to higher-dose (HD) CT by means of supervised pixel-based machine-learning technique. In: Program of Scientific Assembly and Annual Meeting of Radiological Society of North America (RSNA), Chicago, IL, vol. CHS-251 (2014)

11. Chen, H., Zhang, Y., Zhang, W., Liao, P., Li, K., Zhou, J., Wang, G.: Low-dose CT via convolutional neural network. Biomed. Opti. Express **8**, 679–694 (2017)

12. Wolterink, J.M., Leiner, T., Viergever, M.A., Isgum, I.: Generative adversarial networks for noise reduction in low-dose CT. In: IEEE Transactions on Medical Imaging (2017)

13. Suzuki, K., Horiba, I., Ikegaya, K., Nanki, M.: Recognition of coronary arterial stenosis using neural network on DSA system. Syst. Comput. Jpn. **26**, 66–74 (1995)

14. Suzuki, K., Horiba, I., Sugie, N.: A simple neural network pruning algorithm with application to filter synthesis. Neural Process. Lett. **13**, 43–53 (2001)

15. Suzuki, K., Horiba, I., Sugie, N.: Efficient approximation of neural filters for removing quantum noise from images. IEEE Trans. Signal Process. **50**, 1787–1799 (2002)

16. Suzuki, K., Armato 3rd, S.G., Li, F., Sone, S., Doi, K.: Massive training artificial neural network (MTANN) for reduction of false positives in computerized detection of lung nodules in low-dose computed tomography. Med. Phys. **30**, 1602–1617 (2003)

17. Suzuki, K., Horiba, I., Sugie, N.: Neural edge enhancer for supervised edge enhancement from noisy images. IEEE Trans. Pattern Anal. Mach. Intell. **25**, 1582–1596 (2003)

18. Suzuki, K., Horiba, I., Sugie, N., Nanki, M.: Neural filter with selection of input features and its application to image quality improvement of medical image sequences. IEICE Trans. Inf. Syst. **E85-D**, 1710–1718 (2002)

19. Suzuki, K., Horiba, I., Sugie, N., Nanki, M.: Extraction of left ventricular contours from left ventriculograms by means of a neural edge detector. IEEE Trans. Med. Imaging **23**, 330–339 (2004)

20. Suzuki, K., Li, F., Sone, S., Doi, K.: Computer-aided diagnostic scheme for distinction between benign and malignant nodules in thoracic low-dose CT by use of massive training artificial neural network. IEEE Trans. Med. Imaging **24**, 1138–1150 (2005)

21. Suzuki, K., Yoshida, H., Nappi, J., Armato 3rd, S.G., Dachman, A.H.: Mixture of expert 3D massive-training ANNs for reduction of multiple types of false positives in CAD for detection of polyps in CT colonography. Med. Phys. **35**, 694–703 (2008)

22. Xu, J., Suzuki, K.: Massive-training support vector regression and Gaussian process for false-positive reduction in computer-aided detection of polyps in CT colonography. Med. Phys. **38**, 1888–1902 (2011)

23. Suzuki, K., Zhang, J., Xu, J.: Massive-training artificial neural network coupled with Laplacian-eigenfunction-based dimensionality reduction for computer-aided detection of polyps in CT colonography. IEEE Trans. Med. Imaging **29**, 1907–1917 (2010)
24. Rumelhart, D.E., Hinton, G.E., Williams, R.J.: Learning representations by back-propagating errors. Nature **323**, 533–536 (1986)
25. Wang, Z., Bovik, A.C., Sheikh, H.R., Simoncelli, E.P.: Image quality assessment: from error visibility to structural similarity. IEEE Trans. Image Process. **13**, 600–612 (2004)
26. Elad, M., Aharon, M.: Image denoising via sparse and redundant representations over learned dictionaries. IEEE Trans. Image Process. **15**, 3736–3745 (2006)
27. Dabov, K., Foi, A., Katkovnik, V., Egiazarian, K.: Image denoising by sparse 3-D transform-domain collaborative filtering. IEEE Trans. Image Process. **16**, 2080–2095 (2007)

Deep-FExt: Deep Feature Extraction for Vessel Segmentation and Centerline Prediction

Giles Tetteh[2(✉)], Markus Rempfler[2], Claus Zimmer[1], and Bjoern H. Menze[2,3]

[1] Neuroradiology, Klinikum Rechts der Isar, TU München, Munich, Germany
[2] Department of Computer Science, TU München, Munich, Germany
giles.tetteh@tum.de
[3] Institute for Advanced Study, TU München, Munich, Germany

Abstract. Feature extraction is a very crucial task in image and pixel (voxel) classification and regression in biomedical image modelling. In this work we present a feature extraction scheme based on inception models for pixel classification tasks. We extract features under multi-scale and multi-layer schemes through convolutional operators. Layers of Fully Convolutional Network are later stacked on these feature extraction layers and trained end-to-end for the purpose of classification. We test our model on the DRIVE and STARE public data sets for the purpose of segmentation and centerline detection and it outperforms most existing hand crafted or deterministic feature schemes found in literature. We achieve an average maximum Dice of 0.85 on the DRIVE data set which outperforms the scores from the second human annotator of this data set. We also achieve an average maximum Dice of 0.85 and kappa of 0.84 on the STARE data set. Even though these datasets are only 2-D we also propose ways of extending this feature extraction scheme to handle 3-D datasets.

Keywords: Feature extraction · Image and pixel classification and regression · Biomedical image modelling · Inception models · Convolutional Networks · Vessel segmentation · Centerline prediction

1 Introduction

Most recent research in biomedical modelling involves qualitative and quantitative classification of a single pixel (voxel), a region of interest ROI and or an image (volume). These classification tasks mostly involve three main steps: feature extraction, feature selection and classification [1]. Out of these three steps, the feature extraction step is the most crucial since it determines which information will be present or discarded in the next steps.

Feature extraction is the process of generating features to be used in the selection and classification tasks [1]. In whole image or volume classification, feature extraction and selection can serve as a dimensionality reduction where a subset of the extracted features is selected to eliminate redundant features while maintaining the underlying discriminatory information [2]. The newly extracted

© Springer International Publishing AG 2017
Q. Wang et al. (Eds.): MLMI 2017, LNCS 10541, pp. 344–352, 2017.
DOI: 10.1007/978-3-319-67389-9_40

features are normally of lower dimension than the original feature space. However, most pixelwise feature extraction tasks lead to dimensionality extension. That is, a new set of features of high dimension is extracted for each given pixel based on its neighbourhood.

Feature extraction techniques come mainly in three main flavours - hand crafted texture features, supervised learned features and unsupervised feature extraction.

Textures are complex visual patterns composed of entities, or subpatterns, that have characteristic brightness, colour, slope, or size [3]. The local subpattern properties give rise to the perceived lightness, uniformity, density, roughness, regularity, linearity, frequency, phase, directionality, coarseness, randomness, fineness, smoothness, or granulation of the texture as a whole [4]. For a review of texture features, categorization and various uses one can refer to [3].

Other groups of hand crafted features are based on differential geometry and the analysis of gradient and Hessian of pixel intensity. These are mostly used as image enhancement to objects of specific shape of interest in a given image. For example in [5] the multiscale second order local structure of an image (Hessian) is examined with the purpose of developing a vessel enhancement filter. Ultimately, a vesselness measure is obtained on the basis of the eigenvalues of the Hessian. This vesselness measure serves as a measure of the likelihood of the presence of geometrical structures which can be regarded as tubular. Also a curvilinear structure detector, called Optimally Oriented Flux (OOF) finds an optimal axis on which image gradients are projected in order to compute the image gradient flux [6].

The second class of feature extraction techniques are in the form of unsupervised learning and transfer learning. These are mainly autoencoders and its variations like restricted Boltzmann's machine. Autoencoders are simple learning circuits which aim to transform inputs into outputs with the least possible amount of distortion [7]. For detailed discussion of autoencoders, unsupervised learning and deep architectures one can refer to [7]. These architectures though very simple are very important in the field of machine learning and form the base components of deep learning architectures.

Architectures like CNN and other deep networks also extract hierarchical features in a supervised manner through the use of ground truth annotations. Szegedy et al. [8] proposed the inceptions model as a way of building deeper networks capable of learning and extracting dense feature while maintaining acceptable speed and memory usage. This idea has been used in building the GoogLeNET [8] which achieves the state of the art results on image classification tasks.

In this paper we discuss briefly inception models in general and extend the idea to build feature extraction layers in an autoencoder fashion. We will also discuss how to stack these pixelwise feature extraction layers to form a deep architecture which is then fine-tuned for the purpose of supervised learning.

2   Methodology

2.1   Inception Models

The main idea of the Inception architecture is based on finding out how an optimal local sparse structure in a convolutional vision network can be approximated and covered by readily available dense components [8]. Inception based networks replaces convolutional operations with mini-networks which uses less parameters and less computation. A convolution with a filter size of 5×5 can be replaced with a mini-network of two layers of filter sizes 3×3 each as shown in Fig. 1i. This reduces the parameter size from 25 (i.e. 5×5) to 18 (i.e. $3 \times 3 + 3 \times 3$ Similarly a convolutional operation with filter size 3×3 can be replaced with a mini-network of two layers with filters 1×3 and 3×1 respectively as shown in Fig. 1ii.

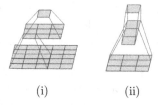

(i)   (ii)

Fig. 1. (i): Mini-network replacing a 5×5 convolutional operation. (ii): Mini-network replacing a 3×3 convolutional operation

By factorizing convolutional operations with bigger filter sizes into mini-networks with smaller filter sizes [9] proposed building a network which make use of filters with sizes not greater than 3×3. This helps to conserve memory and computational time which can be used to increase the depth of the network to improve performance. Inception modules as described in [8,9] form the building layers of the state of the art GoogLeNet network which was presented to the ILSVRC14 competition. Thorough discussion of inception architecture can be found in [8,9]. The original inception models are used in networks meant for full image classification. In the next section we discuss adapting the inception model to form a feature extraction layer in pixel wise classification tasks.

2.2   Pixelwise Feature Extraction Layer

The original inception architecture described in Sect. 2.1 is designed to fit in the domain of full image classification. This therefore leads to feature or dimensionality reduction. However, in this section we are rather interested in extracting features for pixel classification. In order to achieve this aim we first take the following two steps:

1. Remove all pooling operations. Pooling operations are used in image based classification tasks to extract invariant features and to reduce the dimension in the downstream layers of the network. Pooling layers work by replacing a region of an image by a statistic (e.g. mean, or maximum) of that region. This helps in image based classification by removing noise and outliers. However, pooling leads to loss of fine local details which is very crucial in pixelwise (voxelwise) tasks. This is a major problem in applying deep learning to detection problems in medical images. We therefore remove all pooling layers to make our feature extraction layers robust to object of interest of all sizes. Again we note that this is done only in the feature extraction layers not in the classifier which is later stack on the extracted features.

2. All convolution operations result in an output of the same size as the input. Here the idea is to keep the feature extraction layers as simple as possible such that we can stack them. We do this by padding the input to each layer with enough zeros so that it takes care of the number of pixels or voxels that are lost through the convolutional operation. This makes stacking the layers easier without thinking about the output shape of the previous layers.

We then choose a set of scales s e.g. $\{3, 5, 7, 9\}$ design a multiscale layer as shown in Fig. 2i. We then replace all convolutions with bigger than 3×3 filter sizes with mini-networks as described in Sect. 2.1 to obtain our final feature extraction layer in Fig. 2ii. By stacking multiple layers together we build a feature extraction network suitable for pixel classification. We note that the output from each layer is further transformed by a non-linear activation function (rectified linear units - ReLU) before it moves to the next layer. The concatenated output from each layer together with the input image are further concatenated to form the final feature set as shown in Fig. 3. We refer to this deep feature extraction network as Deep-FExt in the rest of the paper.

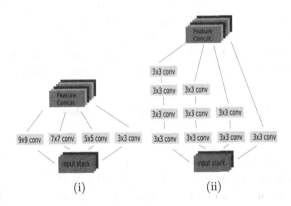

(i)   (ii)

Fig. 2. Feature extraction layers: (i) represents a layer without network factorization and (ii) represents a layer after network factorization.

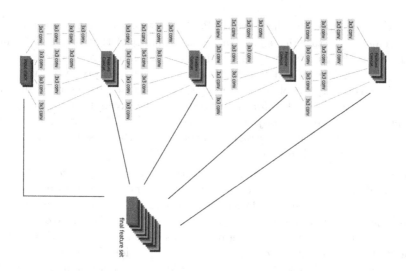

Fig. 3. Feature extraction network with final feature set from multiple layers

3 Experiments

To test Deep-FExt we design a network of 5 feature extraction layers which extract a total of 100 features per pixel (see Fig. 1). We then create a 10×10 feature mesh from each pixel feature set. Hence each pixel is then represented by 2-D image of size 10×10. We first train the feature extraction network in an unsupervised manner and then stack a CNN with 3 layers and randomly initialized parameters on the feature mesh and fine-tune end-to-end using stochastic gradient descent for classification and prediction purposes.

The full network structure is described in Table 1. Qualitative visualizations in Fig. 4 show that Deep-FExt is able to extract hierarchical features ranging from edge detectors, intensity gradients, and curvature at different scales.

Table 1. Feature extraction network structure employed in our experiment.

Layer	Input type and size	Filter sizes (extracted feats)	Total features
1	RGB image with 3 channels	3(5),5(5),7(5),9(3),11(3)	21
2	concat features from layer 1	3(5),5(5),7(5),9(3),11(3)	21
3	concat features from layer 2	3(5),5(4),7(4),9(3),11(3)	19
4	concat features from layer 3	3(4),5(4),7(4),9(3),11(3)	18
5	concat features from layer 4	3(4),5(4),7(4),9(3),11(3)	18
	Total	97 + 3 (input RGB) = 100	

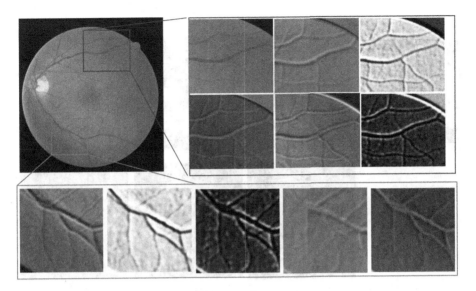

Fig. 4. Actual image (top left). We observe that Deep-FExt is able to learn features that resemble edge detectors, intensity gradients, and curvature at different scales.

3.1 Vessel Segmentation

For vessel segmentation we experiment on the DRIVE [10] and STARE [11] datasets. The DRIVE dataset is made up of 20 training examples and 20 test examples with two annotations in each group. We use the first annotation as the ground truth for training our network and testing. We also compare our results to the second annotation. The STARE dataset is made up of 20 annotated images with two annotations each. We split the data into 10 images for training and the remaining 10 for testing. Our results (See Table 2) show that our Deep-FExt network outperforms most of the existing architecture on the segmentation of the DRIVE and STARE datasets. Results for Deep Retinal Understanding (DRIU) [12] are obtained by evaluating pre-computed probability maps provided on the paper's page. DRIU outperforms Deep-FExt in dice however, DRIU uses VGG as a "base network", which is much deeper, carefully pre-trained and fine-tuned on millions of images. In contrast, Deep-FExt uses a simple SGD and does not employ any pre-training, or special parameter initialization. Yet we achieved results which is less than 3% lower than DRIU in dice. Other results are also stated as reported by [12].

3.2 Centerline Prediction

We again test Deep-FExt on DRIVE and STARE datasets for the purpose of centerline prediction. We generated centerline annotations by applying skeletonization to the the various manual annotations and used the same training and testing splits that were used for the vessel segmentation. We evaluated our

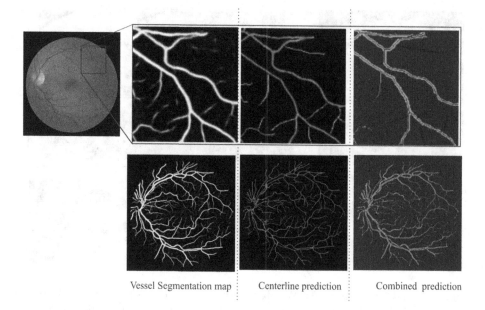

Vessel Segmentation map ┊ Centerline prediction ┊ Combined prediction

Fig. 5. Qualitative predictions from Deep-FExt. Top images show close view of region marked blue in the original image. (Color figure online)

Table 2. Vessel segmentation results on the DRIVE and STARE datasets. AMD refers to the average maximum Dice.

Dataset	Method	Precision	Recall	Dice	AMD	Kappa
DRIVE	Deep-FExt	80.44	80.32	80.38	84.67	78.48
	DRIU [12]	81.59	82.61	82.10	86.02	80.34
	N^4 fields [13]			80.50		
	Kernel Boost [14]			80.00		
	HED [15]			79.60		
	CRFs [16]			78.10		
	2nd Annotator	80.40	77.46	78.90	82.98	76.90
STARE	Deep-FExt	82.04	79.54	80.78	84.87	79.20
	DRIU [12]	82.67	83.80	83.23	86.28	81.84
	HED [15]			80.50		
	2nd Annotator	63.65	94.46	76.05	79.66	73.64

results based on centerline prediction alone (OC) and a combined multi-class prediction of centerline and vessel (B). We compare our results to the second annotator of these datasets (see Table 3).

Table 3. Centerline prediction results on the DRIVE and STARE datasets. Metrics are computed on a pixel level. AMD refers to the average maximum Dice.

Dataset	Method	Precision	Recall	Dice	AMD	Kappa
DRIVE	Deep-FExt(OC)	57.95	82.04	67.92	72.30	66.88
	Deep-FExt(B)	71.38	74.65	72.98	77.20	71.49
	2nd Annotator(OC)	60.38	45.86	52.13	63.95	44.72
	2nd Annotator(B)	70.45	69.35	69.89	69.89	67.31
STARE	Deep-FExt(OC)	53.63	74.27	62.29	75.98	61.45
	Deep-FExt(B)	73.33	75.73	74.51	79.72	72.45
	2nd Annotator(OC)	57.51	52.43	54.85	66.42	40.72
	2nd Annotator(B)	63.23	75.99	69.02	72.27	65.54

4 Conclusion

Deep-FExt outperforms most of the existing architectures on the DRIVE and STARE datasets. We believe Deep-FExt can be used to extract feature for general medical image segmentation tasks. By replacing the 2-D convolutions with 3-D we can also extend Deep-FExt to handle medical volumes. With the idea of mini-networks memory is conserved and speed is also improved. As further research, we consider experimenting with training Deep-FExt in an unsupervised manner similar to autoencoders. This would be valuable for generating features for clustering, or in situations where supervised learning is not feasible due to lack of annotated data.

References

1. Choras, R.S.: Image feature extraction techniques and their applications for cbir and biometrics systems. Int. J. Biol. Biomed. Eng. **1**, 6–15 (2007)
2. Adegoke, B.O., Ola, B.O., Omotayo, M.E.: Review of feature selection methods in medical image processing. IOSR J. Eng. (IOSRJEN) **4**, 1 (2014)
3. Materka, A., Strzelecki, M.: Texture analysis methods - a review. University of Lodz, Institute of Electronics, COST B11 report (1998)
4. Levine, M.: Vision in Man and Machine. McGraw-Hill, New York (1985)
5. Frangi, A.F., Niessen, W.J., Vincken, K.L., Viergever, M.A.: Multiscale vessel enhancement filtering. In: Wells, W.M., Colchester, A., Delp, S. (eds.) MICCAI 1998. LNCS, vol. 1496, pp. 130–137. Springer, Heidelberg (1998). doi:10.1007/BFb0056195
6. Law, M.W.K., Chung, A.C.S.: Three dimensional curvilinear structure detection using optimally oriented flux. In: Forsyth, D., Torr, P., Zisserman, A. (eds.) ECCV 2008. LNCS, vol. 5305, pp. 368–382. Springer, Heidelberg (2008). doi:10.1007/978-3-540-88693-8_27
7. Baldi, P.: Autoencoders, unsupervised learning, and deep architectures. In: Workshop on Unsupervised and Transfer Learning (2012). JMLR: Workshop and Conference Proceedings 50

8. Szegedy, C., et al.: Going deeper with convolutions. In: CVPR (2015)
9. Szegedy, C., et al.: Rethinking the inception architecture for computer vision. In: CVPR (2016)
10. Staal, J., et al.: Ridge-based vessel segmentation in color images of the retina. IEEE T-MI **23**(4), 501–509 (2004)
11. Hoover, A., Kouznetsova, V., Goldbaum, M.: Locating blood vessels in retinal images by piecewise threshold probing of a matched filter response. IEEE T-MI **19**(3), 203–210 (2000)
12. Maninis, K.-K., Pont-Tuset, J., Arbeláez, P., Gool, L.: Deep retinal image understanding. In: Ourselin, S., Joskowicz, L., Sabuncu, M.R., Unal, G., Wells, W. (eds.) MICCAI 2016. LNCS, vol. 9901, pp. 140–148. Springer, Cham (2016). doi:10.1007/978-3-319-46723-8_17
13. Ganin, Y., Lempitsky, V.: N^4-fields: neural network nearest neighbor fields for image transforms. In: Cremers, D., Reid, I., Saito, H., Yang, M.-H. (eds.) ACCV 2014. LNCS, vol. 9004, pp. 536–551. Springer, Cham (2015). doi:10.1007/978-3-319-16808-1_36
14. Becker, C., Rigamonti, R., Lepetit, V., Fua, P.: Supervised feature learning for curvilinear structure segmentation. In: Mori, K., Sakuma, I., Sato, Y., Barillot, C., Navab, N. (eds.) MICCAI 2013. LNCS, vol. 8149, pp. 526–533. Springer, Heidelberg (2013). doi:10.1007/978-3-642-40811-3_66
15. Xie, S., Tu, Z.: Holistically-nested edge detection. In: ICCV, pp. 142–154 (2015)
16. Orlando, J.I., Blaschko, M.: Learning fully-connected CRFs for blood vessel segmentation in retinal images. In: Golland, P., Hata, N., Barillot, C., Hornegger, J., Howe, R. (eds.) MICCAI 2014. LNCS, vol. 8673, pp. 634–641. Springer, Cham (2014). doi:10.1007/978-3-319-10404-1_79

Product Space Decompositions for Continuous Representations of Brain Connectivity

Daniel Moyer[✉], Boris A. Gutman, Neda Jahanshad, and Paul M. Thompson

Imaging Genetics Center, Stevens Institute for Neuroimaging and Informatics, University of Southern California, Los Angeles, USA
moyerd@usc.edu

Abstract. We develop a method for the decomposition of structural brain connectivity estimates into locally coherent components, leveraging a non-parametric Bayesian hierarchical mixture model with tangent Gaussian components. This model provides a mechanism to share information across subjects while still including explicit mixture distributions of connections for each subject. It further uses mixture components defined directly on the surface of the brain, eschewing the usual graph-theoretic framework of structural connectivity in favor of a continuous model that avoids a priori assumptions of parcellation configuration. The results of two experiments on a test-retest dataset are presented, to validate the method. We also provide an example analysis of the components.

Keywords: Brain connectivity · Non-parametric bayes · Unsupervised learning

1 Introduction

Structural brain connectivity is commonly estimated from the distribution of streamline endpoint pairs on the cortical surface. It is known that both this distribution and the underlying biological distribution are non-uniform and highly structured. Further, it can be safely assumed that there is some degree of correspondence between the structures of different (healthy) subjects. However, the recovery, representation, and study of the variation of these structures remains non-trivial. It is thus useful to construct methods for that purpose.

Most connectivity representations rely on discrete graphs of cortical parcels. This places a strong constraint on the structure of the endpoint distributions recovered. In particular, the use of fixed parcels abstracts away the geometry of the surface, so that all endpoints connecting two regions are equivalent and indistinguishable. The discrete topology of the graph and removal of the underlying distance metric removes notions of nearness to a particular region, except within the graph context itself.

Electronic supplementary material The online version of this chapter (doi:10.1007/978-3-319-67389-9_41) contains supplementary material, which is available to authorized users.

© Springer International Publishing AG 2017
Q. Wang et al. (Eds.): MLMI 2017, LNCS 10541, pp. 353–361, 2017.
DOI: 10.1007/978-3-319-67389-9_41

Instead, we model the appearance of these streamline endpoints on the cortical surface directly. We introduce a hierarchical Dirichlet process mixture model for the appearance of streamline endpoints on the white matter/grey matter interface (the inner cortical surface). This model simultaneously learns clusters in each subject's (continuous) connectome yet also learns correspondences between these clusters by organizing subject-wise clusters into prototypical cluster components. This second level of mixture modeling allows further study of the variation across subjects. We use the Bayesian non-parametric frame, which does not enforce a strict choice of the number of clusters.

1.1 Previous Relevant Work

This work directly relies on two models, the hierarchical Dirichlet process (HDP) proposed by Teh et al. [12] and the tangent Gaussian used as mixture components from Straub et al. [11]. The original HDP manuscript applied the model to topic identification in text corpora. Similar models have been used in connectomics before for node clustering, in particular Jbabdi et al. [5], which attempts to cluster cortical regions from connectivity traces using the HDP and a conjugate prior pair. Notably, their proposed method does not use a surface, modeling voxels with only a prior to enforce spatial coherence. Other Bayesian non-parametric methods have also been suggested, including the directed dependent Chinese restaurant process (ddCRP) [1,7], and a Chinese restaurant process stochastic blockmodel (also known as the Infinite Relational Model) [4].

The vast majority of connectomics research uses discrete graph structures instead of a continuous domain [10]. Several works make use of continuous connective representations [6,7], but do not perform streamline clustering. On discrete domains, spatially sensitive edge clustering is less meaningful, as the graph abstracts away the local geometry. We use the continuous domain in order to be able to identify components that do not conform to parcel pairs defined a priori.

Parcellation tasks using connectivity data are also well studied (e.g. [9]), and are often a pre-processing step for functional connectivity; however, such models only consider "half" the space, while the data are observed on the product of the surfaces (i.e. over pairs of surface subsets). Outside of connectomics, streamline clustering has been studied with respect to white matter trajectories. In particular, the work of O'Donnell and Westin [8] and later Wassermann et al. [14] define forms of kernel spaces for tract registration and clustering tasks.

2 Model

We model the observation of streamline intersections with the inner cortical surface as a random Poisson point process on the product of spheres $S^2 \times S^2$, with each hemisphere of the brain being modeled by its spherical inflation, disjoint from the other hemisphere. In this frame each streamline is an independent observation drawn from a latent intensity function. It is in this context that we would like to construct a parametric mixture model for the appearance of streamline pairs on the cortical surfaces. We also would like to share information between subjects' particular mixtures. We do not know a priori the number of mixture components nor their configuration. To this end, we introduce a hierarchical Dirichlet process model with tangent Gaussian components.

We will construct the model in the proceeding sections from the top down, then describe the sampling method. We include in the supplemental material a table of notation, as the bookkeeping and notation of these models is fairly complex.

2.1   Hierarchical Dirichlet Process

We choose a hierarchical Dirichlet process (HDP) [12] to model our mixture distributions. Also known as the Chinese Restaurant Franchise, the HDP model is a hierarchical extension of the Chinese Restaurant Process, a popular nonparametric Bayesian mixture model. In such mixtures, the restaurant process serves as a prior over all possible label assignments (assuming the labels have no order between themselves). In a practical sense this means that they assign a probability to each possible partition of the dataset for any number of partitions (clusters), given a base mixture distribution. The hierarchical extension of this allows each mixture component to be drawn from one of a finite (but not fixed) number of prototypical components.

Let G be a prior distribution on component parameters, and let F be a point-mass distribution of prototypical components drawn from G. For a number of dishes K we sample parameters $\theta_k \sim G$, then for subjects $n \in \{1, \ldots, N\}$, we sample components F_n, from which we sample observed endpoints.

$$g_c^n, \theta_k \sim G(\gamma, G_0) \qquad t_i^n, x_i \sim F_n(\alpha, \theta_k)$$

Here, we also include two sets of association indexes, $t_i^n \in \{1, \ldots, C_n\}$ which tracks the association of data points to clusters, and $g_c^n \in \{1, \ldots, K\}$ which tracks the association of clusters to parameters θ_k. Neither K nor the C_n are fixed. Each of these are Dirichlet processes with concentration parameters γ and α. From a practical standpoint, for each subject we sample component labels over "active" clusters F_n, possibly sampling a new cluster with probability set by α. If a new cluster is sampled, we will sample from θ_k (from which all clusters across subjects have been drawn), possibly adding a new prototypical cluster.

2.2   Tangent Gaussian Mixture Components

Our observed data lie on the white matter/gray matter interface, a surface commonly abstracted to S^2 (e.g. via FreeSurfer [2]). We observe pairs of points on the surface, streamline intersections with the gray matter boundary, so our induced space is $S^2 \times S^2$. The vast majority of connectomics papers further abstract this by dividing the space into regions, conducting their analysis on the discrete graph formed by the set product of the regions. We instead choose to model the data directly in $S^2 \times S^2$.

A recently introduced component distribution for the sphere is the so-called Tangent Gaussian of Straub et al. [11]. Given a cluster mean, each component is modeled by a zero mean Gaussian *in the tangent space* of the sphere at the cluster mean. This allows for anisotropic distributions with, as we show in the supplemental material, a reasonable posterior predictive distribution for certain choices of hyper-prior parameters. We choose to use a product of Tangent Gaussians to model our data.

Define the following functions to and from the tangent space for a mean μ:

$$\mathrm{Log}: S^2 \times S^2 \to \mathbb{R}^2 \qquad \mathrm{Log}(x; \mu) = (x - \mu(x \cdot \mu))\frac{\theta}{\sin(\theta)}$$

$$\mathrm{Exp}: \mathbb{R}^2 \times S^2 \to S^2 \qquad \mathrm{Exp}(x; \mu) = \mu\cos(\|x\|_2) + \frac{x}{\|x\|}\sin(\|x\|_2)$$

Here, $\theta = \arccos(x \cdot \mu)$. For cluster mean and tangent covariance (μ_k, Σ_k), the likelihood of a datapoint $s \in S^2$ is $\mathcal{N}(\mathrm{Log}(s; \mu); 0, \Sigma)$. Our data $x_i = (s_1, s_2)$ are on $S^2 \times S^2$, thus we use the product density

$$p(x_i | \mu, \Sigma) = \mathcal{N}(\mathrm{Log}(s_1; \mu_1); 0, \Sigma_1) \times \mathcal{N}(\mathrm{Log}(s_2; \mu_2); 0, \Sigma_2)$$

which has pairs of parameters (μ_1, μ_2) and (Σ_1, Σ_2). For convenience (and because their respective priors are assumed to be independent) we refer to each pair as simply μ and Σ.

2.3 Full Model and Sampling

Our full model is then

$$\begin{aligned}
g_c^n, \theta_k &\sim G(\gamma, G_0) \\
\theta_k = (\mu_k, \Sigma_k) &\sim \mathrm{Unif}(S^2), \mathrm{Inv.\ Wishart}(\Delta, \nu) \\
t_i^n &\sim F_n(\alpha, \theta_k) \\
x_i = (s_1, s_2)_i^n &\sim \mathcal{N} \times \mathcal{N} \mid t_i^n, \theta_k
\end{aligned}$$

We have four hyper parameters, (Δ, ν) the prior parameters for the Inverse Wishart distribtion, and two concentration parameters α and γ. We use Gibbs sampling to sample model parameters, using multiple layers of sampling. As suggested by Teh et al. [12], we use component indexes to (somewhat) simplify bookkeeping during sampling. For each data point in each subject, we need to sample its component label t_i^n. We then sample component parameters (μ_k, Σ_k), which are across subjects (cohort-wide parameters). Finally, we sample component associations of each subject's clusters to prototypical components, g_c. In practice, we find that due to the particular cluster components and configuration of the data, this last step rarely changes cluster assignments.

We assume a uniform prior on μ and an inverse Wishart prior with parameters (Δ, ν) for Σ. This is G_0 from which we draw new parameters $\theta = (\mu, \Sigma)$. To avoid multiple subscripts, we denote the parameters associated with cluster c as $\mu : g_c^n$ and $\Sigma : g_c^n$. Sampling can then be divided into three steps:

(1) Sample t_i^n for each streamline, adding clusters as dictated by the appearance of c_{new} and deleting clusters if $\sum_n \eta_k^n = 0$. This has marginal distribution

$$p(t_i^n = c|\{\mu, \Sigma\}, G_0) \propto \mathcal{N} \times \mathcal{N}(x)|\mu : g_c^n, \Sigma : g_c^n$$
$$= \mathcal{N} \times \mathcal{N}(\text{Log}(s_1; \mu_1), \text{Log}(s_2; \mu_2))|\mu : g_c^n, \Sigma : g_c^n \quad (1)$$

$$p(t_i^n = c_{new}|\{\mu, \Sigma\}, G_0) \propto \alpha \sum_k \frac{\eta_k}{C_* + \gamma} p(x|\mu_k, \Sigma_k) \quad (2)$$

$$+ \frac{\gamma}{C_* + \gamma} p(x|\mu_k, \Sigma_k, k_{new})$$

If c_{new} is sampled, then we need to choose a corresponding g_c^n. This has marginal distribution

$$P(g_c^n = k|c_{new}, \{\theta\}, G_0) \propto p(x|\mu_k, \Sigma_k) \quad (3)$$
$$P(g_c^n = k_{new}|c_{new}, \{\theta\}, G_0) \propto \gamma p(x|\mu_k, \Sigma_k, k_{new}) \quad (4)$$

$$p(x|\mu_k, \Sigma_k, k_{new}) = \iint p(x|\mu, \Sigma) p(\mu) p(\Sigma|\Delta, \nu) \quad (5)$$

$$= \underbrace{\frac{1}{|Sphere|} \iint p(x|\mu, \Sigma) p(\mu) p(\Sigma|\Delta, \nu) d\mu d\Sigma}_{Constant}$$

We provide a tractable method of computing the double integral in the supplemental material for reasonable priors. This needs only to be computed once.

(2) Sample μ, Σ. Σ has the marginal distribution

$$p(\Sigma|\{x_i\}, \{t_i^n\}, \{g_c^n\}, \Delta, \nu) = \text{IW}(\Delta + A_k, \nu + \sum_{n,c} \eta_c^n) \quad (6)$$

$$\text{with} \quad A_k = \sum_n \sum_{\substack{i:t_i^n=c \\ g_c^n=k}} \text{Exp}(x_i; \mu : g_c^n) \text{Exp}(x_i; \mu : g_c^n)^T$$

Due to the tangent Gaussian approximations, we choose to use a Metropolis-Hastings correction (as suggested by Straub et al. [11]) and rejection step to sample μ:

$$q(\mu_k = \mu|.) = \mathcal{N}(\text{Log}(\mu; \langle x \rangle_c); 0, \frac{\Sigma_k}{N})$$

$$r = \prod_n \prod_{\substack{i:t_i^n=c \\ g_c^n=k}} \frac{p(x_i|\mu_k^{prop}, \Sigma_k) p(\mu_k^{prop}) q(\mu_k^{old}|.)}{p(x_i|\mu_k^{old}, \Sigma_k) p(\mu_k^{old}) q(\mu_k^{prop}|.)}$$

$$= \frac{\mathcal{N}(\text{Log}(\mu_k^{old}; \langle x \rangle_c)|0, \frac{\Sigma_k}{N})}{\mathcal{N}(\text{Log}(x; \mu_k^{prop})|0, \frac{\Sigma_k}{N})} \prod_n \prod_{\substack{i:t_i^n=c \\ g_c^n=k}} \frac{\mathcal{N}(\text{Log}(\mu_k^{prop}; \langle x \rangle_c)|0, \Sigma_k)}{\mathcal{N}(\text{Log}(x; \mu_k^{old})|0, \Sigma_k)}$$

Here, we use the Karcher mean of the cluster to resample μ, denoted $\langle x \rangle_c$.

(3) Sample g_c^n for each cluster, deleting prototypes if no cluster claims them.

$$p(g_c^n = k|\{x_i\}, \{t_i^n\}, \{\theta_k\}) \propto \prod_n \prod_{\substack{i:t_i^n=c \\ g_c^n=k}} \mathcal{N} \times \mathcal{N}(x_i)|\mu : g_c^n, \Sigma : g_c^n$$

3 Experiments

We demonstrate the use of our framework on a test-retest dataset. Our data are comprised of 21 subjects from the Institute of Psychology, Chinese Academy of Sciences sub-dataset of the Consortium for Reliability and Reproducibility (CoRR) dataset [15]. T1-weighted (T1w) and diffusion weighted (DWI) images were obtained on 3T Siemens TrioTim using an 8-channel head coil and 60 directions. Each subject was scanned twice, roughly two weeks apart.

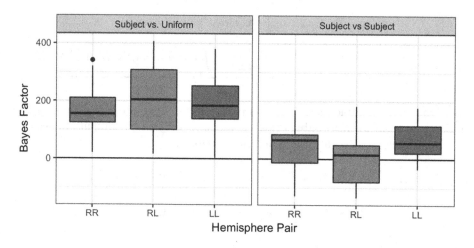

Fig. 1. Plotted above are the likelihood ratios (the Bayes factors) using the trained model on data from the retest scans and two different false datasets. On the **left** are the Retest vs. Uniform random likelihood ratios, on the **right** the Retest vs. other Subjects ratios.

T1-weighted images were processed with FreeSurfer's [2] recon-all pipeline to obtain a triangle mesh of the gray-white matter boundary registered to a shared spherical space. Probabilistic streamline tractography was conducted using the DWI in 2-mm isotropic MNI 152 space, using Dipy's [3] implementation of constrained spherical deconvolution (CSD) [13] with a harmonic order of 6. We retain only tracts longer than 5 mm with endpoints in likely grey matter.

We train our model on the set of subjects' first scans using the proposed sampling method, learning the prototype parameters μ, Σ, the per-subject cluster weights η_c^n (subject encodings), and the cluster assignments. After collecting

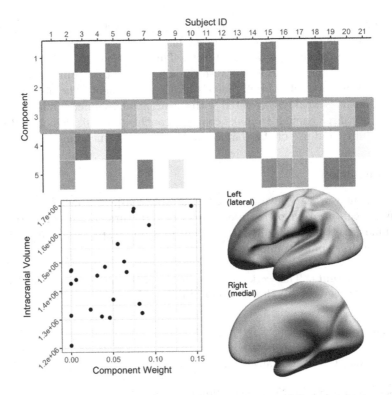

Fig. 2. Top: the top 5 components displayed as a heatmap of their weights across components. Comp. 3 (in Yellow) is displayed below. **Bottom Left**: Component 3 weights vs. Intracranial Volume (each subj. is a point). This plot shows a weak correlation between the appearance of the feature in a subject and cranial volume ($\rho = 0.56$). **Bottom Right**: A plot of the component on a smoothed subject surface, where the red density at approximately the R. post. cingulate connects to the blue density at the temporoparietal junction. The right hemisphere is shown from the medial view. (Color figure online)

samples we find the Maximum a Posteriori (MAP) likelihood parameter set, and then perform evaluations on the subjects' second scans using the MAP parameter values.

We perform two different evaluations of the model. Each measures the posterior predictive probability of two datasets given a subject's particular encoding, one being the subject's second scan. In the first experiment, the second scan's probability is compared to a spatially uniform random dataset. In the second, we compare the subject's second scan to an equal number of randomly selected points from other subjects. Note that a separate model is learned for each pair of hemispheres. We use the Bayes Factor as the evaluation metric.

As can be seen in Fig. 1, in the first task, differentiating between the actual second scan and a uniform random one, the model performs with 100% accuracy. This is a helpful sanity check, as one would expect the structure to be non-uniform. In the second task, the models perform well, though not perfectly. In particular, the crossing streamline (one hemisphere to another) distributions are less distinguishable between subjects. This may be because there is less observable variation, or simply because the model fails to capture it.

In Fig. 2, we present a brief analysis of one component. The observation of this component is weakly correlated with intracranial volume. While this study is clearly not large enough to make concrete conclusions, this demonstrates the interpretability and use of the component/subject-wise encoding.

3.1   Conclusion

In the present work we have constructed a multi-subject model for the locally sensitive decomposition of representations of structural brain connectivity in a continuous setting. This model may be useful for exploratory analysis and parcellation free connectomics.

Acknowledgements. This work was supported by NIH Grant U54 EB020403, as well as the NSF Graduate Research Fellowship Program.

References

1. Baldassano, C., et al.: Parcellating connectivity in spatial maps. PeerJ **3**, e784 (2015)
2. Fischl, B.: FreeSurfer. NeuroImage **2**(62), 774–781 (2012)
3. Garyfallidis, E., et al.: Dipy, a library for the analysis of diffusion MRI data. Front. Neuroinform **8**(8), 1–17 (2014)
4. Hinne, M., et al.: Probabilistic clustering of the human connectome identifies communities and hubs. PLoS ONE **10**(1), e0117179 (2015)
5. Jbabdi, S., et al.: Multiple-subjects connectivity-based parcellation using hierarchical Dirichlet process mixture models. NeuroImage **44**(2), 373–384 (2009)
6. Moyer, D., Gutman, B.A., Faskowitz, J., Jahanshad, N., Thompson, P.M.: A continuous model of cortical connectivity. In: Ourselin, S., Joskowicz, L., Sabuncu, M.R., Unal, G., Wells, W. (eds.) MICCAI 2016. LNCS, vol. 9900, pp. 157–165. Springer, Cham (2016). doi:10.1007/978-3-319-46720-7_19
7. Moyer, D., Gutman, B.A., Jahanshad, N., Thompson, P.M.: A restaurant process mixture model for connectivity based parcellation of the cortex. In: Niethammer, M., Styner, M., Aylward, S., Zhu, H., Oguz, I., Yap, P.-T., Shen, D. (eds.) IPMI 2017. LNCS, vol. 10265, pp. 336–347. Springer, Cham (2017). doi:10.1007/978-3-319-59050-9_27
8. O'Donnell, L., Westin, C.-F.: White matter tract clustering and correspondence in populations. In: Duncan, J.S., Gerig, G. (eds.) MICCAI 2005. LNCS, vol. 3749, pp. 140–147. Springer, Heidelberg (2005). doi:10.1007/11566465_18
9. Parisot, S., et al.: Group-wise parcellation of the cortex through multi-scale spectral clustering. NeuroImage **136**, 68–83 (2016)
10. de Reus, M.A., Van den Heuvel, M.P.: The parcellation-based connectome: limitations and extensions. NeuroImage **80**, 397–404 (2013)
11. Straub, J., Chang, J., Freifeld, O., Fisher III., J.: A Dirichlet process mixture model for spherical data. In: Artificial Intelligence and Statistics, pp. 930–938 (2015)

12. Teh, Y.W., et al.: Sharing clusters among related groups: hierarchical Dirichlet processes. In: Advances in Neural Information Processing Systems (2005)
13. Tournier, J.D., et al.: Resolving crossing fibres using constrained spherical deconvolution: validation using diffusion-weighted imaging phantom data. NeuroImage **42**(2), 617–625 (2008)
14. Wassermann, D., Rathi, Y., Bouix, S., Kubicki, M., Kikinis, R., Shenton, M., Westin, C.-F.: White matter bundle registration and population analysis based on gaussian processes. In: Székely, G., Hahn, H.K. (eds.) IPMI 2011. LNCS, vol. 6801, pp. 320–332. Springer, Heidelberg (2011). doi:10.1007/978-3-642-22092-0_27
15. Zuo, X.N., et al.: An open science resource for establishing reliability and reproducibility in functional connectomics. Sci. Data **1**, 140049 (2014)

Identifying Autism from Resting-State fMRI Using Long Short-Term Memory Networks

Nicha C. Dvornek[1(✉)], Pamela Ventola[2], Kevin A. Pelphrey[3],
and James S. Duncan[1,4,5]

[1] Department of Radiology and Biomedical Imaging, New Haven, CT, USA
nicha.dvornek@yale.edu
[2] Child Study Center, Yale School of Medicine, New Haven, CT, USA
[3] Autism and Neurodevelopmental Disorders Institute,
George Washington University and Children's National Medical Center,
Washington, DC, USA
[4] Department of Biomedical Engineering, Yale University, New Haven, CT, USA
[5] Department of Electrical Engineering, Yale University, New Haven, CT, USA

Abstract. Functional magnetic resonance imaging (fMRI) has helped characterize the pathophysiology of autism spectrum disorders (ASD) and carries promise for producing objective biomarkers for ASD. Recent work has focused on deriving ASD biomarkers from resting-state functional connectivity measures. However, current efforts that have identified ASD with high accuracy were limited to homogeneous, small datasets, while classification results for heterogeneous, multi-site data have shown much lower accuracy. In this paper, we propose the use of recurrent neural networks with long short-term memory (LSTMs) for classification of individuals with ASD and typical controls directly from the resting-state fMRI time-series. We used the entire large, multi-site Autism Brain Imaging Data Exchange (ABIDE) I dataset for training and testing the LSTM models. Under a cross-validation framework, we achieved classification accuracy of 68.5%, which is 9% higher than previously reported methods that used fMRI data from the whole ABIDE cohort. Finally, we presented interpretation of the trained LSTM weights, which highlight potential functional networks and regions that are known to be implicated in ASD.

1 Introduction

Investigating the pathophysiology of autism spectrum disorders (ASD) with functional magnetic resonance imaging (fMRI) holds promise for identifying objective biomarkers of the neurodevelopmental disorder. Discovering biomarkers for ASD would potentially lead to better understanding the underlying causes of ASD. This would have far-reaching implications, aiding in diagnosis, the design of improved therapies, and monitoring and predicting treatment outcomes.

This work was supported in part by T32 MH18268 and R01 NS035193.

Q. Wang et al. (Eds.): MLMI 2017, LNCS 10541, pp. 362–370, 2017.
DOI: 10.1007/978-3-319-67389-9_42

Recent efforts have focused on investigating ASD biomarkers based on measures of functional connectivity, computed from resting-state fMRI (rsfMRI). Functional connectivity measures are used as predictors for classifying ASD v.s. neurotypical control, using popular learning methods such as support vector machines, random forests, or ridge regression [1,3,13]. Pairwise connections deemed important for accurate classification are then potential biomarkers for ASD.

While high accuracies have been reported for identifying ASD from rsfMRI, these results were found using small, homogeneous datasets gathered from a single [15] or a few [13] imaging sites and likely do not generalize well to the larger, heterogeneous ASD population. To aid in discovering more generalizeable fndings, the Autism Brain Imaging Data Exchange (ABIDE) gathered neuroimaging and phenotypic data from 1112 subjects across 17 sites for their first publicly shared dataset, ABIDE I [7]. While larger datasets are usually helpful in achieving higher classification accuracy, the heterogeneity of ASD has proved to be a challenge; recent methods which trained on large portions of this diverse dataset have demonstrated much lower classification accuracy [9,12].

We propose a new approach in which we learn the ASD classification directly from the rsfMRI time-series, rather than from precomputed measures of functional connectivity. Since the fMRI data represents dynamic brain activity, we hypothesize that the time-series will carry more useful information than single, static functional connectivity measures. To learn directly from the rsfMRI time-series, we base our approach on Long Short-Term Memory networks (LSTMs), a type of deep neural network designed to handle very long sequence data [10].

In this paper, we investigate the use of LSTMs for identifying individuals with ASD from rsfMRI time-series. To the best of our knowledge, this is the first use of LSTMs for classifying fMRI data. We train and test the developed LSTM models on the entire ABIDE dataset and compare classification accuracy against previous studies that classified the ABIDE subjects from rsfMRI. Finally, we interpret the best model, identifying brain regions important for distinguishing ASD from typical controls. We hypothesize the learned LSTM weights will encode potential networks that have previously been implicated in ASD.

2   Methods

2.1   Network Architecture

LSTMs are a special type of recurrent neural network, composed of repeated cells that receive input from the previous cell as well as the data input x_t for the current timestep t. Each LSTM cell contains a cell state c_t and hidden state h_t, which are modulated by 4 neural network layers that control the flow of information into and out of cell memory. The equations governing an LSTM are:

$$i_t = \sigma \left(W_i x_t + U_i h_{t-1} + b_i \right) \tag{1}$$

$$f_t = \sigma \left(W_f x_t + U_f h_{t-1} + b_f \right) \tag{2}$$

$$\tilde{c}_t = \tanh \left(W_c x_t + U_c h_{t-1} + b_c \right) \tag{3}$$

$$c_t = i_t * \tilde{c}_t + f_t * c_{t-1} \tag{4}$$

$$o_t = \sigma \left(W_o x_t + U_o h_{t-1} + b_o \right) \tag{5}$$

$$h_t = o_t * \tanh \left(c_t \right) \tag{6}$$

W matrices contain weights applied to the current input, U matrices represent weights applied to the previous hidden state, b vectors are biases for each layer, and σ is the sigmoid function. The input gate i_t (Eq. (1)) decides what information from the current estimated cell state is updated. The forget gate f_t (Eq. (2)) controls what information from the previous cell state is kept. Next, the estimated current cell state (Eq. (3)) and previous cell state are combined with restrictions from the input and forget gates, respectively, to update the cell state (Eq. (4)). Finally, cell state information is filtered with the output gate o_t (Eq. (5)) to update the hidden state (Eq. (6)), which is the output of the LSTM cell.

We propose an LSTM architecture which takes the rsfMRI time-series as input x and connects the output of each repeating cell to a dense layer with a single node (Fig. 1). This gives the signal at every time point a more direct say in how to classify the signal, compared to the traditional approach of looking at the final output after the whole sequence is analyzed (h_T). We believe this will be more robust to the noisy fMRI data. The outputs of the single nodes are then averaged across the entire sequence and fed to a sigmoid activation function to produce the probability of an ASD label. For regularization, during training, we apply dropout to the LSTM weights as described in Gal et al. [8] and add a standard dropout layer between the single-node dense layer and pooling layer. In the following, we also investigate a two-layer LSTM model, in which the hidden states output from the first layer are used as the input sequence into a second LSTM layer, after which the architecture is the same as in the single-layer model.

2.2   Dataset and Preprocessing

The ABIDE I dataset includes rsfMRI for 539 individuals with ASD and 573 typical controls from 17 international sites. To further enhance the data-sharing effort, the Preprocessed Connectomes Project released preprocessed ABIDE data using a number of popular pipelines and several calculated derivatives [5]. We chose the data processed through the Connectome Computation System, without global signal regression but with band-pass filtering. See the ABIDE Preprocessed website [14] for more preprocessing details.

The preprocessed ABIDE data includes extracted mean time-series from regions of interest defined by several atlases. Here, we utilized the mean time-series from the Craddock 200 atlas [6], which was provided for 1100 subjects.

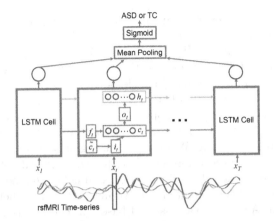

Fig. 1. Diagram of the LSTM network for classifying ASD from rsfMRI. The recurrent neural network is visualized "unrolled" for clarity. Each green square is a neural network layer that takes x_t and h_{t-1} as inputs.

Each time course was normalized to represent percent change from the average signal for that region of interest. Further, since different sites used different acquisition protocols, we resampled each time-series using an interval of 2 s to bring the data to the same time scale. The preprocessed mean time courses from the 200 atlas regions were used as input x into the LSTM.

2.3 Data Augmentation

While the ABIDE dataset has a large number of subjects for a neuroimaging database, training neural networks often requires many more samples to prevent overfitting. Furthermore, the ABIDE time courses have different lengths depending on the site. Thus, we propose cropping the input time courses to a fixed sequence length for all subjects and augmenting the number of inputs for each subject to make the most use of the full time-series. Based on the length of the shortest time-series, we chose a sequence length of $T = 90$, which represents 3 min of imaging. For each subject, we crop 10 sequences of length T from the time-series, randomly varying the starting time of each cropped sequence. This augmented our dataset by a factor of 10 to a total of 11,000 input sequences.

3   Experiments

3.1 Experimental Methods

The LSTM training and testing were performed using Keras [4]. Models were trained using the binary cross-entropy loss function and the Adadelta optimizer with the default parameter values. The dropout rate during training was fixed to 0.5. Models were initialized using default Keras settings.

We explored the impact of parameters and variations of the proposed archi-tecture as well as training conditions. We tested not augmenting data, varying the number of hidden nodes (8, 16, 32, or 64) in the LSTM, and removing dropout. We also tested variations on the base network: connecting only the final LSTM cell's output (h_T) to a single dense node, and stacking LSTM layers.

To validate the performance of the LSTMs, we used stratified 10-fold cross-validation, such that the proportion of subjects from each site was approximately the same in all folds. For each fold, data was split into 85% for training, 5% for validation, and 10% for testing. When using the augmented dataset, all sequences belonging to the same subject appeared in either training, validation, or testing. Training was stopped when the validation loss had not decreased in 20 epochs or when 300 epochs had been executed. The trained model was then tested on the left-out test data. Accuracy was assessed based on classification of each input sequence ("sequence accuracy") as well as classification of each subject using the average score of all input sequences from a subject ("subject accuracy"). Significance tests were performed using two-tailed, paired t-tests with $\alpha = 0.05$. We compared our approach to previous studies that trained on ABIDE rsfMRI. To better compare against these other studies which used different subsets from the ABIDE cohort, we computed the difference between the model's accuracy and the accuracy of assigning classifications by chance within the tested dataset.

Finally, we considered interpretation of the LSTM model which resulted in the highest classification accuracy. Entries in the LSTM weight matrix $W_l(n, r)$ with large magnitude, regardless of sign, should denote that atlas region r has a strong influence on LSTM node n for layer l. We investigated regions that were considered important for each layer and for each node. First, for each layer l, we averaged the absolute values of the weights across all nodes. We then created a binary mask of important regions, defined as those regions with weight magnitudes greater than 2 standard deviations above the mean for the layer. The mask of important regions was then input into Neurosynth, a meta-analysis tool that compares a brain map to a database of approximately 10,000 fMRI studies and assigns correlations between the map and almost 3000 descriptors [16]. Similarly, for each node n, we defined important regions as those with weights greater than 2 standard deviations away from the mean in the node for each layer, aggregated the important regions across all layers into a single binary mask per node, and input the mask into Neurosynth for interpretation.

3.2   Classification Accuracy

Results from previous studies and from our LSTM models are compared in Table 1. The highest accuracy was reported by Plitt et al. [13]; however, only a small, very homogeneous subset (16%) of the ABIDE dataset was used. Chen et al. [3] showed a large improvement compared to chance, but also used a very pruned subset of the data with a single training/validation split. The two stud-ies with the largest datasets [9,12] demonstrated lower accuracy compared to our LSTM model trained on only a single input sequence from each subject. All other LSTM models, which used the augmented dataset, performed even better.

Table 1. Autism classification results from methods that trained on rsfMRI from the ABIDE dataset. Classification accuracies of best LSTM-based model are in bold. LSTM# = LSTM with # hidden nodes, NoAug = No data augmentation, NoDrop = No dropout regularization, Last = Pass only the last hidden state to dense node, LSTM#x2 = Two-layer LSTM with # hidden nodes, Train/Val = Single training and validation set, CV10 = 10-fold cross-validation, LOO = Leave-one-out cross-validation, SD = Standard deviation. [a]Significant difference between sequence and subject accuracies. [b]Significant difference compared to best model LSTM32.

Classification method	Validation method	Number of subjects	Mean (SD) sequence accuracy (%)	Difference from chance (%)	Mean (SD) subject accuracy (%)	Difference from chance (%)
Plitt et al. [13]	CV10	178	-	-	69.7	19.7
Chen et al. [3]	Train/Val	252	-	-	66	16
Abraham et al. [1]	CV10	871	-	-	66.9 (2.7)	13.2
Nielsen et al. [12]	LOO	964	-	-	60.0	6.4
Ghiassian et al. [9]	Train/Val	1111	-	-	59.2	7.6
LSTM8	CV10	1100	65.6 (4.1)	13.7	66.7 (5.3)	14.8
LSTM16	CV10	1100	65.3 (4.8)	13.3	66.8 (5.4)	14.9
LSTM32	CV10	1100	**66.8 (4.5)**	**14.9**	**68.5 (5.5)**[a]	**16.6**
LSTM64	CV10	1100	65.8 (3.8)	13.9	67.5 (4.4)[a]	15.5
LSTM32_NoAug	CV10	1100	-	-	61.4 (4.5)[b]	9.5
LSTM32_NoDrop	CV10	1100	59.7 (2.3)	7.7	61.8 (4.0)[b]	9.9
LSTM32_Last	CV10	1100	62.2 (3.3)	10.3	64.5 (4.5)[a]	12.5
LSTM32x2	CV10	1100	66.3 (4.2)	14.4	67.5 (5.0)[a]	15.5

Subject accuracy was higher than sequence accuracy for all models. Among the single layer models, the highest subject accuracy was achieved for the LSTM with 32 hidden nodes (68.5%). Compared to the most competitive result using the majority of the ABIDE cohort [1], the difference between our accuracy and chance is over 3% higher, while our dataset contained more challenging, heterogeneous data with 25% more subjects. Furthermore, compared to the study with the closest number of subjects to ours [9], our model improved accuracy compared to chance by 9%. Thus, our method would likely generalize best to new data.

All tested variations of the proposed network resulted in degraded accuracy. Removing dropout regularization reduced accuracy by almost 7%. Using only the final hidden state of the LSTM sequence decreased accuracy by 4%. Finally, creating a deeper model with two stacked LSTM layers was not helpful.

3.3 Model Interpretation

We investigated the learned weights of the best model, LSTM32. Table 2 shows, for each layer, the top associated Neurosynth anatomical and functional descriptors. The input and forget gates, which modulate the cell state information, are heavily influenced by regions associated with language and communication; impairment of these functions are primary symptoms of ASD. Functional terms associated with influential regions for the current estimated cell state are important for supporting social interactions, which are difficult for individuals with

Table 2. Top Neurosynth anatomical and functional terms associated with the mask created from the brain regions with the greatest weight magnitudes for each layer.

Layer	Anatomical terms	Functional terms
Input	Superior Temporal Sulcus, Middle Temporal Gyrus, Planum Temporale	Sentence, Comprehension, Linguistic, Audiovisual, Language
Forget	Inferior Frontal Gyrus, Temporal Pole, Planum Temporale	Sentence, Verb, Nouns, Semantically, Sentence Comprehension
Cell	Midbrain, Thalamus, Superior Temporal Sulcus	Reward, Speaker, Voice, Audiovisual, Speech
Output	Hypothalamus, Inferior Parietal Lobe, Medial Prefrontal Cortex	Self, Sexual, Referential, Memory Retrieval, Regulation

autism. The output gate is most influenced by regions associated with self-referential processing, which has been shown to be impaired in autistic individuals [11].

Finally, we explored potential brain networks encoded by each LSTM cell node. The important regions for the four nodes with greatest influence (i.e., with the largest weight magnitudes from the dense layer of the neural network) are shown in Fig. 2. These region groupings highlight neurocognitive functions affected by ASD; e.g., social reward is diminished, face processing and communication skills are impaired, and theory of mind, a leading hypothesis for social impairment in autism, is lacking in autistic individuals [2].

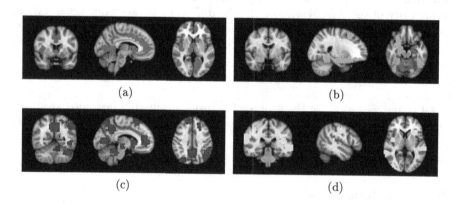

(a)   (b)

(c)   (d)

Fig. 2. Influential brain regions for the 4 most important LSTM nodes. Top associated Neurosynth functional features include: (a) Pain, reward, anticipation, incentive. (b) Faces, objects, word form, emotional, visual. (c) Default mode, reward, listening, mental states, theory of mind. (d) Listening, sounds, theory of mind, social, speech perception.

4 Conclusions

We have presented a method for identifying individuals with ASD from rsfMRI using LSTMs. Our model demonstrated the highest classification accuracy compared to other methods which utilized the majority of the ABIDE cohort. We contend it is important to succeed on large heterogeneous datasets, since ASD covers a wide spectrum, and image quality can be difficult to control for individuals with autism and young children. Data augmentation and choice of network structure were crucial in training an accurate model. More in depth tuning of hyperparameters, training on other parcellations, including demographic information, and combining models would likely lead to higher classification accuracy.

The learned LSTM input weights had meaningful interpretation; anatomical regions with high influence on the network have previously been shown to be abnormal in ASD. Further, meta-analysis highlighted neurocognitive processes that are affected in individuals with ASD. Inspection of network activations and hidden state weights could lead to greater insights into the mechanism of ASD.

References

1. Abraham, A., Milham, M.P., Martino, A.D., Craddock, R.C., Samaras, D., Thirion, B., Varoquaux, G.: Deriving reproducible biomarkers from multi-site resting-state data: an autism-based example. Neuroimage **147**, 736–745 (2017)
2. Baron-Cohen, S., Abraham, A., Leslie, M., Frith, U.: Does the autistic child have a "theory of mind". Cognition **21**, 37–46 (1985)
3. Chen, C.P., Keown, C.L., Jahedi, A., Nair, A., Pflieger, M.E., Bailey, B.A., Müller, R.A.: Diagnostic classification of intrinsic functional connectivity highlights somatosensory, default mode, and visual regions in autism. Neuroimage: Clin. **8**, 238–245 (2015)
4. Chollet, F.: Keras (2015). https://github.com/fchollet/keras
5. Craddock, C., Benhajali, Y., Chu, C., Chouinard, F., Evans, A., Jakab, A., Khundrakpam, B.S., Lewis, J.D., Li, Q., Milham, M., Yan, C., Bellec, P.: The neuro bureau preprocessing initiative: open sharing of preprocessed neuroimaging data and derivatives. In: Neuroinformatics (2013)
6. Craddock, R.C., James, G.A., Holtzheimer, P.E., Hu, X.P., Mayberg, H.S.: A whole brain fMRI atlas generated via spatially constrained spectral clustering, human brain mapping. Hum. Brain Mapp. **33**, 1914–1928 (2012)
7. Di Martino, A., Yan, C.G., Li, Q., Denio, E., Castellanos, F.X., Alaerts, K., Anderson, J.S., Assaf, M., Bookheimer, S.Y., Dapretto, M., Deen, B., Delmonte, S., Dinstein, I., Ertl-Wagner, B., Fair, D.A., Gallagher, L., Kennedy, D.P., Keown, C.L., Keysers, C., Lainhart, J.E., Lord, C., Luna, B., Menon, V., Minshew, N.J., Monk, C.S., Mueller, S., Müller, R.A., Nebel, M.B., Nigg, J.T., O'Hearn, K., Pelphrey, K.A., Peltier, S.J., Rudie, J.D., Sunaert, S., Thioux, M., Tyszka, J.M., Uddin, L.Q., Verhoeven, J.S., Wenderoth, N., Wiggins, J.L., Mostofsky, S.H., Milham, M.P.: The autism brain imaging data exchange: towards a large-scale evaluation of the intrinsic brain architecture in autism. Mol. Psychiatry **19**, 659–667 (2014)
8. Gal, Y., Ghahramani, Z.: A theoretically grounded application of dropout in recurrent neural networks. In: NIPS (2016)

9. Ghiassian, S., Greiner, R., Jin, P., Brown, M.R.G.: Using functional or structural magnetic resonance images and personal characteristic data to identify adhd and autism. PLOS One **11**(12) (2016)

10. Hochreiter, S., Schmidhuber, J.: Long short-term memory. Neural Comput. **9**(8), 1735–1780 (1997)

11. Lombardo, M.V., Barnes, J.L., Wheelwright, S.J., Baron-Cohen, S.: Self-referential cognition and empathy in autism. PLoS One **2** (2007)

12. Nielsen, J.A., Zielinski, B.A., Fletcher, P.T., Alexander, A.L., Lange, N., Bigler, E.D., Lainhart, J.E., Anderson, J.S.: Multisite functional connectivity MRI classification of autism: abide results. Front. Hum. Neurosci. **7**, 599 (2013)

13. Plitt, M., Barnes, K.A., Martin, A.: Functional connectivity classification of autism identifies highly predictive brain features but falls short of biomarker standards. Neuroimage: Clin. **7**, 359–366 (2015)

14. Preprocessed Connectomes Project: ABIDE Preprocessed. http://preprocessed-connectomes-project.org/abide/

15. Uddin, L.Q., Supekar, K., Lynch, C.J., Khouzam, A., Phillips, J., Feinstein, C., Menon, V.: Salience network-based classification and prediction of symptom severity in children with autism. JAMA Psychiatry **70**(8), 869–879 (2014)

16. Yarkoni, T., Poldrack, R.A., Nichols, T.E., Van Essen, D.C., Wager, T.D.: Large-scale automated synthesis of human functional neuroimaging data. Nat. Methods (2011). www.neurosynth.org

Machine Learning for Large-Scale Quality Control of 3D Shape Models in Neuroimaging

Dmitry Petrov[1,2], Boris A. Gutman[1(✉)], Shih-Hua (Julie) Yu[1],
Kathryn Alpert[3], Artemis Zavaliangos-Petropulu[1], Dmitry Isaev[1],
Jessica A. Turner[4], Theo G.M. van Erp[5], Lei Wang[3], Lianne Schmaal[6,7],
Dick Veltman[7], and Paul M. Thompson[1]

[1] Imaging Genetics Center, Stevens Institute for Neuroimaging and Informatics,
University of Southern California, Los Angeles, USA
bgutman@gmail.com
[2] The Institute for Information Transmission Problems, Moscow, Russia
[3] Department of Psychiatry, Northwestern University, Chicago, USA
[4] The Mind Research Network, Albuquerque, USA
[5] University of California, Irvine, USA
[6] Orygen, The National Centre of Excellence in Youth Mental Health,
Melbourne, Australia
[7] Department of Psychiatry, VU University Medical Center,
Amsterdam, The Netherlands

Abstract. As very large studies of complex neuroimaging phenotypes become more common, human quality assessment of MRI-derived data remains one of the last major bottlenecks. Few attempts have so far been made to address this issue with machine learning. In this work, we optimize predictive models of quality for meshes representing deep brain structure shapes. We use standard vertex-wise and global shape features computed homologously across 19 cohorts and over 7500 human-rated subjects, training kernelized Support Vector Machine and Gradient Boosted Decision Trees classifiers to detect meshes of failing quality. Our models generalize across datasets and diseases, reducing human workload by 30–70%, or equivalently hundreds of human rater hours for datasets of comparable size, with recall rates approaching inter-rater reliability.

Keywords: Shape analysis · Machine learning · Quality control

1 Introduction

In recent years, large-scale neuroimaging studies numbering in the thousands and even 10s of thousands of subjects have become a reality [1]. Though automated MRI processing tools [2] have become sufficiently mature to handle large datasets, visual quality control (QC) is still required. For simple summary measures of brain MRI, QC may be a relatively quick process. For more complex

---

D. Petrov and B.A. Gutman—These authors contributed equally.

Q. Wang et al. (Eds.): MLMI 2017, LNCS 10541, pp. 371–378, 2017.
DOI: 10.1007/978-3-319-67389-9_43

measures, as in large studies of voxel- and vertex-wise features [3], the QC process becomes more time-intensive for the human raters. Both training of raters and conducting QC ratings, once trained, can take hours even for modest datasets.

This issue is particularly relevant in the context of multi-site meta-analyses, exemplified by the ENIGMA consortium [1]. Such studies, involving dozens of institutions, require multiple researchers to perform quality control on their cohorts, as individual data cannot always be shared. In addition, for meta-analysis studies performed after data collection, the QC protocols must be reliable in spite of differences in scanning parameters, post-processing, and demographics. In effect, QC has become one of the main practical bottlenecks in big-data neuroimaging. Reducing human rater time via predictive modeling and automated quality control is bound to play an increasingly important role in maintaining and hastening the pace of the scientific discovery cycle in this field.

In this paper, we train several predictive models for deep brain structure shape model quality. Our data is comprised of the ENIGMA Schizophrenia and Major Depressive Disorder working groups participating in the ENIGMA-Shape project [3]. Using ENIGMA's Shape protocol and rater-labeled shapes, we train a discriminative model to separate "FAIL"(F) and "PASS"(P) cases. For classification, we use a support vector classifier with a radial basis kernel (SVC) and Gradient Boosted Decision Trees (GBDT). Features are derived from the standard vertex-wise measures as well as global features. For six out of seven deep brain structures, we are able to reduce human rater time by 30 to 70% in out-of-sample validation, while maintaining FAIL recall rates similar to human inter-rater reliability. Our models generalize across datasets and disease samples.

2   Methods

Our goal in using machine learning for automated QC differs somewhat from most predictive modeling problems. Typical two-class discriminative solutions seek to balance misclassification rates of each class. In the case of QC, we focus primarily on correctly identifying FAIL cases, by far the smaller of the two classes (Table 1). In this first effort to automate shape QC, we do not attempt to eliminate human involvement, but simply to reduce it by focusing human rater time on a smaller subsample of the data containing nearly all failing cases. Our quality measures, described below, reflect this nuance.

2.1   MRI Processing and Shape Features

Our deep brain structure shape measures are computed using a previously described pipeline [4,5], available via the ENIGMA Shape package. Briefly, structural MR images are parcellated into cortical and subcortical regions using FreeSurfer. Among the 19 cohorts participating in this study, FreeSurfer versions 5.1 and 5.3 were used, depending on the institution. The binary region of interest (ROI) images are then surfaced with triangle meshes and parametrically (spherically) registered to a common region-specific surface template [6].

This leads to a one-to-one surface correspondence across the dataset at roughly 2,500 vertices per ROI. Our ROIs include the left and right thalamus, caudate, putamen, pallidum, hippocampus, amygdala, and nucleus accumbens. Each vertex p of mesh model M is endowed with two shape descriptors:

Medial Thickness, $D(p) = \|c_p - p\|$, where c_p is the point on the medial curve c closest to p.

$LogJac(p)$, Log of the Jacobian determinant J arising from the template mapping, $J : T_{\phi(p)}M_t \to T_pM$.

Since the ENIGMA surface atlas is in symmetric correspondence, i.e. the left and right shapes are vertex-wise symmetrically registered, we can combine two hemispheres for each region for the purposes of predictive modeling. At the cost of assuming no hemispheric bias in QC failure, we effectively double our sample.

The vertex-wise features above are augmented with their volume-normalized counterparts: $\{D, J\}_{normed}(p) = \frac{\{D,J\}(p)}{V^{\{\frac{1}{3}, \frac{2}{3}\}}}$. Given discrete area elements of the template at vertex p, $A_t(p)$, we estimate volume as $V = \sum_{p \in vrts(M)} 3A_t(p)J(p)D(p)$. We also use two global features: the shape-wide feature median, and the shape-wise 95th percentile feature threshold.

2.2 Human Quality Rating

Human-rated quality control of shape models is performed following the ENIGMA-Shape QC protocol[1]. Briefly, raters are provided with several snapshots of each region model as well as its placement in several anatomical MR slices (Fig. 1). A guide with examples of FAIL (QC = 1) and PASS (QC = 3) cases is provided to raters, with an additional category of MODERATE PASS (QC = 2) suggested for inexperienced raters. Cases from the last category are usually referred to more experienced raters for second opinions. Once a rater becomes sufficiently experienced, he or she typically switches to the binary FAIL/PASS rating. In this work, all remaining QC = 2 cases are treated as PASS cases, consistent with ENIGMA shape studies.

2.3 Predictive Models

First, we used Gradient Boosted Decision Trees (GBDT). This is a powerful ensemble learning method introduced by Friedman [7] in which subsequent trees correct for the errors of the previous trees. In our experiments we used the Xgboost [8] implementation due to speed and regularization heuristics, with the logistic loss function. Second, we used Support Vector Classifier. Based on earlier experiments and the clustered nature of FAIL cases in our feature space, we used the radial basis function (RBF) kernel in our SVC models. Indeed, in preliminary experiments RBF outperformed linear and polynomial kernels. We used scikit-learn's [9] implementation of SVC.

---

[1] enigma.usc.edu/ongoing/enigma-shape-analysis.

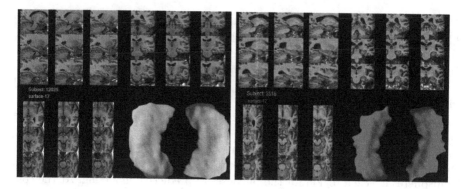

Fig. 1. Example hippocampal shape snapshots used for human QC rating. **Left:** A mesh passing visual QC. **Right:** A mesh failing visual QC.

2.4 Quality Measures

In describing our quality measures below, we use the following definitions. TF stands for TRUE FAIL, FF stands for FALSE FAIL, TP stands for TRUE PASS, and FP stands for FALSE PASS. Our first measure, **F-recall** $= \frac{TF}{TF+FP}$, shows the proportion of FAILS that are correctly labeled by the predictive model. The second measure, **F-share** $= \frac{TF+FF}{\text{Number of observations}}$, shows the proportion of the test sample labeled as FAIL by the model. Finally, we used a **modified F-score**, which allows us to compare models based on the specific requirements of our task, i.e. a very high F-recall and F-share substantially below 1, we use a variation on the standard F-score.

$$\text{F-score}_{\text{mod}} = 2 \times \frac{\text{F-recall} \times (1 - \text{F-share})}{\text{F-recall} + (1 - \text{F-share})}.$$

Note that the modified F-score cannot equal 1, as in the standard case. An ideal prediction leads to F-score$_{\text{mod}} = 1 - $ F-share. The intuition behind our custom F-score is based on the highly imbalanced FAIL and PASS samples. A model that accurately labels all failed cases is only valuable if it substantially reduces the workload for human raters, a benefit reflected by F-share.

3 Experiments

For each of the seven ROIs, we performed eight experiments defined by two predictive models (SVC and GBDT), two types of features (original and normed) and two cross-validation approaches. We tested "Leave-One-Site-Out" and 5-fold stratified cross-validation, as described below.

3.1 Datasets

In our experiments, we used deep brain structure shape data from the ENIGMA Schizophrenia and Major Depressive Disorder working groups.

Table 1. Overview of FAIL percentage mean, standard deviation, maximum and minimum for each site. Sample sizes for each ROI vary slightly due to FreeSurfer segmentation failure.

	FAIL %	Accumbens	Caudate	Hippocampus	Thalamus	Putamen	Pallidum	Amygdala
Train	mean ± std	3.4 ± 4.7	0.9 ± 0.7	2.0 ± 1.1	0.8 ± 1.0	0.6 ± 0.6	2.3 ± 3.6	0.9 ± 0.9
	max	16.4	2.1	4.2	3.4	1.5	13.8	2.6
	min	0.0	0.0	0.5	0.0	0.0	0.0	0.0
	size	10431	10433	10436	10436	10436	10435	10436
Test	mean ± std	4.7 ± 4.5	1.4 ± 1.5	4.9 ± 4.8	1.4 ± 1.5	0.4 ± 0.8	1.9 ± 2.0	0.8 ± 0.9
	max	10.5	3.5	11.4	3.5	1.6	3.8	2.1
	min	0.0	0.0	0.0	0.0	0.0	0.0	0.0
	size	3017	3018	3018	3018	3017	3018	3018

Our predictive models were trained using 15 cohorts totaling 5718 subjects' subcortical shape models from the ENIGMA-Schizophrenia working group. The ENIGMA-Schizophrenia (ENIGMA-SCZ) working group is comprised of over two dozen cohorts from around the world. The goal of the working group is to identify subtle effects of Schizophrenia and related clinical factors on brain imaging features. For a complete overview of ENIGMA-SCZ projects and cohort details, see [10].

To test our final models, we used data from 4 cohorts in the Major Depressive disorder working group (ENIGMA-MDD), totaling 1509 subjects, for final out-of-fold testing. A detailed description of the ENIGMA-MDD sites and clinical questions can be found here [11].

3.2 Model Validation

All experiments were performed separately for each ROI. The training dataset was split into two halves referred to as 'TRAIN GRID' and 'TRAIN EVAL.' The two halves contained data from each ENIGMA-SCZ cohort, stratified by the cohort-specific portion of FAIL cases. Model parameters were optimized using a grid search within 'TRAIN GRID', with either stratified 5-fold or Leave-One-Site-Out cross-validation. Parameters yielding the highest Area Under the ROC-curve were selected from among all cross-validation and feature types.

Both SVC and GBDT produce probability estimates indicating the likelihood that the individual subject's ROI mesh is a FAIL case, P_{FAIL}. Exploiting this, we sought a probability threshold for each model selected during the grid search to optimize the modified F-score in the 'TRAIN EVAL' sample. This amounts to a small secondary grid search. To simplify traversing this parameter space, we instead sample F-score$_{mod}$ at regularly spaced values of P_{FAIL}, from 0.1 to 0.9 in 0.1 increments. This is equivalent to F-share in the 'TRAIN EVAL' sample (Eval F-share, Table 2).

Final thresholds (Thres in Table 2) were selected based on the highest F-score$_{mod}$, requiring that F-recall $\geq$ 0.8 - a minimal estimate of inter-rater reliability. It is important to stress that while we used sample distribution information in selecting a threshold, the final out-of-sample prediction is made on an individual basis for each mesh.

4 Results

Trained models were deliberately set to use a loose threshold for FAIL detection, predicting 0.3–0.8 of observations as FAILs in the TRAIN GRID sample. These predicted FAIL observations contained 0.85–0.9 of all true FAILs, promising to reduce the human rater QC time by 20–70%. These results largely generalized to the 'TRAIN EVAL' and test samples: Table 2 shows our final model and threshold performance for each ROI.

Table 2. Test performance of the models with the best F-score$_{mod}$ on evaluation (TRAIN EVAL). Excepting the thalamus, overall models' performance generalizes to out-of-sample test data.

ROI	Model	CV	Features	Thres	Eval F-recall	Eval F-share	Eval F-score	Test F-recall	Test F-share	Test F-score
Accumbens	GBDT	5-fold	Normed	0.014	0.83	0.2	0.81	0.75	0.27	0.74
Amygdala	GBDT	5-fold	Normed	0.007	0.89	0.4	0.72	0.76	0.40	0.67
Caudate	SVC	LOSO	Original	0.017	0.84	0.3	0.76	0.92	0.45	0.68
Hippocampus	GBDT	5-fold	Normed	0.010	0.85	0.2	0.83	0.91	0.29	0.80
Pallidum	GBDT	5-fold	Normed	0.009	0.86	0.2	0.83	0.86	0.30	0.77
Putamen	SVC	LOSO	Normed	0.007	0.84	0.4	0.70	0.65	0.44	0.60
Thalamus	SVC	LOSO	Original	0.007	0.84	0.4	0.70	1.00	1.00	0.00

With the exception of the thalamus, our final models' performance measures generalized to the test sample, in some cases having better sample F-recall and lower percentage of images still requiring human rating compared to the evaluation sample. A closer look suggests that variability in model predictions across sites generally follows human rater differences. Table 3 breaks down performance by test cohort. It is noteworthy that the largest cohort, Münster (N = 1033 subjects, 2066 shape samples), has the best QC prediction performance. At the same time, the "cleanest" dataset, Houston, with no human-detected quality failures, has the lowest F-share. In other words, Houston would require the least human rater time relative to its size, as would be hoped.

Table 3. Performance of best models for each test site. Models are the same as in Table 2. Symbol '-' indicates that there were no FAILs for particular ROI and test site.

ROI	Berlin F-recall	Berlin F-share	Stanford F-recall	Stanford F-share	Munster F-recall	Munster F-share	Houston F-recall	Houston F-share
Accumbens	0.58	0.21	0.58	0.28	0.88	0.30	-	0.10
Amygdala	1.00	0.36	1.00	0.71	0.74	0.42	-	0.17
Caudate	0.67	0.41	0.88	0.53	0.96	0.51	-	0.16
Hippocampus	0.88	0.21	0.88	0.52	0.92	0.31	-	0.05
Pallidum	1.00	0.23	0.88	0.43	0.86	0.34	-	0.06
Putamen	-	0.47	-	0.71	0.65	0.46	-	0.14
Thalamus	1.00	1.00	1.00	1.00	1.00	1.00	-	1.00

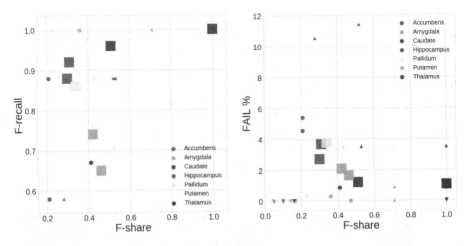

Fig. 2. Scatter plots of F-recall and actual FAIL case percentage vs. proportion of predicted FAIL cases on test datasets. **Left:** F-share vs F-recall. **Right:** Fail F-share vs FAIL percentage. Mark size shows the dataset size. Mark shape represents dataset (site): ○ - **CODE-Berlin (N = 176)**; □ - **Münster (N = 1033)**; △ - **Stanford (N = 105)**; ▽ - **Houston (N = 195)**.

Visualizing the test results in Fig. 2, we see the trend for lower F-share with higher overall dataset quality maintained by the smaller cohorts, but reversed by Münster. This could be a reflection of our current models' bias toward accuracy in lower-quality data due to greater numbers of FAIL examples (i.e., FAILs in high and low quality datasets may be qualitatively different). At the same time, F-recall appears to be independent of QC workload reduction due to ML, with most rates above the 0.8 mark.

5   Conclusion

We have presented a preliminary study of potential machine learning solutions for semi-automated quality control of deep brain structure shape data. Though some work on automated MRI QC exists [12], we believe this is the first ML approach in detecting end-of-the-pipeline feature failure in deep brain structure geometry. We showed that machine learning can robustly reduce human visual QC time for large-scale analyses for six out of the seven regions in question, across diverse MRI datasets and populations. Failure of the thalamus ML QC ratings to generalize out-of-sample may be explained by the region's specific features. Though we have only used geometry information in model training, MRI intensity, available to human raters for all ROI's, plays a particularly important role in thalamus ratings. The most common thalamus segmentation failure is the inclusion of lateral ventricle by FreeSurfer. Geometry is generally altered undetectably in such cases.

Beyond adding intensity-based features, possible areas of future improvement include combining ML algorithms, exploiting parametric mesh deep learning, employing geometric data augmentation, and refining the performance measures. Specifically, mesh-based convolutional neural nets can help visualize problem areas, which can be helpful for raters.

Very large-scale studies, such as the UK Biobank, ENIGMA, and others, are becoming more common. To make full use of these datasets, it is imperative to maximally automate the quality control process that has so far been almost entirely manual in neuroimaging. Our work here is a step in this direction.

References

1. Thompson, P.M., Andreassen, O.A., Arias-Vasquez, A., Bearden, C.E., Boedhoe, P.S., Brouwer, R.M., Buckner, R.L., Buitelaar, J.K., Bulaeva, K.B., Cannon, D.M.: Enigma and the individual: predicting factors that affect the brain in 35 countries worldwide. Neuroimage **145**(Pt B), 389–408 (2015)
2. Fischl, B.: Freesurfer. Neuroimage **62**(2), 774–781 (2012)
3. Gutman, B., Ching, C., Andreassen, O., Schmaal, L., Veltman, D., Van Erp, T., Turner, J., Thompson, P.M., et al.: Harmonized large-scale anatomical shape analysis: mapping subcortical differences across the enigma bipolar, schizophrenia, and major depression working groups. Biol. Psychiatry **81**(10), S308 (2017)
4. Gutman, B.A., Jahanshad, N., Ching, C.R., Wang, Y., Kochunov, P.V., Nichols, T.E., Thompson, P.M.: Medial demons registration localizes the degree of genetic influence over subcortical shape variability: An n = 1480 meta-analysis. In: 2015 IEEE 12th International Symposium on Biomedical Imaging (ISBI), pp. 1402–1406. IEEE (2015)
5. Roshchupkin, G.V., Gutman, B.A., et al.: Heritability of the shape of subcortical brain structures in the general population. Nat. Commun. **7**, 13738 (2016)
6. Gutman, B.A., Madsen, S.K., Toga, A.W., Thompson, P.M.: A family of fast spherical registration algorithms for cortical shapes. In: Shen, L., Liu, T., Yap, P.-T., Huang, H., Shen, D., Westin, C.-F. (eds.) MBIA 2013. LNCS, vol. 8159, pp. 246–257. Springer, Cham (2013). doi:10.1007/978-3-319-02126-3_24
7. Friedman, J.H.: Greedy function approximation: a gradient boosting machine. Ann. Stat. **29**(5), 1189–1232 (2001)
8. Chen, T., Guestrin, C.: XGBoost: a scalable tree boosting system. In: Proceedings of the 22nd ACM SIGKDD International Conference on Knowledge Discovery and Data Mining, KDD 2016, pp. 785–794. ACM, New York (2016)
9. Pedregosa, F., Varoquaux, G., Gramfort, A., et al.: Scikit-learn: machine learning in Python. J. Mach. Learn. Res. **12**, 2825–2830 (2011)
10. van Erp, T.G.M., Hibar, D.P., et al.: Subcortical brain volume abnormalities in 2028 individuals with schizophrenia and 2540 healthy controls via the enigma consortium. Mol. Psychiatry **21**, 547–553 (2015)
11. Schmaal, L., Hibar, D.P., et al.: Cortical abnormalities in adults and adolescents with major depression based on brain scans from 20 cohorts worldwide in the enigma major depressive disorder working group. Mol. Psychiatry **22**(6), 900–909 (2017)
12. Esteban, O., Birman, D., Schaer, M., Koyejo, O.O., Poldrack, R.A., Gorgolewski, K.J.: Mriqc: predicting quality in manual MRI assessment protocols using no-reference image quality measures. bioRxiv (2017)

Tversky Loss Function for Image Segmentation Using 3D Fully Convolutional Deep Networks

Seyed Sadegh Mohseni Salehi[1,2]([✉]), Deniz Erdogmus[1], and Ali Gholipour[2]

[1] Electrical and Computer Engineering Department,
Northeastern University, Boston, USA
ssalehi@ece.neu.edu

[2] Radiology Department, Boston Children's Hospital and Harvard Medical School,
Boston, USA

Abstract. Fully convolutional deep neural networks carry out excellent potential for fast and accurate image segmentation. One of the main challenges in training these networks is data imbalance, which is particularly problematic in medical imaging applications such as lesion segmentation where the number of lesion voxels is often much lower than the number of non-lesion voxels. Training with unbalanced data can lead to predictions that are severely biased towards high precision but low recall (sensitivity), which is undesired especially in medical applications where false negatives are much less tolerable than false positives. Several methods have been proposed to deal with this problem including balanced sampling, two step training, sample re-weighting, and similarity loss functions. In this paper, we propose a generalized loss function based on the Tversky index to address the issue of data imbalance and achieve much better trade-off between precision and recall in training 3D fully convolutional deep neural networks. Experimental results in multiple sclerosis lesion segmentation on magnetic resonance images show improved F_2 score, Dice coefficient, and the area under the precision-recall curve in test data. Based on these results we suggest Tversky loss function as a generalized framework to effectively train deep neural networks.

1 Introduction

Deep convolutional neural networks have attracted enormous attention in medical image segmentation as they have shown superior performance compared to conventional methods in several applications, including automatic segmentation of brain lesions [2,10], tumors [9,15,21], and neuroanatomy [3,14,22] using voxelwise network architectures [9,14,17], and more recently using 3D voxelwise networks [3,10] and fully convolutional networks (FCNs) [4,13,17]. Compared to voxelwise methods, FCNs are fast in testing and training, and use all samples to learn image features. Voxelwise networks, on the other hand, may use a subset of samples to reduce data imbalance issues and increase efficiency [17].

Electronic supplementary material The online version of this chapter (doi:10.1007/978-3-319-67389-9_44) contains supplementary material, which is available to authorized users.

Data imbalance is a common issue in medical image segmentation. For example in lesion detection the number of non-lesion voxels is typically >500 times larger than the number of diagnosed lesion voxels. Without balancing the labels the learning process may converge to local minima of a sub-optimal loss function, thus predictions may strongly bias towards non-lesion tissue. The outcome will be high-precision, low-recall segmentations. This is undesired especially in computer-aided diagnosis or clinical decision support systems where high sensitivity (recall) is a key characteristic of an automatic detection system.

A common approach to account for data imbalance, especially in voxelwise methods, is to extract equal training samples from each class [20]. The downsides of this approach are that it does not use all the information content of the images and may bias towards rare classes. Hierarchical training [5,20,21] and retraining [9] have been proposed as alternative strategies but they can be prone to overfitting and sensitive to the state of the initial classifiers [10]. Recent training methods for FCNs resorted to loss functions based on sample re-weighting [2,10,12,16,18], where lesion regions, for example, are given more importance than non-lesion regions during training. In the re-weighting approach, to balance the training samples between classes, the total cost is calculated based on weighted mean of each class. The weights are inversely proportional to the probability of each class appearance, i.e. higher appearance probabilities lead to lower weights. Although this approach works well for some relatively unbalanced data like brain extraction [17] and tumor detection [15], it becomes difficult to calibrate and does not perform well for highly unbalanced data such as lesion detection. To eliminate sample re-weighting, Milletari et al. proposed a loss function based on the Dice similarity coefficient [13].

The Dice loss layer is a harmonic mean of precision and recall thus weighs false positives (FPs) and false negatives (FNs) equally. To achieve a better trade-off between precision and recall (FPs vs. FNs), we propose a loss layer based on the Tversky similarity index [19]. Tversky index is a generalization of the Dice similarity coefficient and the F_β scores. We show how adjusting the hyperparameters of this index allow placing emphasis on false negatives in training a network that generalizes and performs well in highly imbalanced data as it leads to high sensitivity, Dice, F_2 score, and the area under the precision-recall (PR) curve [1] in the test set. To this end, we adopt a 3D FCN, based on the U-net architecture, with a Tversky loss layer, and test it in the challenging multiple sclerosis lesion detection problem on multi-channel MRI [6,20]. The ability to train a network for higher sensitivity (recall) in the expense of acceptable decrease in precision is crucial in many medical image segmentation tasks such as lesion detection.

2   Method

2.1   Network Architecture

We design and evaluate our 3D fully convolutional network [12,18] based on the U-net architecture [16]. To this end, we develop a 3D U-net based on

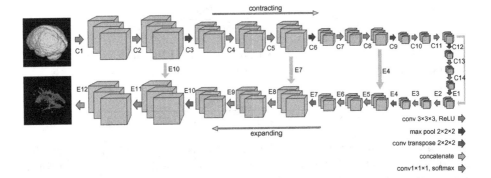

conv 3×3×3, ReLU
max pool 2×2×2
conv transpose 2×2×2
concatenate
conv1×1×1, softmax

Fig. 1. The 3D U-net style architecture; The complete description of the input and output size of each level is presented in Table S1 in the supplementary material.

Auto-Net [17] and introduce a new loss layer based on the Tversky index. This U-net style architecture, which has been designed to work with very small number of training images, is shown in Fig. 1. It consists of a contracting path (to the right) and an expanding path (to the left). To learn and use local information, high-resolution 3D features in the contracting path are concatenated with upsampled versions of global low-resolution 3D features in the expanding path. Through this concatenation the network learns to use both high-resolution local features and low-resolution global features. The contracting path contains padded $3 \times 3 \times 3$ convolutions followed by ReLU non-linear layers. A $2 \times 2 \times 2$ max pooling operation with stride 2 is applied after every two convolutional layers. After each downsampling by the max pooling layers, the number of features is doubled. In the expanding path, a $2 \times 2 \times 2$ transposed convolution operation is applied after every two convolutional layers, and the resulting feature map is concatenated to the corresponding feature map from the contracting path. At the final layer a $1 \times 1 \times 1$ convolution with softmax output is used to reach the feature map with a depth equal to the number of classes (lesion or non-lesion).

2.2 Tversky Loss Layer

The output layer in the network consists of c planes, one per class ($c = 2$ in lesion detection). We applied softmax along each voxel to form the loss. Let P and G be the set of predicted and ground truth binary labels, respectively. The Dice similarity coefficient D between two binary volumes is defined as:

$$D(P, G) = \frac{2|PG|}{|P| + |G|} \tag{1}$$

If this is used in a loss layer in training [13], it weighs FPs and FNs (precision and recall) equally. To give FNs higher weights than FPs in training our network for highly imbalanced data, where detecting small lesions is crucial, we propose a loss layer based on the Tversky index [19]. The Tiversky index is defined as:

$$S(P, G; \alpha, \beta) = \frac{|PG|}{|PG| + \alpha|P \setminus G| + \beta|G \setminus P|} \tag{2}$$

where α and β control the magnitude of penalties for FPs and FNs, respectively. To define the Tversky loss function we use the following formulation:

$$T(\alpha, \beta) = \frac{\sum_{i=1}^{N} p_{0i} g_{0i}}{\sum_{i=1}^{N} p_{0i} g_{0i} + \alpha \sum_{i=1}^{N} p_{0i} g_{1i} + \beta \sum_{i=1}^{N} p_{1i} g_{0i}} \tag{3}$$

where in the output of the softmax layer, the p_{0i} is the probability of voxel i be a lesion and p_{1i} is the probability of voxel i be a non-lesion. Also, g_{0i} is 1 for a lesion voxel and 0 for a non-lesion voxel and vice versa for the g_{1i}. The gradient of the loss in Eq. 3 with respect to p_{0i} and p_{1i} can be calculated as:

$$\frac{\partial T}{\partial p_{0i}} = 2 \frac{g_{0j}(\sum_{i=1}^{N} p_{0i} g_{0i} + \alpha \sum_{i=1}^{N} p_{0i} g_{1i} + \beta \sum_{i=1}^{N} p_{1i} g_{0i}) - (g_{0j} + \alpha g_{1j}) \sum_{i=1}^{N} p_{0i} g_{0i}}{(\sum_{i=1}^{N} p_{0i} g_{0i} + \alpha \sum_{i=1}^{N} p_{0i} g_{1i} + \beta \sum_{i=1}^{N} p_{1i} g_{0i})^2} \tag{4}$$

$$\frac{\partial T}{\partial p_{1i}} = -\frac{\beta g_{1j} \sum_{i=1}^{N} p_{0i} g_{0i}}{(\sum_{i=1}^{N} p_{0i} g_{0i} + \alpha \sum_{i=1}^{N} p_{0i} g_{1i} + \beta \sum_{i=1}^{N} p_{1i} g_{0i})^2} \tag{5}$$

Using this formulation we do not need to balance the weights for training. Also by adjusting the hyperparameters α and β we can control the trade-off between false positives and false negatives. It is noteworthy that in the case of $\alpha = \beta = 0.5$ the Tversky index simplifies to be the same as the Dice coefficient, which is also equal to the F_1 score. With $\alpha = \beta = 1$, Eq. 2 produces Tanimoto coefficient, and setting $\alpha + \beta = 1$ produces the set of F_β scores. Larger βs weigh recall higher than precision (by placing more emphasis on false negatives). We hypothesize that using higher βs in our generalized loss function in training will effectively helps us shift the emphasis to lower FNs and boost recall.

2.3   Experimental Design

We tested our FCN with Tversky loss layer to segment multiple sclerosis (MS) lesions [6,20]. T1-weighted, T2-weighted, and FLAIR MRI of 15 subjects were used as input, where we used two-fold cross-validation for training and testing. Images of different sizes were all rigidly registered to a reference image at size $128 \times 224 \times 256$. Our 3D-Unet was trained end-to-end. Cost minimization on 1000 epochs was performed using ADAM optimizer [11] with an initial learning rate of 0.0001 multiplied by 0.9 every 1000 steps. The training time for this network was approximately 4 h on a workstation with Nvidia Geforce GTX1080 GPU.

The test fold MRI volumes were segmented using feedforward through the network. The output of the last convolutional layer with softmax non-linearity consisted of a probability map for lesion and non-lesion tissues. Voxels with computed probabilities of 0.5 or more were considered to belong to the lesion tissue and those with probabilities <0.5 were considered non-lesion tissue.

2.4 Evaluation Metrics

To evaluate the performance of the networks and compare them against state-of-the-art in MS lesion segmentation, we report Dice similarity coefficient (DSC): $DSC = \frac{2|P \cap R|}{|P|+|R|} = \frac{2TP}{2TP+FP+FN}$, where P and R are the predicted and ground truth labels, respectively; and TP, FP, and FN are the true positive, false positive, and false negative rates, respectively. We also calculate and report specificity, $\frac{TN}{TN+FP}$, and sensitivity, $\frac{TP}{TP+FN}$, and the F_2 score as a measure that is commonly used in applications where recall is more important than precision (as compared to F_1 or DSC): $F_2 = \frac{5TP}{5TP+4FN+FP}$. To critically evaluate the performance of the detection for the highly unbalanced (skewed) dataset, we use the Precision-Recall (PR) curve (as opposed to the receiver-operator characteristic, or ROC, curve) as well as the area under the PR curve (the APR score) [1,7,8]. For such skewed datasets, the PR curves and APR scores (on test data) are preferred figures of algorithm performance.

3 Results

To evaluate the effect of Tversky loss function and compare it with Dice in lesion segmentation, we trained our FCN with different α and β values. The performance metrics (on the test set) are reported in Table 1. The results show that (1) the balance between sensitivity and specificity was controlled by the parameters of the loss function; and (2) according to all combined test measures, the best results were obtained from the FCN trained with $\beta = 0.7$, which performed better than the FCN trained with the Dice loss layer corresponding to $\alpha = \beta = 0.5$.

Figure 2(a) shows the PR curve for the entire test dataset, and Fig. 2(b) and (c) show the PR curves for two cases with extremely high and extremely low density of lesions, respectively. The best results based on the precision-recall trade-off were always obtained at $\beta = 0.7$ and not with the Dice loss function.

Table 1. Performance metrics (on the test set) for different values of the hyperparameters α and β used in training the FCN. The best values for each metric have been highlighted in bold. As expected, it is observed that higher β led to higher sensitivity (recall) and lower specificity. The combined performance metrics, in particular APR, F_2 and DSC indicate that the best performance was achieved at $\beta = 0.7$.

Penalties	DSC	Sensitivity	Specificity	F_2 score	APR score
$\alpha = 0.5, \beta = 0.5$	53.42	49.85	**99.93**	51.77	52.57
$\alpha = 0.4, \beta = 0.6$	54.57	55.85	99.91	55.47	54.34
$\alpha = 0.3, \beta = 0.7$	**56.42**	56.85	99.93	**57.32**	**56.04**
$\alpha = 0.2, \beta = 0.8$	48.57	61.00	99.89	54.53	53.31
$\alpha = 0.1, \beta = 0.9$	46.42	**65.57**	99.87	56.11	51.65

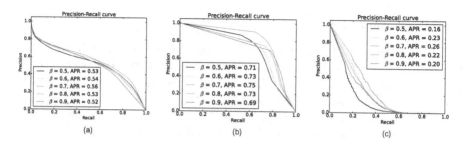

Fig. 2. PR curves with different α and β for: (a) all test set; (b) a subject with high density of lesions (Fig. 3); and (c) a subject with very low density of lesions (Fig. 4).

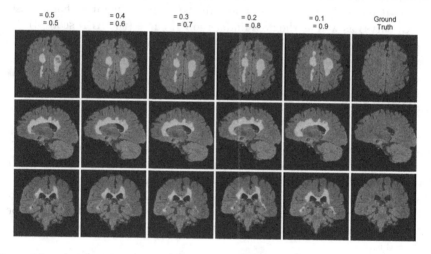

Fig. 3. The effect of different penalties on FP and FN in the Tverskey loss function on a case with extremely high density of lesions. The best results were obtained at $\beta = 0.7$

Figures 3 and 4 show the effect of different penalty magnitudes (βs) on segmenting a subject with high density of lesions and a subject with very few lesions, respectively. These cases, that correspond to the PR curves shown in Fig. 2(b and c), show that the best performance was achieved by using a loss function with $\beta = 0.7$ in training. We note that the network trained with the Dice loss layer ($\beta = 0.5$) did not detect the lesions in the case shown in Fig. 4.

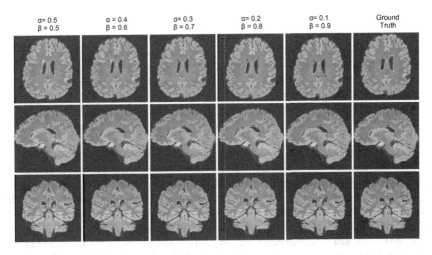

Fig. 4. The effect of different penalties on FP and FN in the Tverskey loss function on a case with extremely low density of lesions. The best results were obtained at $\beta = 0.7$.

4   Discussion and Conclusion

We introduced a new loss function based on the Tversky index, that generalizes the Dice coefficient and F_β scores, to achieve improved trade-off between precision and recall in segmenting highly unbalanced data via deep learning. To this end, we added our proposed loss layer to a state-of-the-art 3D fully convolutional deep neural network based on the U-net architecture [16,17]. Experimental results in MS lesion segmentation show that all performance evaluation metrics (on the test data) improved by using the Tversky loss function rather than using the Dice similarity coefficient in the loss layer. While the loss function was deliberately designed to weigh recall higher than precision (at $\beta = 0.7$), consistent improvements in all test performance metrics including DSC and F_2 scores on the test set indicate improved generalization through this type of training. Compared to DSC which weighs recall and precision equally, and the ROC analysis, we consider the area under the PR curves (APR, shown in Fig. 2) the most reliable performance metric for such highly skewed data [1,8]. To put the work in context, we reported average DSC, F_2, and APR scores (equal to 56.4, 57.3, and 56.0, respectively), which indicate that our approach performed very well compared to the latest results in MS lesion segmentation [6,20]. We did not conduct a direct comparison in the application domain, however, as this paper intended to provide proof-of-concept on the effect and usefulness of the Tversky loss layer (and F_β scores) in deep learning. Future work involves training and testing on larger, standard datasets in multiple applications to compare against state-of-the-art segmentations using appropriate performance criteria.

Acknowledgements. This work was in part supported by the National Institutes of Health (NIH) under grant R01 EB018988. The content of this work is solely the responsibility of the authors and does not necessarily represent the official views of the NIH.

References

1. Boyd, K., Eng, K.H., Page, C.D.: Area under the precision-recall curve: point estimates and confidence intervals. In: Blockeel, H., Kersting, K., Nijssen, S., Železný, F. (eds.) ECML PKDD 2013. LNCS, vol. 8190, pp. 451–466. Springer, Heidelberg (2013). doi:10.1007/978-3-642-40994-3_29

2. Brosch, T., Yoo, Y., Tang, L.Y.W., Li, D.K.B., Traboulsee, A., Tam, R.: Deep convolutional encoder networks for multiple sclerosis lesion segmentation. In: Navab, N., Hornegger, J., Wells, W.M., Frangi, A.F. (eds.) MICCAI 2015. LNCS, vol. 9351, pp. 3–11. Springer, Cham (2015). doi:10.1007/978-3-319-24574-4_1

3. Chen, H., Dou, Q., Yu, L., Qin, J., Heng, P.A.: VoxResNet: deep voxelwise residual networks for brain segmentation from 3D MR images. NeuroImage (2017)

4. Çiçek, Ö., Abdulkadir, A., Lienkamp, S.S., Brox, T., Ronneberger, O.: 3D U-Net: learning dense volumetric segmentation from sparse annotation. In: Ourselin, S., Joskowicz, L., Sabuncu, M.R., Unal, G., Wells, W. (eds.) MICCAI 2016. LNCS, vol. 9901, pp. 424–432. Springer, Cham (2016). doi:10.1007/978-3-319-46723-8_49

5. Cireşan, D.C., Giusti, A., Gambardella, L.M., Schmidhuber, J.: Mitosis detection in breast cancer histology images with deep neural networks. In: Mori, K., Sakuma, I., Sato, Y., Barillot, C., Navab, N. (eds.) MICCAI 2013. LNCS, vol. 8150, pp. 411–418. Springer, Heidelberg (2013). doi:10.1007/978-3-642-40763-5_51

6. Commowick, O., Cervenansky, F., Ameli, R.: MSSEG challenge proceedings: multiple sclerosis lesions segmentation challenge using a data management and processing infrastructure (2016)

7. Davis, J., Goadrich, M.: The relationship between precision-recall and ROC curves. In: Proceedings of the 23rd International Conference on Machine Learning, pp. 233–240. ACM (2006)

8. Fawcett, T.: An introduction to ROC analysis. Pattern Recogn. Lett. **27**(8), 861–874 (2006)

9. Havaei, M., Davy, A., Warde-Farley, D., Biard, A., Courville, A., Bengio, Y., Pal, C., Jodoin, P.M., Larochelle, H.: Brain tumor segmentation with deep neural networks. Med. Image Anal. **35**, 18–31 (2017)

10. Kamnitsas, K., Ledig, C., Newcombe, V., Simpson, J., Kane, A., Menon, D., Rueckert, D., Glocker, B.: Efficient multi-scale 3D CNN with fully connected CRF for accurate brain lesion segmentation. Med. Image Anal. **36**, 61–78 (2017)

11. Kingma, D., Ba, J.: Adam: a method for stochastic optimization. arXiv preprint arXiv:1412.6980 (2014)

12. Long, J., Shelhamer, E., Darrell, T.: Fully convolutional networks for semantic segmentation. In: Proceedings of the IEEE Conference on Computer Vision and Pattern Recognition, pp. 3431–3440 (2015)

13. Milletari, F., Navab, N., Ahmadi, S.A.: V-net: fully convolutional neural networks for volumetric medical image segmentation. In: 2016 Fourth International Conference on 3D Vision (3DV), pp. 565–571. IEEE (2016)

14. Moeskops, P., Viergever, M.A., Mendrik, A.M., de Vries, L.S., Benders, M.J., Išgum, I.: Automatic segmentation of MR brain images with a convolutional neural network. IEEE Trans. Med. Imaging **35**(5), 1252–1261 (2016)

15. Pereira, S., Pinto, A., Alves, V., Silva, C.A.: Brain tumor segmentation using convolutional neural networks in MRI images. IEEE Trans. Med. Imaging **35**(5), 1240–1251 (2016)

16. Ronneberger, O., Fischer, P., Brox, T.: U-Net: convolutional networks for biomedical image segmentation. In: Navab, N., Hornegger, J., Wells, W.M., Frangi, A.F.

(eds.) MICCAI 2015. LNCS, vol. 9351, pp. 234–241. Springer, Cham (2015). doi:10. 1007/978-3-319-24574-4_28

17. Salehi, S.S.M., Erdogmus, D., Gholipour, A.: Auto-context convolutional neural network (Auto-Net) for brain extraction in magnetic resonance imaging. IEEE Trans. Med. Imaging (2017)

18. Shelhamer, E., Long, J., Darrell, T.: Fully convolutional networks for semantic segmentation. IEEE Trans. Pattern Anal. Mach. Intell. **39**(4), 640–651 (2017)

19. Tversky, A.: Features of similarity. Psychol. Rev. **84**(4), 327 (1977)

20. Valverde, S., Cabezas, M., Roura, E., González-Villà, S., Pareto, D., Vilanova, J.C., Ramió-Torrentà, L., Rovira, À., Oliver, A., Lladó, X.: Improving automated multiple sclerosis lesion segmentation with a cascaded 3D convolutional neural network approach. NeuroImage **155**, 159–168 (2017)

21. Wachinger, C., Reuter, M., Klein, T.: DeepNAT: deep convolutional neural network for segmenting neuroanatomy. NeuroImage (2017)

22. Zhang, W., Li, R., Deng, H., Wang, L., Lin, W., Ji, S., Shen, D.: Deep convolutional neural networks for multi-modality isointense infant brain image segmentation. NeuroImage **108**, 214–224 (2015)

Author Index

Printed in the United States
By Bookmasters